Essentials of Nursing Research
Methods and Applications

Essentials of

 J. B. Lippincott Company

Philadelphia

London, Mexico City, New York, St. Louis, São Paulo, Sydney

Nursing Research

Methods and Applications

Denise F. Polit, Ph.D.

Director
Humanalysis, Inc.
Jefferson City, Missouri

Bernadette P. Hungler, B.S.N., M.S.N., M.A.

Boston College School of Nursing
Chestnut Hill, Massachusetts

Sponsoring Editor: Paul Hill
Production Supervisor: Kathleen P. Dunn
Art Director: Tracy Baldwin
Design Coordinator: Susan Caldwell
Designer: Carl Gross
Compositor: University Graphics, Inc.
Printer/Binder: R. R. Donnelley & Sons

3 5 6 4

Library of Congress Cataloging in Publication Data

Polit-O'Hara, Denise F.
    Essentials of nursing research.

    Includes bibliographies and index.
    1. Nursing—Research.   I. Hungler, Bernadette P.
II. Title. [DNLM: 1. Nursing. 2. Research. WY 20.5
P769]
RT81.5.P63 1984   610.73′072   84-7171
ISBN 0-397-54458-8

The authors and publisher have exerted every effort to ensure that drug selection and dosage set forth in this text are in accord with current recommendations and practice at the time of publication. However, in view of ongoing research, changes in government regulations, and the constant flow of information relating to drug therapy and drug reactions, the reader is urged to check the package insert for each drug for any change in indications and dosage and for added warnings and precautions. This is particularly important when the recommended agent is a new or infrequently employed drug.

TO
OUR
PARENTS

Preface

The nursing profession is increasingly involved in the development of a scientific body of knowledge relating to its practice. Not all nurses will engage in a research project of their own, but there is an ever-growing expectation that practicing nurses, nurse administrators, and nurse educators will be able to critically appraise and use the results of research in their work. The purpose of *Essentials of Nursing Research* is to assist those who need to judge the adequacy of a research study in order to come to conclusions about its findings.

Although this text presents most of the fundamentals needed to design and conduct a research investigation, it was written primarily with the consumer of nursing research in mind. To this end, several strategies were adopted. First, step-by-step information on the "how-tos" of research have not been included, although all major topics normally discussed in a more comprehensive text have been covered. Second, the text emphasizes throughout that designing a study is a decision-making process; readers are encouraged to think through the implications of making alternative decisions to address the same research problem. Third, most chapters conclude with a brief description of a fictitious study, which highlights methodological concepts emphasized in that chapter. Then, a critique of the fictitious study is presented to draw attention to some of the more noteworthy strengths and weaknesses of the study's methods.

While we have tried to make our presentation succinct, we felt it important to illustrate many of our points with real or fictitious research examples. We believe that the use of relevant examples is crucial to the development of both an understanding of, and an interest in, the research process. We also hope that the inclusion of many research ideas will stimulate an interest in further reading or pursuing a study of one's own.

To facilitate further learning, each chapter has an accompanying set of study suggestions. A student workbook has also been prepared with this goal in mind. A major section of each workbook chapter presents a fictitious study summary, which the student is asked to evaluate. A series of questions leads the students through the appraisal process.

The content of the text is organized into six main sections that roughly correspond to the steps a researcher takes in conducting a scientific study. Part I consists of three chapters that introduce the reader to the rationale underlying the scientific approach and to some basic research terms and concepts. Chapter 3 is a particularly important chapter because it dissects a study design into five major methodological decisions and then illustrates how alternative decisions affect the conclusions that can be reached.

Part II focuses on the steps that are taken in getting started on a research project. Chapter 4 discusses the development of conceptual contexts for a study problem through literature reviews and theoretical frameworks. Chapter 5 focuses on the formulation of research problem statements and hypotheses.

Various aspects of research design are considered in Part III. Chapter 6 describes the characteristics of experimental and nonexperimental research. The next chapter discusses several types of nursing research studies, such as survey research, evaluations, historical research, and case studies. Chapter 8 presents an overview of important design principles, with particular emphasis on controlling extraneous influences on the outcome of interest. The last chapter of Part III describes various designs for selecting samples of research subjects.

Part IV is devoted to a discussion of the measurement of research concepts. Chapter 10 introduces the reader to the major data-collection methods used by nurse researchers: self-reports, physiological measures, observations, projective techniques, Q sorts, and existing records. Chapters 11 and 12 focus more closely on two of the more widely used techniques, self-report and observational methods, respectively. Chapter 13 deals with various criteria for evaluating measuring tools, with particular emphasis on reliability and validity. The concluding chapter of Part IV describes the fundamentals of measurement theory.

Part V describes the process and rationale of data analysis and related tasks. Chapter 15 begins by discussing the characteristics of qualitative versus quantitative data analysis. Basic descriptive statistical analysis is also reviewed in this chapter. Chapter 16 presents a discussion of bivariate inferential statistics, with emphasis on understanding the purpose and results of statistical tests. Chapter 17 provides an overview of how computers can be used to perform analytic tasks in nursing research.

The final section of the book is concerned with the process of interpreting and communicating research results. Chapter 18 identifies major issues to be considered in evaluating research findings and provides a guide to the critical appraisal of a researcher's methodological decisions. The final chapter discusses what goes into a research report, and concludes with a full fictitious research report and a critique of the report.

It is our hope and expectation that the content, style, and organization of this book will be helpful to those students desiring to become intelligent and thoughtful readers of scientific research studies. We also hope that this text will help to develop an enthusiasm for the kinds of discoveries and knowledge that research can produce.

Denise F. Polit
Bernadette P. Hungler

Acknowledgments

Many individuals played an important role in the preparation and production of this book. We are deeply appreciative of all those involved, and especially of those mentioned below.

First, we would like to thank the many nurses and faculty members in the Boston area who provided helpful suggestions, particularly for research topics. An anonymous reviewer was especially useful in pointing out some shortcomings in an earlier draft. Many thanks, too, to John Burns, without whose guidance in the area of writing, this book would not be possible.

The staff at J. B. Lippincott were instrumental in conceiving this project and seeing it to completion. In particular, we would like to thank Paul Hill for his support and encouragement, and Kathleen Dunn for her helpfulness and care in editing this book.

Pam White typed the bulk of the manuscript and merits special thanks for her efficiency and responsiveness. Susan Hoefener also helped to transform our written pages into a final manuscript.

Finally, we extend our warmest thanks to our friends and families for their ongoing support.

Contents

Essentials of Nursing Research
Methods and Applications

Part I
Introduction
to Scientific Research

Chapter 1
Scientific Research and the Nursing Profession

Have you ever wondered whether the amount of physical contact a nurse has with a patient affects the patient's morale during hospitalization? Or have you ever questioned why one person complies with a medical regimen while another does not? Perhaps you have wondered what obstacles the nurse practitioner faces in gaining a patient's cooperation and trust. You may not have asked these specific questions, but you have undoubtedly wondered about other kinds of issues that confront nurses in their professional lives. These and similar questions are the starting point of scientific inquiry.

There is nothing particularly mysterious or exotic about the conduct of scientific research, nor does it require years and years of specialized training and sophisticated technical skills. True, some research studies are elaborate and sophisticated. Nevertheless, the fundamental skills of research—ones that will allow you to design and conduct a simple but respectable study or that will provide a basis for an intelligent reading of research reports—primarily involve logical reasoning and the mastery of a few major concepts and terms. The purpose of this text is to provide readers with those fundamental skills of scientific research, hopefully with a minimum of anxiety and frustration.

The Scientific Method and Problem Solving

People engage in scientific research to answer questions such as those posed in the opening paragraph above. Researchers strive to make sense of the human experience, to understand regularities, and to predict future circumstances. In short, research is a problem-solving enterprise. But what, after all, is so special about the scientific method? Humans are by nature problem-solvers. Consciously or unconsciously we all ask questions, solve problems, and make decisions daily. So what, one might ask, makes the scientific approach worthy of an entire text or course?

3

First let us consider some of the alternative routes to solving problems and gaining understanding about the world around us:

Tradition. Within our culture and within the nursing profession, certain "truths" are accepted as givens. Many questions are answered and problems solved on the basis of inherited customs or traditions. Tradition is efficient as a basis of knowledge in the sense that each individual is not required to begin from scratch in attempting to deal with daily problems. On the other hand, tradition may pose some obstacles for human inquiry because many traditions are so embedded in our culture that their validity or utility has never been challenged and evaluated.

Authority. In our complex society, there are "authorities," or people with specialized expertise, in every field. Patients turn to nurses or doctors as authorities in the medical field; people with a legal problem rely on lawyers; students depend on their instructors or textbooks in the educational arena. Reliance on authorities is to some degree inevitable: we cannot possibly become experts on every problem with which we are confronted. But, like tradition, authorities as a source of understanding have limitations. Authorities are not infallible, particularly if their expertise is based primarily on personal experience; yet their knowledge often goes unchallenged.

Human Experience. We all solve problems based on prior observations and experiences. Indeed, this is a very important and functional approach. The ability to generalize, to recognize regularities, and to make predictions based on observations are hallmarks of the human mind. Nevertheless, personal experience has two primary limitations as a basis of understanding: first, each person's experience may be too restricted to make valid generalizations to new situations; and second, personal experiences are colored by subjective values and prejudices.

Trial and Error. Sometimes we tackle problems by successively trying out alternative solutions. While this approach may in some cases be practical, it is often fallible and inefficient. The method tends to be haphazard and unsystematic, and the solutions are often idiosyncratic to a particular situation.

Logical Reasoning. We often solve problems by relying on logical thought processes. Indeed, logical reasoning is an important component of the scientific approach, but logical reasoning in and of itself is limited because the validity of deductive logic depends on the accuracy of the "facts" with which one starts, and reasoning itself may be an insufficient basis for evaluating accuracy.

It would be possible to answer the questions posed in the introduction to this chapter by using one or several of the methods just described above. Conceivably, the answers might be correct. But, equally conceivably, the answers might miss the mark. In our personal lives, it may not be of major consequence to base decisions on half-truths or subjective hunches. On the other hand, in our professional lives it is our responsibility to serve clients based on the most solid and dependable information available. The scientific approach is the most advanced method of acquiring knowledge that humans have developed. The scientific method incorporates several procedures and characteristics to create a system of obtaining knowledge that, though not infallible, is generally more reliable than alternative problem-solving approaches.

Characteristics of the Scientific Approach

What, then, are the distinguishing features of the scientific approach? Let us begin by defining scientific research as controlled, systematic investigations that are rooted in objective reality and that aim to develop generalizable knowledge about natural phenomena. Now we can dissect this definition and consider its various components.

Order and Systemization. In a scientific study, the researcher moves in an orderly and systematic fashion from the definition of a problem, through the design of the study and collection of information, to the solution of the problem. By systematic, we mean that the investigator progresses logically through a series of steps, according to a prespecified plan of action. The decisions the researcher makes in developing such a plan are described in Chapter 3.

Control. Control is a key element of the scientific approach. Control involves imposing conditions on the research situation so that biases are minimized and maximum precision and validity are attained. The mechanisms of scientific control are the subject of a large portion of this text.

Empiricism. The term *empiricism* refers to the process whereby evidence rooted in objective reality and gathered directly or indirectly through the human senses is used as the basis for generating knowledge. This requirement causes findings of a scientific investigation to be grounded in reality rather than in the personal biases or beliefs of the researcher. Empirical inquiry imposes a certain degree of objectivity on the research situation because ideas or hunches are exposed to testing in the real-world situation.

Generalization. An important goal of science is to understand phenomena—not in isolated circumstances alone, but in a broad, general sense. The ability to go beyond the specifics of the situation is an important characteristic of the scientific approach. In fact, the degree to which research findings can be generalized is an important criterion for assessing the quality of a research study.

Beyond the features highlighted in the definition of the scientific approach, there are additional characteristics that merit brief mention. The first is that there are some fundamental assumptions that form the cornerstone of scientific inquiry. *Assumptions* refer to basic principles that are assumed to be true without proof or verification. The scientist assumes that nature is basically orderly and regular, and that an objective reality exists independent of human observation. In other words, the world is assumed not to be merely a creation of the human mind. The related assumption of *determinism* refers to the belief that phenomena are not haphazard or random events, but rather that they have antecedent causes. If a person has a cerebral vascular accident, the scientist assumes that there must be one or more reasons that can potentially be identified and understood. Much of the activity in which a scientific researcher is engaged is directed at understanding the underlying causes of natural phenomena.

Another way to describe the characteristics of scientific research is to consider the spirit in which such research is conducted. The scientist is fundamentally a skeptic, challenging unvalidated observations and tentative conclusions. The scientific researcher—and the intelligent consumer of research studies—generally demands evidence in support of conclusions or statements of "fact." Even findings from research studies (particularly if the study has any serious flaws) are regarded as tentative unless they are verified. Such verification generally comes from repeated studies of the same research problem; such studies are called *replications*.

In summary, the scientific approach to inquiry refers to a general set of orderly and disciplined procedures used to acquire dependable and useful information. The term *research* designates the application of this scientific approach to the solution of a problem of interest.

Purposes of Scientific Research

As we have seen, the general purpose of research is to answer questions or solve problems. In this section we examine some of the more specific reasons for conducting research in the context of the nursing profession.

Description. The main objective of many nursing research studies is the description of phenomena relating to the nursing profession. When a scientific approach is employed (i.e., when controlled and systematic empirical observations are made), descriptive studies can be of considerable value. The phenomena that nurse researchers have been interested in describing are varied: stress in patients, pain management, grieving behavior, nutritional habits, rehabilitation success, and time patterns of temperature readings, to mention only a few.

Exploration. Like descriptive research, exploratory research begins with some specific phenomenon of interest, but rather than simply observing and recording incidence of the phenomenon, exploratory research pursues the following question: What factor or factors influence, affect, cause, or relate to this phenomenon? Let us take as an example the level of preoperative stress in patients. The descriptive study would seek to document the degree of stress patients generally experience prior to surgery. The exploratory study would ask the following: What factors are related to a patient's stress level? Is the patient's diagnosis an important factor? Do the patient's age, sex, or prior hospitalization record play a role? Or is a patient's stress related to behaviors of the nursing staff or characteristics of the hospital? Exploratory studies are especially useful when a new area or topic is being investigated.

Explanation. Explanatory research is designed to get at the "why" of natural phenomena. Explanatory research is generally linked to theories. *Theories* represent a method of deriving, organizing, and integrating ideas about the manner in which phenomena are interrelated. It might be said that, whereas descriptive and exploratory research provide new information, explanatory research offers understanding. Leaders in nursing research have increasingly made appeals for more theoretically based studies.

Prediction and Control. With our current level of knowledge, technology, and theoretical progress, there are numerous problems that defy absolute comprehension and explanation. Yet it is frequently possible to make predictions and to control phenomena based on findings from scientific investigations, even in the absence of true understanding. For example, research has shown that the incidence of Down's syndrome in infants increases with the age of the mother. We can *predict* that a woman aged 40 is more at risk of bearing a child with Down's syndrome than is a woman aged 25. We can partially *control* the outcome by educating women about the risks and offering amniocentesis to women over age 35. Note that the ability to predict and control in this example does not depend on an explanation of why older women are at a higher risk of having an abnormal child. There are many examples of nursing and health-related studies in which prediction and control are key objectives.

Sometimes a study is primarily concerned with only one of the goals outlined above. More frequently, however, a study has multiple functions.

The purpose of a scientific inquiry is sometimes classified according to the direct practical utility the findings will have. *Basic research* is concerned with adding information to our store of human knowledge without necessarily having immediate application. Whipple, who studied the bleeding tendency in liver disease, and Dam, who studied cholesterol metabolism, were both engaged in basic research. Yet their independent and seemingly unrelated basic research endeavors led to the practical application of treating bleeding tendencies with vitamin K.

Applied research is focused on finding an immediate solution to a practical problem. Much of the research that has been conducted in nursing has been applied in nature. For example, the question of how long a rectal, oral, or axillary thermometer must be in place to record accurately is a problem for which the solution has immediate application in practice. Yet nursing researchers are demonstrating increasing interest in the conduct of theory-based research designed to enhance a general understanding of the nursing process and the role of nurses.

In many instances the distinction between applied and basic research may be meaningless because of extensive overlap in these two areas. Furthermore, in nursing, as in medicine, the feedback process between basic and applied research seems to operate more freely than in the case of other disciplines. The findings from applied research almost immediately pose questions for basic research, while the results of basic research many times suggest clinical application to a practical problem.

Nursing and the Scientific Approach

Scientific research plays an important role in nursing regardless of what type of position the nurse holds. In recent years one of the primary reasons for conducting nursing research studies has been to improve the practice of nursing. Nursing practice is, as yet, a poorly understood phenomenon. Nurses are increasingly engaging in research to help develop, refine, and extend the scientific body of knowledge fundamental to the practice of nursing. Such a body of knowledge is essential for nursing as it continues to grow as a profession. Nurses who base as many of their clinical decisions as possible on scientifically documented information are being professionally accountable to the clientele served by nursing and are helping nursing achieve its own professional identity.

A second reason nurses engage in research is to help define the parameters of nursing. Nursing is only one of several professions involved in the delivery of health care. Currently, the scope of nursing may be said to be rather broadly and vaguely defined. By conducting research in this area, nurses are assisting in identifying the boundaries of nursing. Such knowledge is beneficial in defining the fairly distinct and unique role that nursing has in the delivery of health care.

The spiraling costs of health care and the cost-containment practices currently being instituted in health-care facilities are a third reason why nurses are engaging in research. Nurses are being asked more than ever before to document the social relevancy and the efficacy of their nursing practices to others, such as consumers of nursing care, administrators of health-care facilities, third-party payers, and governmental agencies. Nurses are focusing their research endeavors in this area on the effectiveness of nursing interventions and actions for various groups of clients. Some of the findings from studies will help nurses eliminate those nursing-care practices that have no effect on the achievement of desired client outcomes. Other findings will help nurses identify the nursing-care practices that make a difference in the health status of individuals and are cost-effective.

It is through research that nurses come to understand the varied dimensions of their profession. Research enables nurses to describe the characteristics of a particular nursing situation about which little is known; to explain phenomena that must be considered in planning nursing care; to predict the probable outcome of certain nursing decisions made in relation to client care; to control the occurrence of undesired client outcomes; and to initiate, with a fair degree of confidence, activities that will achieve desired client behaviors. Nurses also engage in research to develop theories germane to the practice of nursing and to provide nurses with a scientifically based theoretical framework that guides their clinical practice.

Benefits of Nursing Research

The benefits that accrue to a profession as it identifies and extends its knowledge base are many. The findings from nursing research help nurse practitioners, nurse educators, and nurse administrators make more informed decisions in their particular area of functioning. In the clinical arena, research can help to improve the practice of nursing. Current modalities of treatment that produce less than desired effects in clients may be modified or eliminated from practice. Answers may be found to perplexing nursing-care problems, such as why a particular nursing intervention is effective for one client and ineffective for another. The promotion of health or the enhancement of positive health practices in clients may be facilitated by knowing which nursing actions or interventions are the most effective. In addition, as research identifies factors that prevent persons from achieving their optimal level of health, nurse practitioners will be aided in deciding how to thwart the development of undesired behaviors or in deciding how to counter those influences that prevent persons from attaining their highest level of wellness.

Nurse educators also benefit from research that focuses on clinical practice. The findings from such research will assist faculty in structuring nursing curricula and in organizing the content of nursing courses. Nursing actions that have been found to be ineffective may be eliminated from a course. In contrast, as theories emerge, nursing faculty will be able to disseminate to students, with more confidence than is currently possible, the conditions under which particular nursing actions are likely to have a favorable effect on clients. In addition to research based in clinical practice, nursing faculty also profit from research that pertains to teaching methods. Strategies that facilitate student learning in other disciplines may or may not be effective in nursing given its strong clinical component. Nurse educators may engage in research directed toward determining the effectiveness of various teaching methods. The methods that may be most productive for the classroom may differ from the methods found to be most beneficial in the clinical area.

The findings from clinical nursing research benefit nurse administrators as well as nurse practitioners and nurse faculty. Nurse administrators can be assisted by research in planning the nursing-staff requirements necessary to achieve desired client outcomes. Such information is essential in preparing budgets or in documenting the need for alterations in existing staffing patterns. Nurse administrators are also interested in research that focuses on job-related aspects of the nursing role. Such studies help nurse administrators improve the quality of nurses' professional performances by eliminating or reducing factors that prevent job satisfaction and in enhancing those factors known to favorably influence role performance.

Historical Evolution of Nursing Research

Most people would agree that nursing research began with Florence Nightingale during the Crimean War. However, for a number of years following her work, little is found in the nursing literature concerning nursing research. Some have attributed the absence of nursing research during these years to the apprenticeship nature of nursing.

Subsequent to the early years of modern nursing, the pattern that nursing research followed closely paralleled the education of nurses, the staffing pattern of hospitals, and the emergence of nursing as a profession. First, as more nurses received university-based education, studies concerning students—their problems, differential characteristics, satisfactions—became more numerous. Second, as more nurses pursued a college education, the staffing pattern of hospitals changed. Fewer students were available to staff the hospital throughout a 24-hour period. Researchers focused their investigations not only on the supply and demand of nurses, but also on the amount of time required to perform certain nursing activities. It was during these years that nursing struggled with its professional identity, and nursing research took a twist toward studying nurses—who they were, what they did, how other groups received them, and what type of person enters nursing.

It was not until the 1950s that a number of forces combined to put nursing research on the rapidly accelerating upswing it is still experiencing today. An increase in the number of nurses with advanced academic preparation, the establishment of the *Nursing Research* journal, the availability of federal funding to support nursing research, and the upgrading of research skills in faculty are but some of the forces that provided impetus to nursing research.

The major thrust of nursing research today is on the development of a scientific body of knowledge for nursing practice. Clinical studies that explicate nursing practice are encouraged by many national leaders and organizations. For example, the ANA Commission on Nursing Research (1980) has identified several priorities for nursing research in the 1980s. This group recommended that the generation of knowledge for nursing practice should be in the areas of health promotion, prevention of illness, development of cost-effective health-care delivery systems, and development of strategies that provide effective nursing care to groups that are at high risk for the development of particular problems or are culturally different from the majority of health professionals.

Topics of Interest to Nurse Researchers

The topics that interest nurse researchers are as diverse as the types of positions held by nurses, the multiplicity of settings in which nurses practice, the complexity of human nature, and the individuality of each nurse. The following six areas highlight broad categories of topics of current interest to nurse researchers:

Research Concerning the Promotion of Positive Health Behaviors. Studies in this area concern the identification of characteristics associated with the practice of health-enhancing behaviors, such as self-breast examination, exercise, avoidance of smoking, eating nutritional meals, and planned physical examinations.

Research Concerning Compliance or Adherence to Prescribed Programs of Treatment. Nurses are currently interested in learning what associations might exist between various background or psychological characteristics of individuals and their degree of compliance or noncompliance with various therapeutic programs. Such studies involve how coping patterns; family interaction; motivation; locus of control; and personal attributes, such as age, gender, or educational preparation, are related to adherence to alterations in diet, a medication regimen, an exercise program, or alterations in life-style imposed by illness.

Research Concerning the Nursing Process. Research in this area may focus on examining a particular step of the nursing process or on articulating various phases of the process. For example, some studies that focus on the assessment phase of the process examine the degree to which tools such as health-history forms are providing nurses with the kind of information needed to make valid conclusions about a patient's problems. Other studies focus on the defining characteristics or etiologies associated with various nursing diagnoses. Nurses are also evaluating the effectiveness of nursing interventions for particular types of patients with such health problems as alterations in bowel elimination, anorexia, drug abuse, ineffective coping patterns, or alterations in self-esteem. An increasing amount of interest has been directed toward identifying how clinical nursing judgments are made and how these judgments influence subsequent nursing decisions that affect client outcomes.

Research Concerning Minority Groups. Studies in this topic area include the identification of cultural beliefs that influence the health-care practices of various ethnic groups, the availability and frequency of use of health clinics in housing projects for the elderly, the assessment of knowledge possessed by ethnic minorities concerning specific illnesses, and the perceptions of those who are culturally different from the health professionals in their area.

Research Concerning Groups at Risk for Specific Health Problems. Nurses are currently interested in learning how people come to know that they are at risk for developing particular health problems. Do family background, life-style, environmental conditions, or a combination of factors contribute to the developing awareness of the at-risk status? Some important aspects of problems in this area that have interested nurses are how people respond to the knowledge that they have the potential for developing specific health problems, what factors are instrumental in helping reduce the at-risk status, and the satisfaction experienced by altering habits to reduce risk.

In summary, as professionalism has grown in nursing, so has the commitment to apply the scientific approach to nursing problems. In recent years the major focus has turned to delineating a scientific base of knowledge for nursing practice.

Limitations of Scientific Research

The scientific approach has gained widespread acceptance as the highest form of problem solving and knowledge acquisition yet devised. As we have just seen, in the field of nursing the applications of scientific methods have been broad, and the impact of nursing research studies has been considerable. It is increasingly common for nurses and nursing students to conduct their own investigations. It is also increasingly important for nurses to be able to understand and critically evaluate the research reports of others. Despite the rising prominence of scientific research in the nursing profession and despite the problem-solving capabilities of the scientific approach, it is by no means infallible or appropriate to all kinds of human problems. Several limitations deserve special mention.

First, the scientific method cannot be used to answer questions of a moral or ethical nature. Many of our most persistent and intriguing questions about the human condition fall into this area. Consider, for example, the question of the point at which a human life should be construed as starting, or the question of whether or not euthanasia should be practiced. Given the many moral issues that are tied up with medicine and health care, it is inevitable that the nursing process will never rely completely upon scientific information.

A second limitation concerns problems of measurement. In order to study, for example, patient morale, we must be able to measure it; that is, we must be able to assess if a patient's morale is high or low, or higher under certain conditions than under others. While there are reasonably accurate measures of such physiological phenomena as blood pressure, temperature, and cardiac activity, comparably accurate measures of such psychological phenomena as anxiety, pain, self-confidence, or aggression have not been developed. The problems associated with measurement are among the most perplexing in the research process.

A final cautionary note about the entire research process is in order: *virtually every research study contains some flaw.* Perfectly designed and executed studies are unattainable. As we will see in Chapter 3—indeed, throughout this book—every research question can be addressed in an almost infinite number of ways. The researcher must make decisions about how best to proceed. Invariably, there are trade-offs. The best methods are often very expensive and time-consuming. Even when tremendous resources are expended, there are bound to be some flaws. This does not mean that small, simple studies are worthless. It means that *no single study can ever definitively prove or disprove our hunches.* Each completed study adds to a body of accumulated knowledge. If the same question is posed by several researchers, each of whom obtains the same or similar results, increased confidence can be placed in the answer to the question. This is especially true if the researcher's studies have different types of shortcomings.

In summary, scientific methods are extremely powerful tools in helping us understand the world we live in and in helping us solve many practical problems. But our respect for the powers of the scientific approach needs to be tempered by a familiarity with its limitations and fallibility. The findings from research studies are not always right. That is precisely why it is so important for consumers of research to understand the trade-offs and decisions that investigators make, and to evaluate the adequacy of those decisions.

The Ethics of Scientific Research

Most nursing research studies involve the use of human subjects. Whenever human beings are used to answer research questions, the researcher must take care to ensure that the rights of the subjects are protected. The ethical conduct of scientific studies has become a much-discussed topic in scientific circles, not only because of its obvious importance, but also because in certain situations ethical requirements conflict with the rigors of the scientific approach. In this section we briefly discuss some of the major ethical issues that should be considered in designing a research study.

One of the most fundamental ethical principles is that subjects should be protected from harm or discomfort. This principle may seem so obvious as to merit no further discussion, but sometimes harm is very subtle and difficult to anticipate. This is particularly true with respect to psychological consequences. For example, sometimes people are asked questions about their personal views, weaknesses, or fears. Such queries might require individuals to admit to aspects of themselves that they dislike and would perhaps rather forget. The point is not that the researcher should refrain from asking *any* questions but, rather, that it is necessary to think very carefully about the nature of the intrusion upon people's psyches.

Another important principle of ethical conduct in research is that participation in studies should be voluntary. Prospective participants should be informed about the nature of the study, and their voluntary consent secured. Once again, the seemingly straightforward principle of informed consent often conflicts directly with practical considerations or scientific concerns. Suppose one wants to study the behavior of mentally retarded persons, autistic children, or senile older persons. Is informed consent even a meaningful concept with such groups? Or suppose a researcher wants to study the normal behaviors of nurses in intensive care units. Would their behaviors be normal if they knew in advance they were being observed? Furthermore, if we restrict a study to those who cooperate voluntarily, how can we be sure that nonvolunteers are not fundamentally different with respect to the phenomenon under investigation?

Clearly, these are thorny issues. Generally, some kind of compromise must be reached to safeguard the subjects' rights while at the same time not handcuffing the scientist, whose aim is, after all, generally to improve human welfare. When the requirement of voluntary participation threatens the value of a research study, the investigator is forced to evaluate the consequences of involuntary participation and weigh these consequences against the potential contribution of the study. If the scientist believes that the study's findings would be beneficial without making undue impositions on unknowing participants, he or she may feel justified in violating the principle of informed consent.

A third ethical principle concerns the right of individual participants in a study to protect their privacy. Whatever information a researcher obtains in the course of a study should be considered privileged information and should under no circumstances be publicly disclosed in a fashion that would identify any specific person. The two mechanisms for protecting participants' identities are known as anonymity and confidentiality. *Anonymity* can be guaranteed when even the researcher cannot link a participant with the information that has been gathered. For example, if questionnaires were distributed to nursing students and collected without any names or other identifying information, we could say that the anonymity of the respondents had been assured. In many situations, however, anonymity is impossible to achieve, as would be the case if, for example, patients were interviewed about the quality of their nursing care. In such face-to-face situations, the researcher should offer participants a guarantee of *confidentiality*. This means that the researcher promises that any information that the participant divulges will not be publicly reported. Researchers often substitute identification numbers for subjects' names on study records to prevent any accidental breach of confidentiality.

This brief discussion by no means exhausts the issues surrounding the ethical conduct of scientific research. Several considerations were raised here to alert readers to the major moral dilemmas that a researcher must face in carrying out investigations with human subjects. We urge those conducting their own research to pursue this topic in the many books and guidelines that have been devoted to it.

Summary

Scientific research begins with questions about the world around us or with a problem to be solved. The scientific method stands in contrast with several other sources of knowledge and understanding, such as tradition, voices of authority, personal experience, trial and error, and logical reasoning. The scientific method is the most advanced form of inquiry that humans have devised.

The scientific approach may be described in terms of a number of characteristics. It is, first of all, a systematic, disciplined, and controlled process. Scientists base their findings on *empirical observations*, which means that evidence is rooted in objective reality and collected by way of the human senses or their extensions. Unlike many other problem-solving techniques, the scientific approach strives for generalizability and for the development of explanations or theories about the relationships among phenomena.

Essential to the understanding of the scientific approach is a knowledge of the assumptions upon which it is based. The scientist assumes that there is an objective reality that is not dependent upon human observation for its existence. A related belief is that natural phenomena are basically regular and orderly. The assumption of *determinism* refers to the belief that events are not haphazard but, rather, are the result of prior causes. The search for an understanding of underlying causes of phenomena is an activity basic to most scientific endeavors.

Scientific research can be categorized in terms of its functions or objectives. Description, exploration, explanation, prediction, and control of natural phenomena represent the most common goals of a research investigation. It is also possible to describe research in terms of the direct practical utility that it aspires to achieve. *Basic research* is designed to extend the base of knowledge for the sake of knowledge itself. *Applied research* focuses on discovering solutions to immediate practical problems. In reality the distinction is seldom clear-cut, particularly for nursing researchers.

Nurses have increasingly used the scientific approach to solve problems facing the nursing profession and to develop a scientific base of knowledge and theory for nursing practice. Nurse practitioners, administrators, and educators are, more than ever before, committed to understanding the phenomena with which they deal; scientific research helps them to explain, predict, and sometimes control the occurrence of the phenomena. Research also aids nurses to be accountable to clients or patients. While early applications of the scientific approach in nursing focused on nurses themselves or on nursing education, nursing research is increasingly focused on nursing practice. Because of the strengths of the scientific approach, nurses are likely to continue using it as a tool of inquiry in learning about their practice and profession.

Although the scientific approach offers a number of distinct advantages as a system of inquiry over other methods, it is not without its share of difficulties and shortcomings. First of all, the scientific approach is not useful in providing answers to moral or value-laden questions. In addition, there are numerous questions of interest to nurse researchers that are difficult to study because they deal with complex social or psychological functioning, such as pain, fear, guilt, anxiety, motivation, and the like. Such phenomena are difficult to measure (in comparison with aspects of biological functioning, such as blood pressure or body temperature) and difficult to control in a natural setting.

In dealing with human beings in research situations, a number of ethical issues must be raised. Three common ethical requirements are voluntary participation, freedom from physical or psychological harm and distress, and anonymity or confidentiality of information. Ethics in research is a continually perplexing concern, because ethical demands often conflict with scientific requirements.

Study Suggestions

1. Consider one or two nursing "facts" that you possess and then trace the fact back to some source. Is the basis for your knowledge tradition, authority, experience, or scientific research?

2. How does the ability to predict phenomena offer the possibility of their control?

3. Below are a few research problems. For each problem, specify whether you think it is essentially a basic or applied research question. Justify your response.

a. Is the stress level of patients related to the level of information they possess about their medical status?

b. Do students who get better grades in nursing school become more effective nurses than students with lower grades?

c. Does the early discharge of maternity patients lead to later problems with breastfeeding?

d. Can the incidence of decubitus ulcers be affected by a certain massaging technique?

e. Is individual contraceptive counseling more effective than group-based instruction in minimizing unwanted pregnancies?

4. Point out the ethical considerations that might emerge in the following studies:

a. A study of the relationship between sleeping patterns and acting-out behaviors in hospitalized psychiatric patients

b. A study of the effects of a new drug on human subjects

c. An investigation of a person's psychological state following an abortion.

Chapter 2
Basic Concepts and Terms in Scientific Research

Like the field of nursing, or any other discipline, scientific research has its own language and terminology. New terms (or new definitions of familiar terms) are introduced throughout this text. A glossary has also been included at the end of this book for easy reference. Some terms and concepts are so fundamental to the research process, however, that a firm understanding of their meaning is essential before more complex ideas can be reasonably grasped. The purpose of this chapter is to make the rest of the text more manageable by familiarizing readers with the basics of scientific parlance and thought.

Variables

Conceptualization refers to the process of formulating abstract ideas. Scientific research almost always is concerned with abstract rather than tangible phenomena. For example, the terms "good health," "emotional disturbance," and "empathy" are all abstractions derived from the manifestation of specific behaviors or characteristics. These abstractions are referred to as *concepts*, which are the building blocks of scientific inquiry.

Within the context of a research investigation, concepts are generally referred to as *variables*. A variable is, as the name implies, something that varies. Weight, nursing specialty areas, blood pressure readings, preoperative anxiety levels, and body temperature are all variables. That is, each of these properties varies or differs from one person to another. When one considers the variety and complexity of human and situational characteristics, it becomes clear that nearly all aspects of people and our environment can be considered variables. If everyone had black hair and weighed 125 pounds, hair color and weight would not be variables. If it rained continuously and the outdoor temperature were a constant 70° F, weather would not be a variable. But it is precisely because people and conditions do vary that most research is conducted. The bulk of all research activity is aimed at trying to understand how or why things vary in order to gain insights into how differences in one variable are related to differences in another. For example, lung cancer research is concerned with the variable of lung cancer. It is a variable because not everybody has the disease. Researchers in this area are concerned with learning what other variables can be linked to lung cancer. They have discovered that cigarette smoking appears to be related to the disease. Again, this is a variable because not everyone smokes.

A variable, then, is any quality of a person, institution, or situation that varies or takes on different values. Sometimes a variable can take on a range of different values (e.g., height or weight) while other variables take on as few as two values (e.g., pregnant/not pregnant, smoker/non-smoker, male/female). Variables are often characteristics inherent to individuals, such as sex, age, blood type, ethnicity, or grip strength. When a researcher is studying such *attribute variables*, as they are sometimes called, the researcher's task is to observe, measure, and record the value of the variable for each participant in the study. However, variables are not restricted to preexisting attributes of persons or situations. In many research situations the investigator creates or designs a variable. For example, if a researcher is interested in testing the effectiveness of drug A as opposed to drug B in lowering the blood pressure of hypertensive patients, some persons would be given drug A while others would receive drug B. In the context of this study, drug type has become a variable, because different persons will be administered different drugs.

Thus, scientific research is all about the study of variables and how they are interrelated. The variability of the human condition is the basis for most research questions of interest to nurse researchers.

Dependent and Independent Variables

An important differentiation is generally made between two types of variables in a research study, and it is a distinction that the reader should master before proceeding to later chapters. The distinction is between the *dependent variable* and the *independent variable*. Many research studies are aimed at unravelling and understanding the causes underlying phenomena. Does a nursing intervention cause more rapid recovery? Does smoking cause lung cancer? The presumed cause is referred to as the independent variable, while the presumed effect is referred to as the dependent variable. Variability in the dependent variable is presumed to depend upon variability in the independent variable. For example, the researcher investigates the extent to which lung cancer (the dependent variable) depends upon smoking behavior (the independent variable). In another study, a researcher might examine the effects of two special diets (the independent variable) on weight gain in premature infants (the dependent variable). Or, an investigator may be concerned with the extent to which a patient's perception of pain (the dependent variable) is dependent upon different kinds of nursing approaches (the independent variables).

The terms "independent variable" and "dependent variable" are also used even when causality between variables cannot be inferred. Frequently these terms are used to designate the direction of influence rather than cause and effect. For example, let us say that a researcher is studying nurses' attitudes toward abortion and finds that older nurses hold less favorable opinions about abortion than younger nurses. The researcher might be unwilling to take the position that the nurses' attitudes were caused by their age. Yet, the direction of influence clearly runs from age to attitudes. That is, it would make little sense to suggest that the attitudes influenced age. Even though in this example the researcher does not infer a causal relationship between age and attitudes, it is appropriate to conceptualize attitudes toward abortion as the dependent variable and age as the independent variable.

The dependent variable usually is the variable the researcher is interested in understanding, explaining, or predicting. In lung cancer research, it is the carcinoma that is of real interest to the research scientist, not smoking behavior *per se.* As another example, in studies of the effectiveness of different kinds of therapeutic treatment for alcoholics, it is the drinking behavior of the subjects that is under investigation, and that is considered the dependent variable. Although a great deal of time, effort, and resources may be devoted to designing new therapies (the independent variable), they are of no interest in and of themselves but, rather, as they relate to improvements in drinking behavior and overall functioning of alcoholics.

Many of the dependent variables that are studied by researchers have multiple causes or antecedents. If we are interested in studying the factors that influence the weight of a person, for example, we might consider the sex, age, height, physical activity, and eating habits of the person as the independent variables. Note that some of these independent variables are attribute variables (sex, age, and height), while others (activity and eating patterns) can be influenced by the investigator. Just as a study may examine more than one independent variable, two or more dependent variables may be of interest to the researcher. For example, an investigator may be concerned with comparing the effectiveness of two methods of therapy for children with cystic fibrosis. Several dependent variables could be designated as measures of treatment effectiveness, such as the length of stay in the hospital, the number of recurrent respiratory infections, the presence of cough, dyspnea on exertion, and so forth. In short, it is quite common to design studies with multiple independent and dependent variables.

The reader should not get the impression that variables are inherently dependent or independent. A variable that is classified as dependent in one study may be considered an independent variable in another study. For example, a researcher may find that the religious background of a nurse (the independent variable) has an effect on his or her attitude toward death and dying (the dependent variable). Another study, however, may analyze the extent to which attitudes of nurses toward death and dying (the independent variables) have an impact on their job performance (the dependent variable). To illustrate this point with another example, consider a study that examines the effect of contraceptive counseling (the independent variable) or unwanted pregnancies (the dependent variable). Yet another research project could study the effect of unwanted pregnancies (the independent variable) on the incidence of child abuse (the dependent variable). In short, the designation of a variable as independent or dependent is a function of the role that the variable plays in a particular investigation. Table 2-1 presents some additional examples of research questions and specifies the dependent and independent variables.

Before concluding, it should be pointed out that some researchers use the term *criterion variable* (or criterion measure) rather than dependent

Table 2-1. Examples of Independent and Dependent Variables

RESEARCH QUESTION	INDEPENDENT VARIABLE	DEPENDENT VARIABLE
Does the frequency of sleep interruptions during hospitalization affect patients' morale?	Frequency of sleep disturbance	Patients' morale
Are men or women more susceptible to urinary infection following catheterization?	Patients' sex	Incidence of urinary infection
Is turnover higher among intensive care unit nursing staff than among other kinds of staff?	Nursing staff assignment	Nurses' turnover rate
Does exposure to cats during pregnancy increase the likelihood of toxemia?	Exposure to cats	Incidence of toxemia in pregnancy
Does the number of hours nursing students engage in clinical work affect their sense of professionalism?	Number of clinical hours	Students' sense of professionalism
Does circumcision reduce the risk of cervical cancer for men's sexual partners?	Circumcision vs. absence of circumcision	Incidence of cervical cancer

variable. In studies that analyze the consequences of a treatment, therapy, or some other type of intervention, it is usually necessary to establish criteria against which the success of the intervention can be assessed and, hence, the origin of the expression criterion variable. The term "dependent variable," however, is broader and more general in its implications and applicability. Therefore, we generally use the term "dependent variable" in this text, although in many situations the terms "dependent variable" and "criterion variable" are equivalent and interchangeable.

Operational Definitions

Before a study can progress, the researcher must be able to clarify and define the variables under investigation. In order to be really useful, the definition must specify how the variable will be observed and measured in the actual research situation. Such a definition has a special name. An *operational definition* of a concept is a specification of the operations that the researcher must perform in order to collect the required information.

Variables differ considerably in the facility with which they can be operationalized. The variable weight, for example, is easy to define and measure. We may use the following as our definition of weight: the heaviness or lightness of an object in terms of pounds. Note that this definition designates that weight will be determined according to one measuring system (pounds) rather than another (grams). The operational definition might specify that the weight of participants in a research study would be measured to the nearest pound using a spring scale with subjects fully undressed after 10 hours of fasting. This operational definition clearly indicates to both the investigator and to others interested in the study what is meant by the variable weight.

Unfortunately, many of the variables of interest in nursing research are not operationalized as easily and straightforwardly as weight. Often there are multiple methods of measuring a variable and the researcher might choose the method that best captures the variable as he or she conceptualizes it. For example, patient well-being may be defined in terms of both physiological and psychological functioning. If the researcher chooses to emphasize the physiological aspects of patient well-being, the operational definition may involve a measure such as heart rate, white blood cell count, blood pressure, vital capacity, and so forth. If, on the other hand, well-being is conceptualized for the purposes of research as primarily a psychological phenomenon, the operational definition will need to identify the method by which emotional well-being will be assessed, such as the responses of the patient to certain questions or the behaviors of the patient as observed by the researcher.

Not all readers of a research report may agree with the way that the investigator has conceptualized and operationalized the variables. Nevertheless, precision in defining the terms has the advantage of communicating exactly what the terms mean. Operational definitions may often appear to limit the richness of concepts by reducing them to measurable phenomena. No single definition is likely to capture the fullness and complexity of patient well-being, for example. Yet if the researcher is reluctant to be explicit, it will be impossible for others to gauge the full meaning and implications of the research findings.

Relationships

Researchers are rarely interested in single, isolated variables, except perhaps in some descriptive studies. For example, a study might focus on the percentage of women who elect to breast-feed their babies. In this example, there is only one variable: breast-feeding versus bottle-feeding. Generally, however, researchers study two or more variables simultaneously. What scientists are generally interested in is the *relationship* between the independent and dependent variables of a study.

But what exactly is meant by the term "relationship" in scientific terms? Generally speaking, a relationship refers to a bond or connection between two entities. Let us consider as a possible dependent variable a person's body weight. What other variables are related to (associated with) a person's weight? Figure 2-1 graphically presents some possibili-

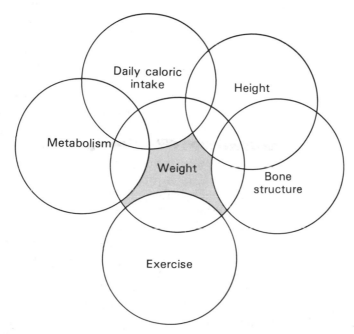

Figure 2-1. Hypothetical representation of factors related to body weight

ties—height, bone structure, metabolism, caloric intake, and exercise. For each of these five independent variables we can make a tentative relational statement:

Height: Tall people, in general, weigh more than short people.

Bone Structure: The finer the bone structure, the lower the person's weight.

Metabolism: The lower a person's metabolic rate, the more he or she will weigh.

Caloric Intake: People with high caloric intake are heavier than those with lower caloric intake.

Exercise: The greater the amount of exercise, the lower the person's weight.

Each of these statements expresses a presumed relationship between weight and an independent variable. The terms "more than" and "lower than" imply that as we observe a change in one variable, we are likely to observe a corresponding change in the other. If Jane were taller than Jean, we would expect (in the absence of any other information) that Jane was also heavier than Jean.

Research is essentially devoted to establishing that relationships do or do not exist among variables. We do not need a scientific study to determine that height and weight are related; sufficient information on this point already exists. But how about a relation between nursing shift assignments and absentee rates? Or between the frequency of turning patients and the incidence and severity of decubiti? One might predict that relationships would exist, but one would need to verify these hunches empirically.

The concept of relations among variables is so fundamental to the research process that it is worth pursuing a bit further. Variables can be related to one another in different ways. Scientists are often interested in what is referred to as *cause-and-effect relationships*. As noted in the introductory chapter, the scientist assumes that natural phenomena are not random or haphazard, but rather that all phenomena have antecedent factors or causes, which are discoverable. If variable X causes the occurrence or manifestation of variable Y, then it can be said that those variables are causally related; there exists a causal relationship between variables X and Y. For instance, in the example presented in Figure 2-1 we might say that there is a causal relationship between caloric intake and weight: eating more calories causes weight gain.

Causality, however, is a tricky business. We are unfortunately only rarely in a position to make definitive assertions concerning cause-and-effect relationships. However, two variables can be related to one another in a noncausal way if there is a systematic connection between their values. There is a relationship, for example, between a person's sex and weight; men tend to be heavier than women, on the average. The relationship is not perfect; some women are heavier than some men. Nevertheless, if we had to guess whether Keith Jones or Debbie Jones were heavier, we would be likely to say Keith, because men generally weigh more than women. We cannot really say, however, that a person's sex causes his or her weight, despite the relationship that exists between the two variables. This type of relationship is sometimes referred to as a *functional* rather than a causal relationship.

Control

The concept of *research control* is central to scientific inquiry. It is a topic to which much of this text is devoted. Chapter 8, in particular, discusses methods of achieving control in scientific research. The concept is so important, however, that some basic ideas about control are presented here.

Essentially, research control is concerned with holding constant possible influences on the dependent variable under investigation so that the true relationship between the independent and dependent variable can be understood. In other words, research control attempts to eliminate any contaminating factors that might otherwise obscure the relationship between the variables that are really of interest. A detailed example should clarify this point.

Let us suppose that a researcher is interested in studying whether teenage women are at higher risk to having low-birthweight infants than are older mothers because of their age. In other words, the researcher wants to test whether there is something about the physiological development of women that causes differences in the birthweights of their babies. Existing studies have shown that, in fact, teenagers have a higher rate of low-birthweight babies than women in their 20s. The question, however, is whether age itself causes this difference or whether there are other mechanisms that mediate the relationship between maternal age and infant birthweight.

The researcher in this example must design the study in such a way that these other factors are controlled. But what are the other variables that must be controlled? To answer this, one must ask the following critical question:

What variables could affect the dependent variable under study while at the same time be related to the independent variable?

In the present study the dependent variable is infant birthweight and the independent variable is maternal age. Two variables are prime candidates for concern (although there are several other possibilities): the nutritional habits of the mother and the amount of prenatal care received.

Teenagers are not always as careful as older women about their eating patterns during pregnancy and are also less likely to obtain adequate medical care. Both nutrition and the amount of care could, in turn, affect the baby's birthweight. Thus, if these two factors are not controlled, then any observed relationship between the mother's age and her baby's weight at birth could be caused by the mother's age itself, her diet, or her prenatal care.

These three possible explanations are shown schematically below:

1. Mother's age → infant birthweight
2. Mother's age → prenatal care → infant birthweight
3. Mother's age → nutrition → infant birthweight

The arrows here symbolize a causal mechanism or an influence. The researcher's task is to design a study in such a way that the true explanation is made clear. Both nutrition and prenatal care must be controlled in order to see if explanation 1 is valid.

How can the researcher impose such control? There are a number of ways, as discussed in Chapter 8, but the general principle underlying each alternative is the same: the competing influences—often referred to as *extraneous variables*—must be held constant. The extraneous variables needing to be controlled must somehow be handled in such a way that they are not related to the independent or dependent variable. Again, an example should help make this point more clear. Let us say we want to compare the birthweights of infants born to two groups of women: those aged 15 to 19 and those aged 25 to 29. We must then design a study in such a way that the nutritional and health-care practices of the two groups are comparable, even though, in general, the two groups are not comparable in these respects. Table 2-2 illustrates how groups could be selected in such a way that both older and younger mothers have similar eating habits and amounts of prenatal attention. By building this comparability into the two groups, we are holding nutrition and prenatal care constant. If

Table 2-2. Fictitious Example of Controlling Two Variables in a Research Study

AGE OF MOTHER	RATING OF NUTRITIONAL PRACTICES	NUMBER OF PRENATAL VISITS	INFANT BIRTHWEIGHT
15–19	33% Good	33% 1–3 visits	
	33% Fair	33% 4–6 visits	20% ≤ 2500 grams
	33% Poor	33% > 6 visits	80% > 2500 grams
25–29	33% Good	33% 1–3 visits	9% ≤ 2500 grams
	33% Fair	33% 4–6 visits	91% > 2500 grams
	33% Poor	33% > 6 visits	

thc babics' birthweights in the two groups continue to differ (as they in fact did in Table 2-2), we will be in a position to conclude that age (and not diet or prenatal care) influenced the birthweight of the infants. If the two groups do not differ, however, we will be left to tentatively conclude that it is not their age *per se* that causes young women to have a higher percentage of low-birthweight babies, but either nutrition, prenatal care, or both variables.

By exercising research control in this example, we have taken a step toward one of the most fundamental aims of science, which is to explain the relationship between variables. Control is essential because the world is extremely complex and many variables are interrelated in complicated ways. When studying a particular problem, it is almost never possible to examine this complexity directly: we must be content to analyze a couple of relationships at a time and put the pieces together like a jigsaw puzzle. That is why even modest research studies can make important contributions to science. The extent of the contribution, however, is strongly related to how well a researcher is able to control contaminating influences. A controlled study allows a researcher to understand the nature of the relationship between the dependent and independent variables.

In the present example, we identified three variables that could affect a baby's birthweight, but dozens of others could have been suggested, such as maternal stress, mothers' use of drugs or alcohol during the pregnancy, and so on. Researchers need to isolate the independent and dependent variables in which they are interested and then pinpoint from the dozens of possible candidates those that need to be controlled. It is not generally possible to control all the variables that affect the dependent variable, nor is it necessary to do so. It is essential to control a variable only if it is simultaneously related to both the dependent and independent variable.

Figure 2-2 illustrates this notion. In this figure, each circle represents the variability associated with a particular variable. The large circle in the center represents the dependent variable, infant birthweight. Overlapping variables indicate the degree to which the variables are related to each other. In this hypothetical example, four variables are shown as possibly being related to infant birthweight: the mother's age, the amount of prenatal care she receives, her nutritional practices, and her use of alcohol during pregnancy. The first three variables are also related to each other: this is shown by the fact that these three circles overlap not only with infant birthweight but also with each other. That is, younger mothers tend to have different patterns of prenatal care and nutrition than older mothers. The mother's prenatal use of alcohol, however, is unrelated to these three variables. In other words, women who drink during their pregnancies (according to this hypothetical representation) are as likely to be young as old, to eat properly as not, and to get a lot of prenatal

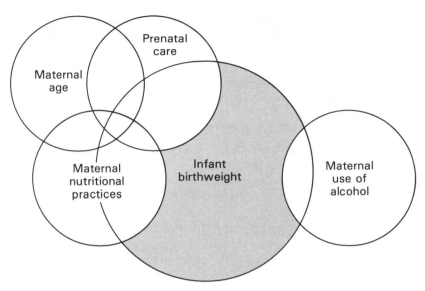

Figure 2-2. Hypothetical representation of factors affecting infant birthweight

care as not. If this representation is accurate, then it would not be essential to control alcohol use in a study of the effect of maternal age on infant birthweight. If this scheme is incorrect—if teenage mothers drink more or less alcohol than older mothers—then the mother's consumption of alcohol should be controlled.

Figure 2-2 does not represent infant birthweight as being totally determined by the four other variables. The darkened area of the birthweight circle designates unexplained variability in infant birthweight. That is, other "circles" or determinants of birthweight are needed in order for us to fully understand what causes babies to be born weighing different amounts. Genetic characteristics, events occurring during the pregnancy, and medical treatments administered to the pregnant woman are all examples of other factors contributing to an infant's weight at birth. Dozens, and perhaps hundreds, of circles would need to be sketched onto Figure 2-2 in order for us to fully understand the complex interrelationships between infant birthweight and other variables. In designing a study we might be interested in the effect of only one variable (such as maternal age) on the dependent variable. This is perfectly respectable—indeed, often necessary. However, researchers need to control those variables that overlap with both the independent and dependent variable. In Figure 2-2, if there are other variables that belong in the darkened area that are also related to maternal age, then those extraneous variables should be controlled. Since uncontrolled extraneous variables can lead to erroneous or misleading conclusions, the researcher designing a study must plan how best to control these extraneous variables to maximize the usefulness of the research. Also, the careful consumer of research studies needs to question whether the investigator has properly designed the study so that the true relationship between the independent and dependent variables is not obscured by the influence of contaminating factors.

Data

The *data* (singular, datum) of a research study are the pieces of information obtained in the course of the investigation. The researcher identifies the variables of interest, develops operational definitions of those variables, and then collects the necessary data. The variables, because they vary, take on different values. The *actual* values of the study variables constitute the data for a research project.

For example, suppose we were interested in studying the relationship between sodium consumption and blood pressure. That is, we want to learn if people who consume more sodium are particularly susceptible to high blood pressure, or whether these variables are unrelated. The data for this study would consist of three pieces of information for all participants: their average daily intake of sodium (in milligrams), their diastolic blood pressure, and their systolic blood pressure. Some hypothetical data for ten subjects are shown in Table 2-3. These numerical values associated with the variables of interest represent the data for a research project. The collection and analysis of data are typically the most time-consuming parts of a study.

Table 2-3. Hypothetical Data for Blood Pressure Study

SUBJECT NUMBER	DAILY SODIUM INTAKE (MILLIGRAMS)	SYSTOLIC BLOOD PRESSURE	DIASTOLIC BLOOD PRESSURE
1	8125	130	90
2	7530	126	80
3	1000	140	90
4	4580	118	78
5	2810	114	76
6	4150	112	78
7	6000	120	80
8	2250	110	70
9	5240	114	76
10	3330	116	74

Summary

This chapter introduced several of the terms and concepts that are the cornerstones of scientific methods.

Scientific research focuses on abstract *concepts.* In research studies, the concepts under investigation are referred to as *variables.* A variable is a characteristic or quality that takes on different values; that is, a variable is something that varies from one person or object to another. The blood type, blood pressure, grip strength, and hair color of a person are variables. These variables, which are inherent characteristics of a person that the researcher only measures or observes, are referred to as *attribute variables.* In some situations, a researcher actively creates or manipulates a variable, as when a drug is administered to some research subjects and a placebo is administered to others.

An important distinction for researchers is differentiation between the dependent and independent variables of a study. The *dependent variable* is the behavior, characteristic, or outcome that the researcher is interested in understanding, explaining, predicting, or affecting. The dependent variable (or criterion variable) is the presumed consequence or effect of the *independent variable.* The independent variable is the presumed cause of, antecedent to, or influence on the dependent variable.

In an actual investigation, the variables must be clarified and defined in such a way that they are amenable to observation or measurement. The *operational definition* of a concept is the specification of the procedures and tools required to make the needed measurements.

Except in rare cases, researchers are not interested in studying variables in isolation, but rather in learning about the *relationship* between two or more variables simultaneously. A relationship refers to a bond or connection between two variables. Researchers focus on the relationship between the independent and dependent variables. When the independent variable causes the occurrence, manifestation, or alteration of the dependent variable, a *cause-and-effect* relationship is said to exist. Variables that are not causally related can be linked by a *functional relationship.*

In attempting to understand how variables are related, researchers need to design a study that controls contaminating factors. Research *control* involves holding constant contaminating influences, known as *extraneous variables,* that might otherwise mask the true relationship between the independent or dependent variables.

The term *data* is used to designate the information that is collected during the course of a study. Since variables take on different values, the record of those values for the subjects in the study constitutes the data. Data collection generally is one of the most time-consuming phases of a research project.

Study Suggestions

1. Name 15 attribute characteristics of students in your class.

2. In the following research problems, identify the independent and dependent variables:

   a. How do nurses and physicians differ in the way they view the extended-role concept for nurses?

   b. Does problem-oriented recording lead to more effective patient care than other recording methods?

   c. Do elderly patients have lower pain thresholds than younger patients?

   d. How are the sleeping patterns of infants affected by different forms of stimulation?

   e. Can home visits by nurses to released psychiatric patients reduce readmission rates?

3. Suggest ways of operationally defining the following concepts: nursing competency; patients' time to first voiding after surgery; aggressive behavior; patients' level of pain; home health hazards; psychogenic sterility; social class; and body image.

4. Suppose you were interested in studying factors affecting attrition from nursing school programs.

   a. Identify an independent variable on which you would want to focus.

   b. Identify at least two extraneous variables you would need to control.

   c. Draw a diagram that shows how these variables might be interrelated, similar to that in Figure 2-2.

5. Read a study in a recent issue of *Nursing Research*. Identify the independent, dependent, and extraneous variables.

Chapter 3
Research as a
Decision-Making Process

The research process begins with a question of interest to the researcher and ends when the question has been answered. A researcher might ask, for example, "Does the method of tracheotomy care affect the incidence of pulmonary infection?" or "Is a patient more satisfied with his or her nursing care if the nurse is from the same ethnic or racial background as the patient?" These questions could form the basis for two research studies. Between the posing of the question and the obtaining of the answer lie many steps and many decisions.

Research Alternatives

Beginning researchers are not always aware of how much flexibility there is in designing and conducting a study. It is not unusual for students to read a report of a scientific investigation and more or less accept the decisions that the researcher made unquestioningly. One of the purposes of this chapter is to demonstrate that the researcher must choose from a number of alternative strategies in designing a study, and that each decision has crucial implications for the quality and integrity of the results.

One thing must be clear from the start: *every study, no matter how sophisticated or well done, has some flaws or limitations.* There is no such thing as a perfect study, and there is no single study that provides unchallengeable answers to research questions. Nevertheless, there is a tremendous range in the quality of studies—from nearly worthless to exemplary. The quality of the research is closely tied to the kinds of decisions the researcher makes in designing the investigation.

While no single study is infallible, the scientific method continues to provide us with the best possible means of answering certain questions. Knowledge accumulates not by conducting a single, isolated study, but rather through an aggregation of findings from many studies. Each study tends to have its own peculiar flaws, because each researcher, in addressing the same or a similar research question, makes somewhat different decisions about how the study should be done.

Let us look at an example that builds on concepts presented in the previous chapter. Suppose researcher A studied the relationship between patients' age and levels of preoperative stress and concluded, based on the data, that older patients experience higher levels of stress than younger ones. Researcher B believes that researcher A made a bad decision in not first controlling for the type of surgical procedure. In controlling this extraneous variable, researcher B found that older patients still had higher levels of preoperative stress than younger ones. Researcher C reviews both studies and decides that the number of prior hospitalizations should also be controlled; the results of the third investigation lead to the same conclusion.

It is in this fashion that knowledge advances. When many different studies—done at different times and places with different methodological decisions—yield similar findings, then we gain confidence in the answers to the research question.

Knowledge accumulation is not always as smooth as this example suggests. Researcher A, in failing to control for extraneous variables, might have come to the conclusion that patients' age and preoperative stress were unrelated. Researcher B might have made a faulty decision in some other aspect of the study and might have come to the same, perhaps incorrect, conclusion. It is not uncommon for researchers to make different decisions and to arrive at different answers.

It is precisely for this reason that consumers of research must be knowledgeable about the research process. As consumers, we must be able to evaluate the decisions that investigators made so that we can determine how much faith should be put in their conclusions. And, in conducting our own research, we must attempt to make the best possible decisions so that our research findings have a good chance of adding to the store of human knowledge.

Much of this book is designed to acquaint the reader with a range of methodological options for the conduct of research—options on how to control extraneous variables, options on how to collect and analyze data, options on how to operationalize variables, and so on. As you read the material in this text, you will become better prepared to challenge a researcher's decisions and to suggest alternative methods. You will also be better prepared to make your own decisions in designing a research project. At this point, however, it is important to recognize that there *are* options and that the choices affect the validity of a study's results.

The next section of this chapter presents an overview of how a researcher progresses from the posing of a research question to the arrival at an answer. Then we turn to a discussion of a researcher's major decisions, illustrated by two hypothetical studies.

Major Steps in the Research Process

A researcher typically moves from the beginning point of a study (the posing of a question) to the end point (the obtaining of an answer) in a logical sequence of steps. True, in some cases the steps overlap; in other cases some steps are interchangeable; in yet other cases some are unnecessary. Still, there is a general flow of activities that is typical of a scientific investigation. That flow is briefly described below. The remainder of the text provides more detail about these research activities in roughly the same sequential order.

1. Formulating and Delimiting the Problem

The first step in the scientific process is to develop a research problem. Good research depends to a great degree on good questions. Sometimes the importance of securing an interesting and meaningful topic gets lost in the concern for utilizing appropriate and sophisticated research procedures. Yet without a good, workable, significant topic, the most carefully and skillfully designed research project will be of little value. Once a general topic is selected, the specific problem to be investigated and the variables it encompasses should be defined as precisely as possible. Initial statements of the problem are typically too broad and too vague. Problem statements that are hazy and broad, however, will ultimately lead to confusion in that they cannot provide direction to the project.

2. Reviewing the Related Literature

Good research does not exist in a vacuum. In order for research findings to be useful, they should be an extension of previous knowledge and theory as well as a guide for future research activity. In order for a researcher to build on existing work, it is essential to understand what is already known about a topic. A thorough review of the literature provides a foundation upon which to base new knowledge.

3. Developing a Theoretical Framework

A *theory* is a generalized, abstract explanation about the interrelationship among phenomena, with the primary purpose of explaining and predicting those phenomena. Theory is the ultimate aim of science in that it transcends the specifics of a particular time, place, and set of persons and aims to identify regularities in the relationships among variables.

When research is performed within the context of a theoretical framework, it is more likely that its findings will be useful in improving our ability to understand or control events, situations, and persons.

4. Formulating Hypotheses

A *hypothesis* is a statement of the researcher's expectations about relationships between the variables under investigation. A hypothesis, in other words, is a prediction of expected outcomes; it states the relationships that the researcher anticipates finding as a result of the study. The problem statement identifies the phenomena under investigation; a hypothesis predicts how those phenomena will be related. For example, a problem statement might be phrased as follows: Is preeclamptic toxemia in pregnant women associated with stress factors present during pregnancy? This might be translated into the following hypothesis or prediction: Pregnant women with preeclamptic toxemia will report a higher incidence of emotionally disturbing or stressful events during pregnancy than asymptomatic pregnant women. Thus, problem statements represent the initial effort to give a research project direction; hypotheses represent a more formalized focus for the collection and interpretation of data.

5. Selecting a Research Design

The research design is the overall plan for how to obtain answers to the questions being studied and how to handle some of the difficulties encountered during the research process. The design should specify which of the various types of research approach will be adopted and how the researcher plans to implement a number of scientific controls to enhance the interpretability of the results.

A wide variety of research approaches are available to nurse researchers. A basic distinction is the difference between *experimental* designs (in which the researcher actively introduces some form of intervention) and *nonexperimental* designs (in which the researcher passively collects data without trying to make any changes or introduce any treatments). For example, if the researcher administered a new drug to one group of people and a placebo to another, the study would involve an intervention and would be considered experimental. If the researcher compared vital sign measurements for a group who normally consumed aspirins with another group who did not, the study would not involve an intervention and would be considered nonexperimental. Experimental designs generally offer the possibility of greater control over extraneous variables than nonexperimental designs.

6. Specifying the Population

The term *population* refers to the aggregate or totality of all the objects, subjects, or members that conform to a set of specifications. For example, we may specify "nurses" (RNs) and "living in the United States" as the attributes of interest; our population would then consist of all licensed RNs who reside in the United States. We could in a similar fashion define a population consisting of all children under 10 years of age with muscular dystrophy in the state of California, or all the patient records in a particular hospital, or all persons who had a fatal coronary during a particular year.

The requirement of defining a population for a research project arises from the need to specify the group to which the results of a study can be applied. It is seldom possible to study an entire population, unless it is quite small. Research studies typically use as subjects only a small fraction of the population, referred to as a *sample*. Before one selects actual study participants (often referred to as *subjects*), it is essential to know what characteristics the sample should possess in order to be able to generalize the findings to the broader population.

7. Operationalizing and Measuring the Research Variables

In order to meaningfully test a research hypothesis, some method must be developed to measure the research variables as objectively and accurately as possible. The researcher should first carefully define the research variables to clarify exactly what each one means. Then the researcher needs to select or design an appropriate tool to measure the variables—that is, to collect the data. A variety of measurement tools exist. *Physiological measurements* often play an important role in nursing research. Another popular form is *self-reports*, wherein subjects are directly asked about their feelings, behaviors, attitudes, and personal traits. Another method of measuring variables is through *observational techniques*. Here the researcher collects data by observing people's behavior and recording relevant aspects of it. In short, the task of operationalizing research variables is a complex and challenging process that permits a great deal of creativity and choice.

8. Conducting a Pilot Study

Unforeseen problems often arise in the course of a project. The effects of such problems may be negligible but in other cases may be so severe that the study has to be stopped so that modifications can be introduced. Whenever possible, therefore, it is advisable to carry out a *pilot study*, which is a small-scale version, or trial run, of the major study. The function of the pilot study is to obtain information for improving the project or for assessing its feasibility. For example, the pilot study may provide information suggesting that the target population was defined too broadly. From a more practical point of view, a trial run may reveal that it will not be possible to secure the cooperation of people by the intended procedures or that the study is more costly than anticipated. Very often, however, the principal focus of a pilot study is the assessment of the adequacy of the measurement instruments or the development of a new measure.

9. Selecting the Sample

Data are generally collected from a sample rather than from an entire population. The advantage of using a sample is that it is more practical and less costly than collecting data from the population. The risk is that the sample selected might not adequately reflect the behaviors, traits, symptoms, or beliefs of the population.

Various methods of obtaining a sample are available to the researcher. These methods vary in cost, effort, and level of skills required, but their adequacy is assessed by the same criterion: the representativeness of the selected sample. That is, the quality of the sample is a function of how typical, or representative, the sample is of the population with respect to the variables of concern in the study. Sophisticated sampling procedures can produce samples that have a high likelihood of being representative. The most sophisticated sampling methods are referred to as *probability sampling*, which employs random procedures for the selection of the sample. In a probability sample, every member of the population has the possiblity of being included in the sample. With *non-probability sampling* techniques, by contrast, there is no way of assuring that each member of the population could be selected; consequently, the risk of a biased (unrepresentative) sample is greater.

10. Collecting the Data

The actual collection of data should proceed according to a preestablished plan in order to minimize confusions, delays, and mistakes. That is, the procedures to be used in describing the study to the participants, in administering the measuring instruments, in answering the questions of participants, and so forth, should be specified in advance. This step may sometimes involve the training of research personnel in the case of complicated experiments or detailed interview studies. The collection of data is typically the most time-consuming phase of a study, although the actual amount of time spent varies considerably from project to project.

11. Preparing the Data for Analysis

Generally, the data collected in a study are not directly amenable to analysis. Some preliminary steps are usually necessary before the analysis can proceed. One such step that is typically needed is known as *coding*, which refers to the process of "translating" verbal data into categories or numerical form. For example, patients' responses to a question about the quality of nursing care they received during hospitalization might be coded into positive reactions, negative reactions, neutral reactions, and mixed reactions.

Another preliminary step that is increasingly common is the preparation of data for computer analysis. The procedures involved in the use of computers are briefly discussed in Chapter 17.

12. Analyzing the Data

The data themselves do not provide us with answers to our research questions. Ordinarily, the amount of data collected in a study is too extensive to be reliably described by mere perusal. In order to meaningfully test the research hypotheses, the data must be processed and analyzed in some orderly, coherent fashion so that patterns and relationships can be discerned. *Statistical procedures* are methods of dealing with quantitative information in such a way as to make that information meaningful and interpretable.

Statistical analyses cover a broad range of techniques, including some very simple procedures as well as complex and sophisticated methods. The underlying logic of statistical tests, however, is relatively simple and should be no cause for concern to the beginning researcher. Computers and pocket calculators have virtually eliminated the need to get bogged down with detailed arithmetical operations.

13. Interpreting the Results

Before the results of a study can be communicated effectively, they must be organized and interpreted in some systematic fashion. By interpretation, we refer to the process of making sense of the results and of examining the implications of the findings within a broader context. The process of interpretation begins with an attempt to explain the findings.

If the research hypotheses have been supported, an explanation of the results is usually straightforward, since the findings fit into a previously conceived argument. If the hypotheses are not supported, the investigator must develop some possible explanations. Is the underlying conceptualization wrong, or perhaps inappropriate for the research problem? Or do the findings reflect problems with the research methods rather than the theory (*e.g.*, was the sample biased)? In order to provide sound explanations for obtained findings, then, the researchers must not only be familiar with the literature on a topic and with the conceptual underpinnings of the problem, but must also be able to understand the methodological weaknesses of the study design. In other words, a researcher should be in a position to critically evaluate the decisions he or she made in designing the study and to recommend alternatives to others interested in the same research problem.

14. Communicating the Findings

The results of a research investigation are of little utility if they are not communicated to others. Even the most compelling hypothesis, the most careful and thorough study, the most dramatic results are of no value to the scientific community if they are unknown. The final task of a research project, therefore, is the preparation of a research report. There are various forms of research reports: term papers, dissertations, journal articles, books, and so on. Journal articles—that is, short reports appearing in such professional journals as *Nursing Research*—are generally the most useful because such reports are available to a broad audience.

Major Decision Points in the Research Process

The steps described above represent a fairly standard progression of activities in conducting a scientific investigation. Mere adherence to these steps, however, is insufficient to guarantee that an important contribution will be made to the store of knowledge on a topic. Several of the steps compel the researcher to make important decisions regarding the conduct of the study. If the investigator does not—or cannot—design the study in such a way that biases or distortions are minimized, then the results of the research may be worthless.

Even people with sophisticated research skills design studies that are imperfect. Indeed, virtually no study is flawless, as we explained earlier in the chapter. One limitation is that even if a "perfect" study could be designed in the abstract, it would be too costly or too impractical to implement in the real world. Conducting large-scale studies generally requires an enormous amount of resources. Research investigations also require people's cooperation, which in some cases may be difficult to obtain. In short, the researcher must strive to design the best study possible with available resources but should be alert to the possibility that different decisions might have improved the quality of the research.

The remainder of this text describes the major options available to researchers designing scientific studies. It also discusses the strengths and weaknesses of the various alternatives, so that both consumers of research and those who wish to conduct their own studies will be better equipped to understand and evaluate key decisions in the research process. In the remainder of this chapter, however, we highlight what the primary methodological decision points are by "walking through" a hypothetical study as designed by two fictitious researchers.

We begin with the statement of the research problem. Let us suppose that the two researchers (nurse A and nurse B) are interested in answering the following question: Does the use of sonography during the first trimester of a pregnancy affect maternal–infant bonding? Both nurses hypothesize that women who "see" their infants in utero during the first trimester will develop stronger (and earlier) attachments to their babies than women who have not had this opportunity. Both researchers begin at the same point, with a question they would like to answer. The two nurses differ, however, in the decisions they make in designing a study to answer the question. And, as we shall see, the confidence that can be placed in the validity of the results hinges on the researchers' decisions.

The first major decision that the researcher makes concerns the design*:

- *Decision I:* What design should be used that will yield the most unambiguous and meaningful results about the relationship between the independent and dependent variables?

The research design is, essentially, the plan for controlling extraneous variables. Some designs exert some very tight controls, while others exercise virtually none. In our present example, the independent variable is the pregnant woman's exposure or nonexposure to sonography during the first trimester; the dependent variable is maternal–infant bonding. The research design is the plan for examining the degree to which these two variables are systematically related to each other. Here is a description of what our two fictitious researchers decided about the research design:

Nurse A: A sample of mothers who have recently delivered a baby will be asked whether they had a sonogram performed during the

---

*Not all of the steps or activities described in the previous section represent critical decision points, even though each step may be important with respect to the overall quality of the research. For example, reviewing related research (step 2) is essential if the researcher wants to extend knowledge, but this task does not itself involve a decision about how to conduct the study. (The review may, however, provide information that helps the researcher to make better decisions.)

first trimester of their pregnancy. Two groups of mothers will be formed on the basis of the women's responses (an early sonogram group and a nonearly sonogram group), and the degree of bonding in the two groups will be compared.

Nurse B: A sample of women who have just been diagnosed as being pregnant (within the first 10 weeks of pregnancy) will be asked to participate in a study of maternal–infant bonding. Half of the sample will randomly be assigned (*i.e.*, be assigned by some nonbiased method such as a coin flip) to the group that will have a sonogram performed in the first trimester, while the second half will be randomly assigned to a group that will not have an early sonogram. The degree of maternal–infant bonding in the two groups will later be compared.

Nurse A chose a nonexperimental design to test the research hypothesis. Researcher A plays a passive role, collecting data after the fact to examine the relationship between early sonography and maternal bonding. Nurse B, by contrast, has chosen an experimental design. This researcher intervenes and controls whether or not an early sonogram is given to some women.

Nurse B has selected a far stronger design than Nurse A. Several comments should help to clarify why the second design is better, though material presented later in this text should make this even clearer. First, nurse B will know for certain that her independent variable is accurate. That is, the researcher controls whether or not the patient receives a sonogram in the first trimester. Nurse A, by contrast, must rely on the memory of the women in the sample. Some women may not understand or remember what a sonogram is; others may not remember exactly when the sonogram was performed; still others may, for one reason or another, falsify their answers.

Second, and most important, the first design does nothing to control extraneous variables. There may be many differences between women who did or did not have an early sonogram, and these differences may themselves be related to maternal infant bonding, rather than the act of having a sonogram. For example, the no-sonogram group in nurse A's study may contain a disproportionately high number of women who did not want or plan for a pregnancy and who did not seek prenatal care in the first trimester. Or, this group may have many very young women who could not afford sonography and whose own developmental status has an effect on their ability to bond with their infants. The second design has the potential to control virtually all extraneous variables because the two groups are formed by chance (randomly). Young women and old women, those who want a pregnancy and those who do not, have an equal chance of being in the experimental group—that is, of obtaining a first-trimester sonogram. Therefore, researcher B can be more confident that any observed relationship between early sonography and bonding is not the result of the extraneous variables. Nurse A does not have the same assurance. Note, however, that nurse A may not really have had the option of using an experimental design. Many practical constraints may interfere with the selection of the strongest design. The first design, while the weaker of the two, does not necessarily result in a worthless study, but its limitations must be kept in mind.

The second major decision concerns the identification of the population:

- *Decision II:* Who are the people (or institutions, groups, etc.) to whom the research question can reasonably be applied?

The research question itself usually suggests the general characteristics of the population. In the present example, we know that the population includes mothers and pregnant women. However, a more precise definition of the population is needed, not only to clarify the nature of the research, but also as a means of designing a more rigorous study. This second decision is really an extension of the first: by a careful specification of the population, the researcher can control extraneous variables. To see why this is so, let us consider what the two fictitious researchers decided regarding the populations they planned to study:

Nurse A: The population consists of women who have delivered infants.

Nurse B: The population consists of married primigravid women between the ages of 20 and 35.

These two specifications differ in two important respects. First, the two researchers are dealing with overlapping but nonidentical populations by virtue of the research design. Nurse A has designed the study in such a way that the study group consists of mothers. Nurse B, on the other hand, is studying pregnant women. As we shall see, this distinction has some implications for the collection of data.

The second difference concerns the degree of specificity. Nurse A implies, with a broad specification, that the results of the research can be generalized to all mothers. Nurse B has delimited the study population in three respects: the women must be pregnant for the first time; they must be married; and they must be neither in their early childbearing years at the time of their first pregnancy nor at the end of their childbearing years. Nurse B is essentially augmenting her research design by a thoughtful definition of the population. This researcher has identified three variables that could potentially affect maternal–infant bonding (pregnancy history, marital status, and age) and has controlled the effect of these variables by eliminating them as variables. Thus, if single and married pregnant women differ in their attachment to a newborn child, the inclusion of only married women eliminates this difference. Marital status is no longer a variable in this study, but rather a constant: the population consists only of those who are married. Nurse A, with a broad specification of the population, has missed an opportunity to control contaminating influences on the dependent variable.

Some of you may be wondering why nurse B needed to delimit the population, given the overall research design. After all, researcher B is randomly assigning women to a sonogram or no-sonogram group. Married and single women, young and old women, primigravida and multi-gravida would be equally likely to be assigned to either group. Therefore, the design has already controlled these extraneous variables.

Researcher B realizes that randomly assigning subjects to groups does not guarantee a perfect balance. For example, if you were to toss a coin ten times, you might get seven heads and three tails rather than five of each. In the long run, after thousands of coin tosses, you would get an even split between heads and tails; but researchers typically work with relatively small samples, and "uneven splits" can happen. The risk of getting a bias (an uneven distribution of some characteristic in the groups being formed) is particularly great when the characteristic itself is uneven in the population.

An example should clarify this point. Let us suppose that we have 20 subjects (10 men and 10 women) to randomly assign to two groups. Ideally, each group would consist of five men and five women; but it would not be unusual for one group to have six men and the other group four. Still, a six–four split is not a very biased distribution. A ten–zero split or even a nine–one split would be strongly biased, but these distributions are highly improbable if random procedures are used. Now let us suppose, as in the present example, that we have 20 pregnant women to assign to two groups; 2 are single and 18 are married. It is quite possible, even using random assignment, for both single women to be assigned to one group (let's say the no-sonogram group). To the extent that marital status influences maternal–infant bonding, this distribution could bias the results and lead to erroneous conclusions. Thus, when a characteristic is unevenly distributed in a population, it may be useful to control it by delimiting the study population, especially if the study sample is relatively small.

Perhaps you have concluded that a careful, precise specification of the population is a painless and "cheap" means of controlling extraneous variables. True, the researcher's decision regarding the population is an efficient method of control, but it is not gratuitous. Once the population is specified, the study findings can be generalized only to that population. Thus, nurse B's results cannot be applied to pregnant teenagers, to unmarried mothers, to women who have had miscarriages, and so on. Nurse A can generalize the study findings to all these groups, but nurse A also runs a greater risk that the results are erroneous.

It should be noted that both researchers failed to delimit their populations in terms of geographical region. This omission is common. By implication, the populations in these examples consist of all pregnant women or mothers throughout the world. In most cases, it is unrealistic to assume that relationships among variables are consistent across cultures, climates, or political divisions. Therefore, it is recommended that some thought be given to defining the geographical boundaries of the target population.

The next major division concerns how the variables will be measured:

- *Decision III:* How should the key variables be operationalized and reliably and validly measured for each participant in the study?

This decision involves choosing a method for the actual collection of data. In the present example, the two researchers must elaborate on what they mean by maternal–infant bonding; they must then spell out the procedures they will use to determine the degree of maternal–infant bonding for each of the women in their sample. Both researchers have hypothesized that bonding is greater among women who had an early sonogram. The task now is to find a good way to capture differences in mothers' bonding with their newborns to see if these differences can be linked to the women's experiences with sonography during pregnancy. While both our fictitious researchers have conceptualized maternal–infant bonding as the psychological rapport established between a mother and her child, they have made different decisions regarding the measurement of this dependent variable:

Nurse A: The degree of maternal–infant bonding will be assessed by summing the women's responses to a 20-question psychological test given to the women within 48 hours of delivering their babies. Two examples of the true/false questions on this test are as follows: (1) "I already feel a strong, binding attachment to my child." and (2) "My baby and I are still strangers who need to get to know one another better." The higher the scores on this test, the greater the degree of maternal–infant bonding.

Nurse B: The degree of maternal–infant bonding will be assessed using several indicators of the women's behavior: (1) whether or not the woman continues her pregnancy or seeks an abortion; (2) the woman's eating, drinking, and smoking patterns during pregnancy; (3) whether or not the woman, after delivery, elects a rooming-in arrangement; and (4) ratings by an objective observer of the quality of the mother's interaction with her child during the first mid-morning feeding following delivery.

Here again we find that although the two researchers were testing the same hypothesis, they have made quite different decisions about the conduct of the research. Nurse A has chosen one single measure of maternal–infant bonding—the summed responses on a self-report instrument. True/false tests such as the one nurse A adopted depend on the cooperation of the study's participants. Each mother is asked to report about her own feelings and beliefs, hence the term "self-report."

Nurse B, by contrast, has decided to use several indicators of maternal–infant bonding and to use indicators that are manifested by the women's behaviors rather than their interpretations of their own attitudes and feelings. Nurse B, once again, has chosen a sounder approach. The use of more than one indicator of the dependent variable indicates the researcher's recognition that any single measure of a variable, particularly variables that are psychological in nature, is imperfect. The woman with the greatest amount of attachment to her infant may not get the highest score on nurse A's test or the highest rating by nurse B's observer. All measures contain some error; hopefully, the amount of error is small. The use of more than one measure in nurse B's study is commendable because different measures generally contain different kinds of error.

The second important difference between the two studies concerns the nature of the data collection. Nurse A has relied exclusively on the mothers' self-reports. Self-reports are an extremely useful and flexible method of collecting data about human beings, but they can, nevertheless, be problematic. The subjects must be interested in cooperating; they must understand the questions; they must all interpret the words in the question the same way; and they must be willing to divulge their innermost feelings, even though the answers may not be flattering or socially acceptable. Given all of these demands, self-report measures are subject to many sources of error that can reduce their accuracy and meaningfulness.

Nurse B has operationalized maternal–infant bonding in terms of behaviors rather than self-reported attitudes. Nurse B believes that women with greater attachment to their infants will begin manifesting it during their pregnancy: they will be less inclined to seek an abortion, and they will take better care of themselves prenatally by eating well and avoiding alcohol and cigarettes. Furthermore, nurse B plans to collect behavioral data by several methods: through patient records (the abortion and rooming-in variables); through self-reports (the nutritional, smoking, and drinking variables); and through observation by an objective party (the quality of the mother's interaction during feeding). Thus, nurse B might be expected to gather sounder and more reliable data about maternal–infant bonding than nurse A.

The next important decision that the researchers face concerns the selection of the research sample:

- *Decision IV:* How large should the sample of subjects be, and what method should be used to select that sample?

Here, the decision for our fictitious researchers involves the identification and recruitment of pregnant women/mothers from the population specified earlier. Often, this decision is one that is subject to many constraints, such as the researcher's resources, the time available for completion of the study, and the accessibility of persons meeting the population specifications. The two researchers in the present example did the following with respect to sample selection:

> *Nurse A:* The sample will consist of 50 women delivering infants at the Cole County Hospital Center. Subjects for the sample will be recruited from the groups attending the prenatal classes given at the hospital. Women will be asked to volunteer to participate in the study following the delivery of their infants.

> *Nurse B:* The sample will consist of 200 married primigravida who are no more than 10 weeks pregnant and who are between the ages of 20 and 35. Women meeting these sampling criteria will be selected from five Ob/Gyn practices that have agreed to assist the researcher in the study. Each practice will invite a randomly selected group of women to participate in the research. Forty women from each practice will be included: 20 will be assigned to an early sonogram condition, and the remaining 20 will have no sonogram in the first trimester of pregnancy.

Once again the two fictitious researchers have opted for different approaches in designing their studies, and again nurse B has a stronger plan. First of all, the second researcher has a larger sample. One of the most common flaws of research studies in nursing and other fields is the inadequate size of the samples. Unfortunately, there is no easy rule of thumb to determine what is an adequate number of subjects. But, in general, large samples run less of a risk of distortion and bias than small samples.

An example might help to clarify this point. Suppose you wanted to know if men or women were more likely to obtain an annual physical checkup. Suppose further that you randomly picked the names of ten men and ten women from the phone book, called them, and asked about their last checkup; you might find that 50% of the women and 10% of the men had had a checkup in the past 12 months. Could you conclude that women practice better preventive health care based on this sample? By chance alone, the sample might have overrepresented men who are especially negligent about health care, or women who are hypochondriacs. But now suppose your sample consisted of 500 men and 500 women, and the same results were obtained. The risk of distortions in the percentages obtaining a checkup decreases as the sample size increases.

The second difference between the samples selected by nurses A and B concerns the method of selection. Nurse A used what is referred to as a *sample of convenience*. The selection process does nothing to assure that the sample is truly representative of the population. Only one hospital is used, and there may be many reasons why women delivering at this particular hospital are nonrepresentative of all women. For example, the Cole County Hospital Center may serve primarily white, well-educated, middle-class women. Furthermore, by going through prenatal classes to recruit subjects, the researcher has automatically excluded women who do not obtain prenatal instruction. Finally, by relying on people to come forward and volunteer, it is likely that yet another bias will be introduced.

Nurse B's sampling plan, though not perfect, is more likely to yield a representative sample than that of nurse A. The use of five different Ob/Gyn practices reduces the risk that the women will come primarily from one religion or ethnic group or social class and so on. The resulting sample may not be totally representative of married primigravida aged 20 to 35, but the biases are likely to be less serious than would be the case if a single practice were used. Furthermore, nurse B's plan does not depend on volunteers. A *random sample* of women (*i.e.*, chosen by some procedure such as drawing names from a hat) will be individually invited to participate. True, some may decline, but a smaller percentage is likely to refuse to cooperate in nurse B's study than is likely to fail to volunteer for nurse A's study. Here again, this means that the likelihood of bias is reduced. In short, nurse B has designed her sample in such a way that the risk of gross distortions has been minimized; nurse A, by contrast, has selected a sample with considerable potential for yielding misleading results.

The final important decision concerns the choice of analytic procedures:

- *Decision V:* What analyses will provide the most rigorous and appropriate tests of the research hypotheses.

The design of a study is not complete until a plan for analyzing the study data has been developed. Generally, the analysis involves the use of a statistical test, and there are many tests from which to choose. The choice of an appropriate test depends on such considerations as the size of the sample, the type of data that have been collected, the availability of a computer for the analysis, and the sophistication of the researcher. There are some simple tests that can easily be computed manually and require little statistical training. Other statistical tests, however, are so computationally laborious that the use of a computer and strong technical skills on the part of the researcher are essential.

Because the factors governing analytic decisions are too complex to briefly describe in this chapter, we do not present a discussion of two hypothetical statistical plans for nurse A and nurse B here. Suffice it to say that there are so many different alternatives that the two plans could be widely divergent in terms of yielding unambiguous and trustworthy results. Some of these analytic alternatives are described in Chapter 16.

We have now reviewed the five major decisions that a researcher must make in designing a research investigation. As we have seen, these decisions lead to substantial differences in the quality of the research. Nurse A's decisions yielded a considerably weaker plan than did nurse B's. The consequence is that we would have less confidence in the findings of nurse A's study.

Suppose that nurse A, on the basis of the investigation as described above, concludes that the hypothesis is not supported. In other words, nurse A's findings indicate that maternal–infant bonding is just as high among women who did not have a first-trimester sonogram as among those who did. Would we be justified in concluding that this is true of all women? There are sufficient flaws in nurse A's study that it would be rash to come to this conclusion without more verification from additional research. Nurse A's finding might not reflect the "truth" for a number of reasons, such as the following: (1) nurse A's failure to control important extraneous variables; (2) too broad a specification of the population; (3) the use of a measuring tool that might be insensitive and subject to distortions; and (4) too small a sample, drawn from a potentially biased source.

Despite these weaknesses, it would be unwise to decide that nurse A's study is worthless. It might, in fact, be true that an early sonogram has no effect on maternal–infant bonding. If later researchers also conduct studies that yield the same result, nurse A's investigation will be an additional piece of evidence that no relationship between bonding and first-trimester sonography exists. And even if nurse A is wrong, the shortcomings of this researcher's investigation are likely to lead to improvements in the design of a new study as other investigators seek to test the same hypothesis. In short, we must learn to be critical of the decisions researchers make so that we can assess the believability of the results. But we should also recognize that virtually all studies have the potential to make some contribution to human knowledge, if only because they spur a desire for further scrutiny of a problem.

Summary

Researchers designing a scientific study must make a number of important decisions that determine the quality and integrity of the research. There are many alternative strategies from which to choose, and decisions generally depend on such factors as the researcher's time, resources, scientific sophistication, and access to subjects, as well as on ethical and practical considerations. It is important to recognize that a researcher's design decisions are inevitably bound by some of these constraints, and that every study is, therefore, subject to some flaws or limitations.

While the quality of studies varies widely as a result of the researcher's study design, the steps involved in the conduct of a scientific investigation are fairly standard. The following steps are often performed in a roughly sequential fashion:

1. Formulating and delimiting the problem
2. Reviewing the related literature
3. Developing a theoretical framework
4. Formulating a hypothesis
5. Selecting a research design
6. Specifying the population
7. Operationalizing and measuring the research variables
8. Conducting a pilot study
9. Selecting a sample
10. Collecting the data
11. Preparing the data for analysis
12. Analyzing the data
13. Interpreting the results
14. Communicating the findings

While all of these steps need to be pursued with great care and attention, five of them represent critical decision points that will have a major effect on the validity of the study's findings. These are steps 5, 6, 7, 9, and 12. Consumers of nursing research should focus critical attention on these decisions in evaluating studies; and those who conduct their own investigations must attempt to make the best decisions possible within the constraints of their circumstances and to understand the limitations to which their decisions give rise.

Study Suggestions

1. Suppose that you were interested in testing the hypothesis that having a sonogram in the first trimester of pregnancy would increase the bonding between a mother and her infant. Describe how you would design the study using women from your own community as subjects.

2. How would you operationalize and measure the following variables: preoperative stress; children's degree of fear of hospitalization; cardiovascular function; pain tolerance; attitudes toward the mentally ill; smoking behavior; and women's reaction to a mastectomy.

3. Read an article in a recent issue of *Nursing Research*. Evaluate the researcher's decisions regarding the conduct of the research.

PART II
Preliminary Steps
in the Research Process

Chapter 4
Contexts for
Research Problems

A scientific study often begins with a vague question, or with an idea about a general topic of interest. Among nurse researchers, nursing experience frequently provides a starting point for a study. Whatever the source for the idea, it is important to recognize that good research generally builds upon existing knowledge. The more developed the network linking one's study with other research, the more of a contribution it is likely to make. The accumulation of scientific knowledge is very much analogous to the fitting together of a jigsaw puzzle. Every piece of the puzzle, small though it may be, may help to link together other parts of the puzzle.

Linkages with an existing body of knowledge are generally developed in two ways. The first is to perform a thorough review of the prior research on a topic. The second is to develop a theoretical framework for the research problem. Both of these activities are important not only because they provide a conceptual context for a scientific investigation, but also because they may help the researcher to refine and delimit the problem to be studied. This chapter discusses these two activities, which generally precede the design and execution of the research.

The Literature Review

A review of related research on a topic has become a standard and virtually essential activity of scientific research projects. A literature review involves the systematic identification, location, scrutiny, and summary of written materials that contain information on a research problem.

A literature review can play a number of important roles. First, as suggested above, a review of work conducted in an area of general interest can help in the formulation or clarification of a research problem. Second, a study of previous work acquaints the researcher with what has been done in a field, thereby minimizing the possibility of unintentional duplication. Third, the review provides a conceptual context or framework for the researcher and for the research community, thereby facilitating the accumulation of scientific knowledge. Fourth, the researcher may be in a better position to assess the feasibility of a proposed study by familiarity with related work. Finally, the review can be highly useful in pointing out the research strategies and specific procedures, measuring instruments, and statistical analyses that might be productive in pursuing one's problem. In short, there is considerable value in conducting a thorough investigation of existing research before embarking on a new scientific endeavor.

The literature review generally begins with a library search. The beginning researcher is undoubtedly familiar with locating library documents and organizing them. However, inasmuch as a review of research literature differs in a number of respects from other kinds of term papers or summaries that students are often called upon to prepare, we present below some general guidelines for the preparation of a literature review.

Types of Information to Seek

Written materials vary considerably in their quality, their intended audience, and the kind of information they contain. The researcher performing a review of the literature ordinarily comes in contact with a wide range of materials and, thus, has to be selective in deciding what to include. How are such decisions to be made? There is, unfortunately, no easy answer to this question, but we can offer a number of suggestions that might prove useful.

The first step in selecting appropriate materials is to make sure that you have been thorough in tracking down all (or most) of the relevant references. In other words, in making decisions about what to include, it is wise to have a good idea about the materials that are available. It is irksome (and embarrassing) to learn of ideal references after the completion of a study. Some hints for locating good source materials are provided later in this chapter.

The type of information included in academic or other nonfictional documents can be classified roughly into five categories: (1) facts, statistics, or findings; (2) theory or interpretation; (3) methods and procedures; (4) opinions, beliefs, or points of view; and (5) anecdotes, clinical impressions, or narrations of incidents and situations.

The first category constitutes the most important source of information for a research review. This category of information represents the results of other research efforts and documents the progress on a specific topic or problem. Normally, research findings are available in a variety of sources, including textbooks, encyclopedias, reports, conference proceedings, publications, and, especially, scholarly journals such as *Nursing Research* and *Research in Nursing and Health*. The review should draw more heavily on primary rather than secondary sources. A *primary source*, from the point of view of the research literature, is the description of an investigation written by the person who conducted it. For example, most of the articles appearing in the journal *Nursing Research* are original research reports and, therefore, are primary sources. A *secondary source* is a description of a study or studies prepared by someone other than the original researcher. Review articles, which summarize the literature on a topic, are secondary sources. There is a tendency for beginning researchers to rely too heavily on secondary sources, and this tendency can greatly affect the quality of the review. Secondary sources are useful in providing bibliographical information on relevant primary sources. However, secondary descriptions of studies should not be considered substitutes for the primary sources. Secondary sources typically fail to provide sufficient detail about research studies; furthermore, secondary sources may distort some aspects of the research. The reviewer should use primary sources whenever possible.

The second category of information—theoretical writings—deals with broader issues that provide a more conceptual orientation for a specific problem. Sometimes discussions of theories are briefly presented in research reports and journal articles, but they are more likely to be found in developed form in books. The second part of this chapter discusses the role of theory in scientific research.

The third type of information that should be sought in a literature review concerns the methods of conducting a study on the topic of interest. That is, in reviewing the literature the researcher should pay attention not only to what has been found, but also to how it was found. What approaches have other researchers used? How have they operationalized or measured their variables? How have they controlled the research situation to enhance interpretation? What statistical procedures have they used to analyze their data? Fortunately, there is no need to "reinvent the wheel" every time we conduct a study. Although we may have to greatly modify existing approaches and instruments, it usually is possible to find techniques that can serve as a foundation for our research activities. Articles and reports concerning similar research problems should be useful in this regard.

There remain two information categories that we have not yet examined: (1) opinions, beliefs, or points of view; and (2) anecdotes, clinical impressions, or narrations of incidents and situations. Usually there are numerous papers and articles that focus on an author's opinions or attitudes concerning the topic of interest. Such articles are inherently value-laden and subjective, presenting the suggestions and points of view of one

or more persons. In the fifth category are the many reports of an anec-
dotal nature that appear frequently in nursing, medical, and health-
related literature. These articles relate the experiences and clinical
impressions of the authors.

Both opinion articles and anecdotes or other types of nonresearch literature may serve to broaden the researcher's understanding of the problem, particularly if the researcher is relatively unfamiliar with the underlying issues. Such sources may also illustrate a point or demonstrate a
need for rigorous research. However, these two categories have limited
utility in literature reviews for research studies because of their highly
subjective nature. Beginning researchers should avoid the temptation of
relying very heavily on such sources in their review of the literature. This
is not to say that such materials are uninteresting or unimportant, but generally they are inappropriate in summarizing scientific knowledge and
theories about a research question.

Locating Existing Information on a Problem

The number of individual books, journals, and reports that could be
consulted in compiling information on a nursing research topic is overwhelming. Fortunately, there are various indexes, abstracting services,
and other retrieval mechanisms that facilitate the process of locating pertinent references. Several major sources that can be consulted in performing the review of the literature are identified here. However, these materials by no means exhaust the possibilities. Librarians are a particularly
valuable resource inasmuch as they are knowledgeable about the literature, literature retrieval tools, and services in their own libraries. Librarians usually are familiar with additional resources available through the
community, state, and regional libraries and the National Library of Medicine, which make up the Health Science Library Network in the United
States.

Indexes. Health-science indexes are the key that unlocks the vast
stores of health-science literature. If indexes were unavailable, the
researcher would have a difficult and time-consuming task in locating
books, periodical articles, pamphlets, and other kinds of literature pertaining to a research problem. It is a wise practice in using any index to
begin the search for relevant references with the most recent issue of the
index and proceed backwards. Several indexes particularly useful to
nurse researchers are the *International Nursing Index, Index Medicus,
Nursing Research Index,* and *Nursing Studies Index,* each of which is
briefly described below.

The *International Nursing Index* is one of the major sources for locating references from both nursing and nonnursing journals. Articles from over 200 nursing journals as well as nursing articles appearing in more than 2000 nonnursing journals are listed alphabetically by subject heading and author. Although the *International Nursing Index* is primarily a periodical index, it also lists in special appendices publications of professional organizations and agencies, nursing books published during the year, and doctoral dissertations by nurses. It is published quarterly with an annual cumulative index and covers articles beginning with 1966 to the present.

The *Nursing Studies Index* is a four-volume index prepared by Virginia Henderson and others. It is an annotated guide to reported studies, research methods, and historical and biographical materials in periodicals, books, and pamphlets published in English. The *Nursing Studies Index* constitutes the only means of access to nursing literature for the period between 1900 and 1959.

The *Index Medicus* is one of the most well-known biomedical indexes. Over 2000 worldwide biomedical journals are indexed. A small number of nursing journals are also indexed. It is published monthly and cumulated annually. A feature included as a separate entity in both the monthly and annual cumulated volumes is the *Bibliography of Medical Reviews*, an index to the latest review articles that have appeared in biomedical journals.

The *Nursing Research Index* appears annually in the last issue of *Nursing Research*. It contains alphabetical listings of research studies by subject heading and author. The index is more selective than the *International Nursing Index* because only research investigations having pertinence to nursing are listed. Because of its focus solely on research, it has been singled out from other journals such as the *American Journal of Nursing* and *Nursing Outlook*, which also have annual cumulated indexes.

Abstracts. Abstract journals summarize articles that have appeared in other journals. They are particularly useful in enabling the researcher to keep track of pertinent information being published in a particular area. Abstracting services are generally more useful than indexes in that they provide a summary (abstract) of a study rather than just a title. The title of an article often is not fully indicative of its contents. Having an abstract helps in deciding whether a particular reference is worth pursuing. Two relevant abstract sources for the nursing literature are described below.

Each issue of *Nursing Research* for the period between 1960 and 1978 contained abstracts of research studies having relevance to nursing. The articles are classified alphabetically by author under alphabetical subject headings. The subject headings are listed at the beginning of the abstract section. The journals from which articles are abstracted are listed in the September–October issue each year. Sometimes only the title of a particular article is given and the reader is referred to the journal in which the original article appears. There is an author–subject guide to these abstracts in the annual index.

Abstracts of books and journal articles in the field of psychology and other behavioral and social sciences appear in *Psychological Abstracts*. Articles from selected nursing journals, such as *Nursing Research*, that are psychologically oriented are abstracted. To use this tool, the researcher first employs the cumulative index and looks up the appropriate subject heading. Under each subject heading are listed, in alphabetical order, the titles of research reports pertaining to the subject area of interest and an abstract number. The abstract number can then be located in the abstract section of this work.

Computer Searches. As an alternative to searching indexes or abstracts manually, a researcher may decide to request a computer literature search. A computer search provides the researcher with a list of references with complete bibliographical information and, in many cases, abstracts as well. References to new literature may be available by way of the computer up to 1 month before their appearance in the printed index or abstract. In addition, computer searches often save some of the researcher's time and energy, thereby providing more time for reading the original publications.

No knowledge of computers is necessary for requesting a computer literature search. The researcher typically fills out a request form indicating the topic of interest and any limitations on the search, such as dates of publication. If the researcher has done some manual searching of the literature, subject headings found to be useful can be indicated. The librarian confers with the researcher, devises the best search strategy, and then performs the actual search.

Most computer searches are able to produce an immediate search, generating references at the time the request is received. This is called an *on-line search*. Generally, if more than a small number of citations is obtained, the bulk of them will be printed off-line because this process is less expensive. The *off-line print* is sent by mail and usually arrives 3 to 5 days after the computer search is conducted. The cost of a computer search varies depending on the type of search (the extensiveness of the bibliography requested) and the data base used in the search.

MEDLINE is the data base most commonly used by nurse researchers. MEDLINE centers are located at the libraries of major research centers, medical schools, nursing schools, and hospitals. It covers all areas of biomedical literature and corresponds to *Index Medicus* with added coverage of nursing and dental literature. All journals currently indexed in the *International Nursing Index* are included in MEDLINE. Other data bases that might be useful to nurse researchers include ERIC (educational

materials); PSYCHOLOGICAL ABSTRACTS (psychological literature); and
SOCABS (sociological literature).

Books. Books should not be overlooked by the researcher conducting
a literature search. While it is true that periodicals contain more up-to-
date information than books, books do provide more extensive coverage
of a particular topic by treating in depth more than one facet or aspect of
the issue. Books are a particularly valuable resource for locating discussions of theoretical issues. Books are also useful in that they usually contain numerous references to other sources of information.

Bibliographies. Bibliographies are compilations of references found in
books, periodicals, and reports on some particular topic. Annotated bibliographies provide comments about the purposes or findings of the references and, sometimes, about their quality. Examples of bibliographies
include *Bibliography on Bioethics, Bibliography* on *Suicide and Suicide
Prevention, International Bibliography of Studies on Alcoholism, Selected
Bibliography on Death and Dying,* and *A Classified Bibliography of Ger-
ontology and Geriatrics.*

Writing a Review of Research Literature

Once a researcher has located, read, and made notes on all of the
major references relevant to the problem of interest, the final task is to
organize and report the material covered. Writing a review of the literature can be rather difficult, particularly if there has been little planning
and organization while the materials were being gathered. Lack of organization is perhaps the most common weakness of students' first attempts
at reviewing the literature. Working from an outline—written or mental—is strongly recommended. The guiding principle is to prepare a
review that, by summarizing what is known on a topic, lays the groundwork for some new research.

The writer also needs to consider the content of the review, as well
as its organization. A review of the literature should be neither a series of
quotes nor a series of abstracts. The central task is to summarize the references so as to lay a systematic foundation for new research. The review
should point out both consistencies and contradictions in the literature as
well as offer possible explanations for the inconsistencies in terms of, say,
different conceptualizations or methods.

Studies that are particularly relevant to the study should be described
in detail, including information about the study design, findings, and conclusions. However, it is neither necessary nor desirable to provide such
extensive coverage for every reference. Reports that result in comparable

findings can usually be grouped together and briefly summarized, as in the following fictitious example:

A number of studies have found that the incidence of phlebitis is directly related to the method of administering intravenous infusions and to certain parameters of materials used in the infusions. (Holcomb, 1984; Hartmann, 1983; Sterling, 1979)

It is important to paraphrase, or summarize, a report in one's own words. The review should demonstrate that thoughtful consideration has been given to the significance of the materials as they relate to the research problem. Stringing together quotes from various documents fails to show that previous research and thought on the topic have been assimilated and understood.

Another point to bear in mind is that the review should be as objective as possible. Studies that fail to support the reviewer's hypotheses or that conflict with personal values should not be omitted. It is not unusual to find studies with conflicting results. The review should not deliberately ignore a study simply because its findings contradict other studies. Analyze inconsistent results and evaluate the supporting evidence as objectively as possible.

The literature-review section should conclude with a summary or overview of the "state of the art" of the problem under consideration. The summary should point out not only what has been studied and how adequate the investigations have been, but should also make note of any gaps or areas of research inactivity. In other words, the summary requires some critical judgment about the extensiveness and dependability of information on a topic. This critical summary should lay the groundwork for hypotheses to be tested in a new study.

One of the most frequent problems for the student researcher preparing a literature review for the first time is adjusting to the style of writing found appropriate for reviews. There is a tendency, for example, for students to accept the results of previous research as a fact or as proof that a theory is correct. This tendency is understandable; it is the style of presentation commonly used in many texts, opinion articles, and other non-research-related papers. This style probably stems partly from a desire for clarity and unambiguity for pedantic purposes, but it is also, in part, the result of a common misunderstanding about the degree of conclusiveness that results from empirical research. *No hypothesis or theory can be definitively proved or disproved by empirical testing.* As we saw in the previous chapter, every study has some limitations, the severity of which depends on the researcher's design decisions. The fact that theories and hypotheses cannot be ultimately proved or disproved does not, of course, mean that we must disregard evidence or challenge every idea we encounter. The problem is partly a semantic one: hypotheses are not proved, but are supported by research findings; theories are not verified, but they may be tentatively accepted if there is a substantial body of evidence demonstrating their legitimacy. The researcher must learn to adopt this language of tentativeness in presenting the review of the literature.

A related stylistic problem is the inclination of beginning researchers to liberally intersperse opinions (their own or someone else's) with the findings of research investigations. The review should use statements of opinions sparingly, if at all, and should be explicit about the source of the opinion. A description of the point of view of a knowledgeable or influential person may be useful in establishing the need to investigate the problem or in providing a perspective on the topic, but it should occupy a relatively small section of the review. The researcher's own opinions do not belong in a review section, with the exception of an assessment of the quality of existing studies.

The left-hand column of Table 4-1 presents several examples of the kinds of stylistic difficulties we have been discussing in this section. The right-hand column offers some recommendations for rewording the sen-

Table 4-1. Examples of Stylistic Difficulties for Research Reviews

INAPPROPRIATE STYLE OR WORDING	RECOMMENDED CHANGE
1. It is known that unmet expectations engender anxiety.	1. A number of commentators have asserted that unmet expectations engender anxiety (Smith, 1981; Thomas, 1980).*
2. The woman who does not undertake preparation for childbirth classes tends to manifest a high degree of stress during labor.	2. Previous studies have demonstrated that women who participate in preparation for childbirth classes manifest less stress during labor than those who do not (Andrew, 1981; Chase, 1978).
3. Studies have proven that doctors and nurses do not fully understand the psychobiological dynamics of breast-feeding.	3. The studies by O'Hara (1982) and Morris and Day (1984) suggest that doctors and nurses do not fully comprehend the psychobiological dynamics of breast-feeding.
4. Attitudes cannot be changed overnight.	4. Attitudes presumably are enduring attributes that cannot be changed overnight.
5. Responsibility is an intrinsic stressor.	5. Responsibility is an intrinsic stressor, according to Doctor A. Cassard, an authority on stress (Cassard, 1982).

*All references are fictitious.

tences to conform to a more generally acceptable form for a research literature review. Many alternative phrasings are possible.

Example of a Literature Review

The following excerpt was taken from a literature review in connection with a study by Joan Austin and colleagues (1984).* In this study, reported in *Nursing Research*, the aim was to assess parental attitudes and adjustments to childhood epilepsy. Austin and her co-authors provided a context for the study with the following review:

Research regarding parenting the school-age child with epilepsy is almost nonexistent in the nursing literature ... The majority of nursing articles on epilepsy focus on the different types of seizures, their treatment, and physical nursing care (Muehl, 1979; Norman & Browne, 1981; Willis & Oppenheimer, 1977). The remainder describes the psychosocial problems associated with epilepsy, including parental reactions believed to lead to emotional problems in children with epilepsy (Ozuna, 1979; Slimmer, 1979).

The few research studies found in related professional literature suggest that parenting may be adversely affected by childhood epilepsy. In a study of 12 families, Mulder and Suurmeijer (1977) found evidence of disruption in every family and that the parents experienced stress due to the epilepsy. In a study of 19 families, Long and Moore (1979) found that parents expected their child with epilepsy to have more emotional problems, to be more unpredictable, and to be more highly strung ($p < .05$) than a sibling without epilepsy. Ferrari, Matthews, and Barabas (1983) reported families of children with epilepsy to have less cohesion and poorer communication patterns than those families of healthy children or children with diabetes.

Only three empirical studies purported to investigate parental attitudes to epilepsy in a child. In two of the studies (Hartlage & Green, 1972; Hartlage, Green, & Offutt, 1972), the Parental Attitude Research Instrument (PARI), developed by Schaeffer and Bell (1958), was used to measure parental attitudes. Unfortunately, the PARI lacks validity because of response-set problems (Becker & Krug, 1965). Hartlage and Green (1972) did, however, find support for a positive relationship between parental attitudes and social maturity in children with epilepsy. Parental attitudes were not found to be significantly correlated with dependency in the Hartlage, Green, and Offutt study (1972), but children with epilepsy were found to be more dependent ($p < .001$) than children who had had recent tonsillectomies or cystic fibrosis.

In the third study, Bagley (1971) conducted interviews with parents of 118 children with epilepsy in order to measure parental attitudes and behavior. Bagley, however, did not use a theoretical model to measure parental attitude and subsequently conflated parental attitude and adjustment. Psychiatric social workers conducted extensive interviews with one or both parents. Information on parental attitude and behavior, including manifestation of anxiety, coping ability, evidence of depression and guilt, support of the child, family dynamics, understanding and response to the implications of epilepsy, discipline, and overprotection, were extracted from the interviews to operationalize attitude and behavior. No attempt was made to separate parental attitude from behavior. Results did show negative parental attitude and behavior to be strongly correlated with behavior disorders in children with epilepsy . . .

In the literature there is a confluence of opinion that negative parental attitudes lead to negative parental adjustment to epilepsy. The increased incidence of emotional problems in children with epilepsy is assumed to be caused by negative parental attitude and adjustment. Available research in this area is both sparse and of limited value due to small samples, invalid measures of parental attitudes, or the failure to differentiate between attitude and adjustment. Descriptive research on parental attitude and adjustment to childhood epilepsy is needed as a first step toward better understanding parental influence on the increased incidence of emotional problems in children with epilepsy.

Theoretical Contexts

While a synthesis of existing knowledge is a critical task in doing scientific research, a literature review in and of itself does not integrate research findings into an orderly, coherent system. Theories are the primary mechanism by which researchers organize empirical findings into a meaningful pattern.

A *theory* is an abstract generalization that presents a systematic explanation about the relationships among phenomena. Theories embody principles for explaining, predicting, and controlling phenomena. Thus, theory construction and testing are intimately related to the advancement of scientific knowledge, and it may even be claimed that theory is the ultimate goal of science. Theoretical and conceptual systems represent the highest and most advanced efforts of humans to understand the complexities of the world in which they live.

Regardless of the discipline, theory serves essentially the same functions in scientific endeavors. The overall purpose of theory is to make scientific findings meaningful and generalizable. Theories allow scientists to knit together observations and facts into an orderly system. They are efficient mechanisms for drawing together and summarizing accumulated facts from separate and isolated investigations. The linkage of findings into a coherent structure makes the body of accumulated knowledge more accessible and, thus, more useful both to practitioners who seek to implement findings and to researchers who seek to extend the knowledge base.

In addition to a summarization function, theories serve to explain scientific findings. Theory guides the scientist's understanding of not only the "what" of natural phenomena, but also the "why" of their occurrence. The power of theories to explain lies in their specification of which variables are related to one another and the nature of that relationship. Finally, theories help to stimulate research and the extension of knowledge by providing both direction and impetus. On the basis of a theory, scientists draw inferences (formulate hypotheses) about what will occur in specific situations. These hypotheses are then subjected to empirical testing in research studies. Theories, thus, serve as a springboard for scientific advances.

The Nature and Characteristics of Theory

Nursing instructors and students frequently use the term "theory" to refer to the content covered in classrooms, as opposed to the actual practice of performing nursing activities or the application of knowledge learned nonexperientially. This usage is not incorrect in that it connotes the involvement of abstraction and generalization. However, in its broader scientific meaning, the term "theory" refers to a series of propositions regarding the interrelationships among variables, from which a large number of empirical observations can be deduced. In this section we will attempt to make this distinction clearer by describing various aspects of a scientific theory.

Theories consist, first of all, of a set of concepts. Examples of nursing concepts are pain, health, interaction, and professionalism. Concepts are the basic ingredients in the formulation of a theory. Secondly, theories consist of a set of statements or propositions, each of which indicates a relationship. Relationships are denoted by such terms as "is associated with," "varies directly with," or "is contingent upon." Thirdly, the propositions must form a logically interrelated deductive system. This means that the theory must provide a mechanism for logically arriving at new statements from the original propositions.

Let us consider an example to illustrate these three points. Selye (1978) developed a theory of adaptation to stress. This theory postulates that a person's body responds to the nonspecific demands of stress by means of the General Adaptation Syndrome, which continues until adaptation occurs or death ensues. Stress may be internal or external and is manifested by the syndrome, which consists of nonspecifically induced changes occurring within the person's body. The General Adaptation Syndrome consists of three phases—the alarm phase, the phase of adaptation or resistance, and the phase of exhaustion—all of which are reversible if adjustment to stress occurs. A greatly simplified construction of Selye's theory might consist of the following propositions, which correspond to the various phases:

1. Humans seek to attain a desired state (*e.g.*, the reduction of stress) by mobilizing the body's general defense mechanisms to overact in order to maintain life.

2. When the specific defense mechanism is identified by the body for dealing with the sources of stress (such as increased muscular activity), the overactivity of the general mechanisms subsides and the specific mechanisms overact (such as increasing the oxygen supply in muscular activity).

3. If the specific defense mechanisms are unable to cope with the stress, then the general defense mechanisms reactivate to help the body adjust, or death ensues.

4. During the alarm and exhaustion phases, there is an increase in the production of adrenocortical hormones, which subsides during the resistance phase when specific defense mechanisms come into play.

The concepts that form the basis of Selye's theory include stress, General Adaptation Syndrome, the body's general defense mechanisms, and specific defense mechanisms. His theory postulates that relationships occur between stress and the body's defense mechanisms, which are activated to cope with the stress. For example, the theory claims that the level of adrenocortical hormones varies with the stage of the General Adaptation Syndrome. Selye's propositions readily lend themselves to empirical verification by providing a mechanism for deductive hypothesis generation. We might hypothesize on the basis of Selye's theory that the level of ACTH will be greater before a meal than it is after a meal or that there is less ACTH production during an intravenous infusion than immediately prior to its inception. On the basis of his theory, we should be able to identify how well the person is coping with the stress by measuring changes in ACTH production.

Two additional characteristics of theories should be emphasized. The first concerns their origin. Theories are not discovered by scientists; they are created and invented by them. The building of a theory depends not only upon the observable facts in our environment but also on the scientist's ingenuity in pulling those facts together and making sense of them. Theory construction, in short, is a creative and intellectual enterprise that can be engaged in by anyone with sufficient imagination. But imagination alone is not an adequate qualification; theories must be congruent with the realities of the world around us and with existing knowledge.

The second characteristic—one that we noted earlier—is the tentative nature of theories. It cannot be stressed too strongly that a theory can never be "proven" or "confirmed." A theory represents a scientist's best efforts to describe and explain phenomena; today's successful theory may be relegated to tomorrow's intellectual garbage dump. It is not only that new evidence or observations "disprove" a previously useful theory; it is also possible that a new theoretical system can integrate new observations with the observations that the old theory made. Furthermore, the theories that are not congruent with a culture's values and philosophical orientation may be discredited. This link between theory and values may surprise those who think of science as being completely objective. It should be remembered, however, that theories are deliberately invented by humans; they can, thus, never be freed totally from the human perspective, which is amenable to change over time. In sum, no theory, no matter what its subject matter, can ever be considered final and verified. There always remains the possibility that a theory will be modified or discarded. Many theories in the physical sciences have received considerable empirical support, and their well-accepted propositions are often referred to as laws, such as Boyle's law of gases. Nevertheless, we have no way of knowing the ultimate accuracy and utility of any theory and should, therefore, treat all theories as tentative. This caveat is nowhere more relevant than in the emerging sciences, such as nursing.

Conceptual Frameworks and Models

The terms "theory," "theoretical framework," "conceptual framework," "conceptual scheme," "conceptual model," and "model" are sometimes used synonymously in the research literature. We have been careful in the preceding discussion to restrict our terminology to "theory" and "theoretical framework" and to use these terms to refer to a well-formulated deductive system of abstract formal statements. In this section we distinguish theories from conceptual frameworks and models.

Conceptual frameworks or *schemes* (we will use the two terms interchangeably) represent a less formal and less well-developed attempt at organizing phenomena than do theories. As the name implies, conceptual frameworks deal with abstractions (concepts) that are assembled by virtue of their relevance to a common theme. Both conceptual schemes and theories use concepts as building blocks. What is absent from conceptual schemes is the deductive system of propositions that assert a relationship between the concepts.

Most of the conceptual work that has been done in connection with nursing practice is more rightfully designated as conceptual frameworks or schemes than as theories. This label in no way diminishes the importance and value of these endeavors. Indeed, many existing conceptual frameworks will undoubtedly serve as the preliminary steps in the construction of more formal theories. In the meantime, conceptual frameworks can serve to guide research that will further support theory development. Conceptual frameworks, like theories, can serve as a springboard for the generation of hypotheses to be tested. For example, King (1971,

1981) has presented a conceptual framework for nursing that includes three types of interacting systems. King also identified concepts relevant for understanding each of the systems. The first type of system, personal systems, is represented by individuals. Concepts included in personal systems are perception, self, body image, growth and development, time, and space. Interpersonal systems are the second type in the network of interacting systems. Any group, large or small, with whom the nurse interacts is considered a component of the interpersonal system. Concepts relevant to interpersonal interactions include role, interaction, communication, transaction, and stress. The third major category in the framework is social systems. Any social system, such as family or hospital, in which the nurse interacts with health-care consumers belongs to this category of systems. Concepts relevant for functioning in social systems include organization, role, power, authority, and decision making. King's framework, then, consists of a multiplicity of concepts and systems that are loosely organized into a structural whole. It does not, however, contain formally stated propositions about the interrelations among concepts that exist, in contrast with Selye's theory. However, the framework does suggest many hypotheses, which can operate within a broader context than might otherwise be the case.

Models, like conceptual frameworks, are constructed representations of some aspect of our environment; they use abstractions (concepts) as the building blocks. However, models attempt to represent reality with a minimal use of words. Language is, and probably always will be, a problem for scientists. A word or phrase that designates a concept can convey different meanings to different people. A visual or symbolic representation of a theory or conceptual framework often helps to express abstract ideas in a more readily understandable or precise form than the original conceptualization.

Schematic models are quite common and undoubtedly are familiar to all readers. A schematic model or diagram represents the phenomenon of interest figuratively. Concepts and the linkages between them are represented diagrammatically through the use of boxes, arrows, or other symbols. An example of a schematic model is presented in Figure 4-1. This model is described by its designer as "a human interaction diagram showing nurse and client interactions" (King, 1981, p. 145). Schematic models of this type can be quite useful in the research process in clarifying concepts and their associations, in enabling researchers to place a specific problem into an appropriate context, and in revealing areas of inquiry.

In summary, it may not always prove possible to identify a formal theory that is relevant to a nursing research problem, but conceptual schemes and models of the type discussed here can also be used to clarify concepts and to provide a context for findings that might otherwise be isolated and meaningless. Conceptual schemes in nursing are very much in need of testing if theories for nursing are to be formulated.

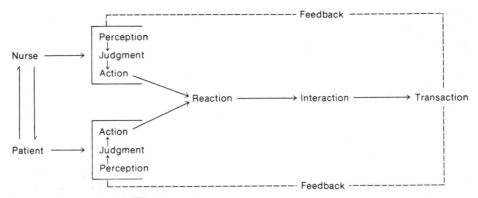

Figure 4-1. Examples of a schematic model: the human interaction process. (After King, IM. *A Theory for Nursing*. New York: John Wiley & Sons, 1981, p. 145. Copyright © 1981 by John Wiley & Sons, Inc. Reprinted by permission of John Wiley & Sons, Inc.)

Testing and Using a Theory/Conceptual Framework

The process of theory testing normally begins with the derivation of implications of the theory (or conceptual framework) in the form of research hypotheses. These hypotheses are predictions about the manner in which variables would be related, if the theory were correct and useful. The hypotheses are then subjected to empirical testing through controlled research. A theory is never tested directly. It is the hypotheses deduced from a theory that are subjected to scientific investigations. Comparisons between the observed outcomes of research and the relationships predicted by the hypotheses are the major focus of the testing process. Through this process, the theory is continually subjected to potential disconfirmation. Repeated failures of research endeavors to disconfirm a theory result in increasing support for and acceptance of a theoretical position. The testing process continues until some piece of evidence cannot be interpreted within the context of the theory but can be explained by a new theory that also accounts for all previous findings.

If a researcher decides to base a research project on an existing theory or conceptual scheme, deductions from the theory must be developed. Essentially, the researcher must ask the following questions: (1) If this theory is correct, what kind of behavior would I expect to find in certain situations or under certain conditions? and (2) What kind of evidence could be found to support this theory? Let us look at an example of how a problem can be derived from a conceptual system. Levine (1969) has postulated a conceptual framework for nursing that concerns conservation. She explains nursing as conserving the patient's energy, structural integrity, personal integrity, and social integrity. From this conceptual framework, the researcher could formulate specific predictions. For example, it might be hypothesized that primary nursing is more effective in conserving the patient's energy and social integrity than team nursing. By developing measures of energy expenditure and social integration, this hypothesis could be tested scientifically.

Circumstances sometimes arise in which the problem is formulated before consideration is given to a theoretical/conceptual framework. Even in such situations researchers may strive to (or may be required to) devise a theoretical context to enrich the value and meaningfulness of their inquiry. It should be recognized that, while such efforts may prove useful, an after-the-fact linkage of theory to a research question is considerably more problematic than the testing of hypotheses deduced from a theory. This is particularly true for neophyte researchers who may lack a thorough grounding in the theoretical positions of their own or related disciplines.

The search for relevant existing theories can be greatly facilitated by first conceptualizing on a sufficiently abstract level what the nature of the problem is. For example, take the following problem statement: Do daily telephone conversations between a psychiatric nurse and a patient for 2 weeks following discharge from the hospital result in lower rates of readmission by short-term psychiatric patients? This is a relatively concrete research problem but might profitably be viewed as relevant to a theory of reinforcement, a theory of social influence, a theory of crisis resolution, or a personality theory, such as Murray's need-press theory. Part of the difficulty in finding a theory is that a problem of interest can be conceptualized in a number of ways and may refer the researcher to conceptual schemes from a wide range of disciplines.

Once the reseacher has abstracted from the problem a generalized issue or idea, the search for existing theories or conceptual frameworks can proceed relatively efficiently because the difficult part of the task will have been completed. Textbooks, handbooks, and encyclopedias in the chosen discipline usually are a good starting point for the selection of a theory. These sources usually summarize the status of a theoretical position and document the efforts to confirm and disconfirm it. When a theoretical position has been developed at length or has been supported by extensive empirical observations, whole books may be devoted to their description; such is the case with King's *A Theory for Nursing*, Roy and Robert's *Theory Construction in Nursing: An Adaption Model*, or Lefcourt's *Locus of Control: Current Trends in Theory and Research*.

The task of fitting a problem to a theory should be done with caution. It is true that having a theoretical content enhances the meaningfulness of a research study, but artificially cramming a problem into a theory is not the route to scientific utility. There is a need for balance at this point in a research project: researchers should not shirk their intellectual duties by failing to make an attempt to link their problem to broader theoretical concerns, but there is no point fabricating such a link when it really does not exist.

Example of the Use of Theory in Research

The psychologist Leon Festinger developed a theory known as cognitive dissonance theory that has generated extensive research interest in a number of disciplines, including nursing. Cognitive dissonance theory postulates that the presence of dissonance motivates a person both to seek consonance and to avoid situations that will likely increase the dissonance. The term "dissonance" refers to an incongruity or disagreement between some aspects of a person's experiences, while "consonance" implies mutual consistency.

Stillman (1977) used cognitive dissonance theory as a base for investigating the health beliefs about breast cancer and the practice of breast self-examination as a preventive measure in women. The independent variables of the study were perceived susceptibility and perceived benefit from breast self-examination. The sample consisted of 122 women and the data were collected by means of a questionnaire. The results revealed that the majority of women who believed themselves to be highly susceptible to breast cancer or who perceived benefits to be gained by performing breast self-examination practiced the technique more frequently than did those women who perceived themselves to have low susceptibility to breast cancer. These findings are consistent with the theory of cognitive dissonance.

Cognitive dissonance theory was the basis for a study by Keiser and Bickle (1980) that investigated the effect of attitude change in nurses on implementing primary nursing. The participants, 60 VA nurses, held a relatively consonant view that primary nursing was not feasible for their institutions. A 2½-day training program aimed at positively affecting staff attitudes toward primary nursing introduced successful examples of primary nursing that already existed in the institutions. Three months following training the nurses reported on their implementation of primary nursing. Consistent with cognitive dissonance theory, the researchers found that nurses who had experienced a greater degree of attitude change had implemented primary nursing to a greater extent than nurses who reported little or no attitude change.

Summary

Scientific research cannot add to human knowledge if it is conducted in isolation from other scientific efforts. Studies need to be given a context if they are to be meaningful. Two mechanisms for providing such a context are the development of linkages with earlier relevant research via a literature review and the integration of the research problem into a theoretical framework.

The task of reviewing literature involves the identification, selection, critical analysis, and reporting of existing information on the topic of interest. It is almost always necessary to examine previous literature on a subject before actually undertaking a research project. The kinds of information available in written documents can be categorized into five broad classes: facts, findings, or results; theory; research procedures or methods; opinions; points of view or personal commentaries; and anecdotes or impressions of a particular event or situation. For most literature reviews, the last two categories are of limited usefulness because of their highly subjective nature.

The search for existing writings on a topic is greatly facilitated by the use of various abstracting and indexing services. Since more than a million scientific and technical articles are published in hundreds of journals, reports, and periodicals annually, it is obvious that the location of all the papers on a given topic would be impossible without such services. An important bibliographic development to emerge in recent years is the increasing availability of various computerized information retrieval systems.

In writing the review of the literature, the researcher should devote a considerable amount of effort to the organization of materials. The literature should be linked in some meaningful fashion and should be presented in such a way that the rationale for conducting new research clearly emerges. The review should not be a succession of quotes or abstracts. The role of the reviewer is to point out what has been studied to date, how adequate and dependable those studies are, what gaps there are in the existing body of research, and what contribution the new study will make. The reviewer should present "facts" and "findings" in the tentative language that befits scientific inquiry and should remember to identify the source of opinions, points of view, and generalizations.

The second step in developing a context for a research problem is to link it to a theory or conceptual framework. A *theory* is an abstract generalization that explains systematically the relationships among phenomena. The overall objective of theory is to make scientific findings meaningful and generalizable. In addition, theories help to summarize existing knowledge into coherent systems, stimulate new research by providing both direction and impetus, and explain the nature of relationships between or among variables. The basic components of a theory are concepts. Theories consist of a set of statements, each of which expresses a relationship. The statements are arranged in a logically interrelated system that permits new statements to be derived from them.

Conceptual schemes are less well-developed attempts at organizing phenomena than are theories. As in the case of theories, concepts are the basic elements of a conceptual scheme. However, the concepts are not linked to one another in a logically ordered deductive system. Much of the conceptual work in nursing is more rightfully described as conceptual schemes than as theories. Conceptual frameworks are highly valuable in that they often serve as the springboard for theory development.

Models are symbolic representations of phenomena. Models depict a theory or conceptual scheme through the use of symbols or diagrams. They are useful to scientists because they use a minimal amount of words, which tend to be ambiguous, in representing reality.

Conceptual schemes and theories can be integrated with empirical research in a number of ways. The investigator may design a scientific study specifically to test a theory of interest. In other situations, a problem may be developed first and a theory selected to "fit" the problem. An after-the-fact selection of a theory usually is more problematic and less meaningful than the systematic testing of a particular theory.

Study Suggestions

1. Suppose that you were planning to study contraception practices and programs for the urban poor. Make a list of several key words relating to this topic that could be used with indexes or information retrieval systems for identifying previous work.

2. Below are five sentences from fictitious literature reviews that require stylistic improvements. Rewrite these sentences to conform to considerations mentioned in the text. (Feel free to give fictitious references if desired.)

a. Parents who abuse their children have psychopathological disturbances.

b. Young adolescents are not prepared to cope with complex issues of sexual morality.

c. More structured programs to use part-time nurses are needed.

d. Intensive care nurses need so much emotional support themselves that they can provide insufficient support to patients.

e. Most nurses have not been adequately educated to understand and cope with the reality of the dying patient.

3. Suppose you are studying factors relating to the discharge of chronic psychiatric patients. Obtain five bibliographical references for this topic. Compare your references and sources with those of other students.

4. Four researchable problems are listed below. Abstract a generalized issue or issues for each of the problems. Search for an existing theory that might be applicable and appropriate.

a. What is the relationship between angina pain and alcohol intake?

b. What effect does rapid weight gain during the second trimester have on the outcome of pregnancy?

c. Do multiple hospital readmissions affect the achievement level of children?

d. To what extent do people's coping mechanisms differ in health and illness?

Chapter 5
Research Problems
and Hypotheses

The selection of a general topic and development of an appropriate context for a research problem are important first steps in the research process. However, researchers must go a bit further before being in a position to design the actual study. Research problems generally need to be narrowed down, refined, and assessed for feasibility. It is simply not possible to proceed in an orderly, intelligent fashion on a research project unless a clear description of the problem has been developed. The most focused specification of a research problem is articulated in the form of a hypothesis. This chapter discusses the formulation and evaluation of problem statements and hypotheses.

The Research Problem

Beginning researchers typically develop problems that are too broad in scope or too complex and unwieldy for their level of methodological expertise. The transformation of the general topic into a workable problem is typically accomplished in a number of uneven steps, involving a series of successive approximations. Each step should result in progress toward the goals of narrowing the scope of the problem and sharpening and defining the concepts.

Let us consider an example. Suppose you were working on a medical unit and observed that some patients always complained about having to wait for pain medication when certain nurses were assigned to them, and yet these same patients offered no complaints when other nurses were assigned to them. You wonder why this phenomenon occurs. The general problem area is discrepancy in complaints from patients regarding pain medications administered by different nurses. You might ask "What accounts for this discrepancy?" or "How can I improve the situation?" Such questions are not actual research questions because they are too broad and vague. They may, however, lead you to ask other questions, such as "How do the two groups of nurses differ?" or "What characteristics are unique to each group of nurses?" or "What characteristics do the group of complaining patients share?" At this point you may observe that the cultural background of the patients and nurses appears to be a relevant factor. This may direct you to a review of the literature for studies concerning ethnic subcultures and their effect on nursing interventions, or it may provoke you to discuss the observations with peers. The result of these efforts may be several researchable problems, such as the following:

Is there a relationship between the ethnic background of nurses and the frequency with which they dispense pain medication?

Is there a relationship between the ethnic background of patients and their complaints of having to wait for pain medication?

Does the number of patient complaints increase when the patients are of dissimilar ethnic backgrounds as opposed to when they are of the same ethnic background as the nurse?

Do nurses' dispensing behaviors change as a function of the similarity between their own ethnic background and that of the patients?

All of these problems have a similar theme, yet each would be studied in a different manner. How does one choose the final problem to be studied? Tentative problems usually vary considerably in their feasibility and worth. Some guidelines for evaluating research problems are presented below.

Criteria for Evaluating Research Problems

Whether you are developing your own research study or critiquing someone else's, there are several considerations that should be kept in mind in assessing the value of a research problem. For those conducting their own research, a critical factor is personal interest in the problem area. Genuine interest in and curiosity about the chosen research problem are important prerequisites to a successful study. A great deal of time and energy are expended in any scientific investigation, and interest as well as enthusiasm ebb and flow throughout the time required for completion of the project. The problem selected should be of sufficient importance that the findings will extend the researcher's personal knowledge as well as the base of knowledge for others.

For both consumers and producers of research, another key consideration in evaluating a research problem is its significance to nursing. The research question should have the potential of contributing to the body of knowledge in nursing in a meaningful way. The following kinds of questions should be posed: Is the problem an important one? Are there practical applications? Does the possibility exist that patients, nurses, or the broader health-care community will benefit by the knowledge produced? Can the findings potentially help to formulate or alter nursing practices or policies? If the answer to all of these questions is "no," the worth of the research problem is probably quite low.

Another consideration in evaluating a problem is its "researchability." Not all questions are amenable to study through scientific investigation. Problems or issues of a moral or ethical nature, although provocative, are not capable of being researched. An example of a philosophically oriented question is "Should nurses join unions?" The answer to such a question is ultimately based on a person's values. There are no "right" or "wrong" answers, only points of view. The question as stated is more suitable to a debate than to scientific research. To be sure, it is possible to modify the question so that aspects of the issue could be researched. For instance, each of the following questions could be investigated in a research project:

What are nurses' attitudes toward unionization?

Does a person's role (nurse vs. nursing administrator vs. hospital administrator) affect his or her perceptions of the consequences of unions on the delivery of health care?

Is opposition to unionization for nurses based primarily on perceived outcomes to patients and clients or on outcomes to the nursing profession?

The findings from these hypothetical projects would have no bearing, of course, on the answer to the original question of whether or not nurses should join unions, but the information could be useful in developing a comprehensive understanding of the issues and in facilitating decision making regarding unionization.

In addition to the significance and researchability of a problem, its feasibility needs to be considered. While most of the factors that determine the feasibility of studying a problem are relevant primarily to producers of research, consumers should also review whether a researcher paid adequate consideration to these factors. Several issues are related to the question of feasibility.

Time. Most studies have deadlines or at least informal goals for their completion. Therefore, the problem must be one that can be adequately studied within the time allotted. This means that the scope of the problem should be sufficiently restricted that enough time will be available for the various steps reviewed in Chapter 3. It is usually wise to allocate more time to the performance of the tasks than originally anticipated. Research activities almost always require more time to accomplish than one thinks.

Availability of Subjects. The second issue concerns the question of whether or not the researcher will be in a position to obtain a sufficient number of subjects to investigate the problem. In any study involving human beings, the researcher needs to consider whether people with the desired characteristics will be available and willing to cooperate. Securing cooperation may be relatively easy, but it could also be problematic. Some people may not have the time or interest to participate in a study that has little personal relevance or benefit, and others may be suspicious of the researcher's motives or even hostile to research in general.

Cooperation of Others. Often it is not sufficient to obtain the cooperation of prospective subjects alone. If the sample includes children, the mentally retarded or mentally incompetent, or senile persons, it is almost always necessary to secure the permission of parents or guardians. In institutional settings, such as hospitals, clinics, public schools, or industrial firms, access to clients, members, personnel, or records usually requires administrative approval.

Facilities and Equipment. All research projects have some resource requirements, though in some cases the needs will be modest. It is prudent to consider what facilities and equipment will be needed, and whether or not they will be available, before embarking on a project in order to prevent disappointments and frustration. Here is a partial list of considerations that fall into this category:

Will space be required and can it be obtained?

Will telephones, typewriters, or other office supplies be required?

If technical equipment and apparatus are needed, can they be secured and are they functioning properly?

Are reproducing or printing services available and are they reliable?

Will transportation needs pose any difficulties?

Will a computer be required for the analysis of the data, and are computing facilities easily obtainable?

The researcher who has given some thought to the feasibility of the study in terms of these requirements usually will be rewarded for his or her efforts.

Money. Where there is a need for facilities and equipment, there is usually a need for some expenditures. Monetary requirements for research projects vary widely, ranging from $10 to $20 for small student projects to hundreds of thousands of dollars for large-scale, federally sponsored research. The investigator on a limited budget should think very carefully about projected expenses before the final selection of a problem is made. In assessing the feasibility of a study in terms of monetary considerations, researchers should ask themselves not only "Will I have enough money to complete this project?" but also "Does the anticipated cost outweigh the value of the expected findings?"

Experience of the Researcher. The problem should be chosen from a field about which the investigator has some experience or knowledge. The researcher will have a difficult time in adequately preparing and designing a study on a topic that is totally new and unfamiliar. In addition to substantive knowledge of existing concepts, findings, or theories, the issue of technical expertise should not be overlooked. A beginning researcher usually has limited methodological skills and should, therefore, avoid research problems that require the development of sophisticated measuring instruments or that involve complex statistical analyses.

Ethical Considerations. A research problem may not be feasible if the investigation of the problem would pose unfair or unethical demands on the participants. An overview of major ethical considerations should be reviewed in considering the feasibility of a prospective topic.

Statement of the Research Problem

A research report that contains a carefully and concisely worded problem statement is clearly helpful in orienting the readers to the research being described. Although this assertion sounds obvious, a surprisingly high percentage of research reports fail to state unambiguously the problem under investigation.

A formal statement of the problem is usually useful to the producer as well as the consumer of research. Conceptual flaws are more easily and objectively identified when they are on paper than when they are in one's head. A good statement of the problem should serve as a guide to the researcher in the course of designing the study. The statement should identify the key variables in the study, specify the nature of the population being studied, and suggest the possibility of empirical testing.

Researchers differ in their opinion of the form the problem statement should take. The two basic alternatives are declarative and interrogative. The following example illustrates these two options:

Declarative: The purpose of this research is to investigate the relationship between the dependency level of renal transplant patients and their rate of recovery.

Interrogative: What is the relationship between the dependency level of renal transplant patients and their rate of recovery?

The question form has the advantage of simplicity and directness. Questions invite an answer and help psychologically to focus the researcher's attention on the kinds of data that would have to be collected in order to provide that answer. We recommend the interrogative form for the statement of the problem.

In order to familiarize the reader with researchable problem areas and appropriate forms for the problem statement, several examples are presented in Table 5-1. The left-hand column of this table gives examples of the original topics, while the right-hand column presents the more formal statements of the problem. In real-life situations, the transition from the broad topic to the final statement usually requires many intermediary attempts. Problem statements such as those presented in Table 5-1 should be accompanied by a set of definitions of the variables involved. The definitions should imply or specify the method of operationalizing (observing and measuring) the variables. For example, in the first problem statement

Table 5-1. Examples of Problem Statements for Nursing Research

GENERAL TOPIC	FORMAL PROBLEM STATEMENT
Early discharge	Is early discharge for hemorrhoidectomy patients related to postoperative problems?
Chloasma gravidarum	Are women with chloasma gravidarum more likely to have premature infants than those who do not?
Bladder catheterization	Is there a relationship between bladder catheterization and urinary infection in patients?
Decubitus ulcers	Is there a relationship between the incidence of decubitus ulcers in comatose patients and the frequency of turning?
Blood-pressure variations	Are month-to-month blood-pressure variations predictive of cerebral vascular accidents in the elderly?
Effects of visitors	Do hospitalized patients who have daily visitors express fewer somatic complaints than patients without daily visitors?
Attitudes toward the mentally ill	Are nurses' attitudes toward the mentally ill related to the nurses' length of experience in working with them?
Nursing performance	Is the on-the-job performance of nurses as evaluated by their supervisor related to their scores on their licensure examination?
Malpractice risks	How aware are nurses of their liabilities with respect to malpractice?
Children's hospital adjustment	Do children who are instructed about pain manifest better adjustment to hospitalization than those who are not?

in Table 5-1, "early discharge" might be defined as "discharged on the first postoperative day"; "postdischarge problem" might be defined, in part, as "the patient's inability to have a bowel movement within 3 postoperative days." When adequate definitions are appended to a well-formulated problem statement, there should be little confusion as to what is being studied.

The Research Hypothesis

A hypothesis is a tentative prediction or explanation of the relationship between two or more variables. A hypothesis, in other words, translates the problem statement into a precise, unambiguous prediction of expected outcomes. It is the hypothesis, rather than the problem statement, that is subjected to empirical testing through the collection and analysis of data.

Research problems, as we have seen, are typically phrased in the form of questions concerning how phenomena are related and interact. Hypotheses, on the other hand, are tentative solutions or answers to such research queries. For instance, the problem statement might ask "Does room temperature affect the optimal placement time of rectal temperature measurements in adults?" As a tentative solution to this problem, the researcher might predict the following: Cooler room temperatures will require longer placement times for rectal temperature measurements in adults than warmer room temperatures. Hypotheses should always be developed *before* the conduct of the study itself, because it is the hypothesis that gives direction to the gathering and interpretation of data.

Hypotheses often follow directly from a theoretical framework. The scientist reasons from theories to hypotheses and tests those hypotheses in the real world. The validity of a theory is never examined directly. Rather, it is through hypotheses that the worth of a theory can be evaluated. Let us take as an example the general theory of reinforcement. This theory maintains that behavior or activity that is positively reinforced (rewarded) will tend to be learned or repeated. Since nurses play an important teaching and guiding role in hospitals or clinical settings, there are many opportunities for this general theory to be incorporated into the context of nursing practice. However, the theory itself is too abstract to be put to an empirical test. Nevertheless, if the theory is valid, then it should be possible to make accurate predictions (hypotheses) about certain kinds of behavior in hospitals. For example, the following hypotheses have been deduced from reinforcement theory: (1) Elderly patients who are praised (reinforced) by nursing personnel for self-feeding will require less assistance in feeding than patients who are not praised; and (2) Hyperactive children who are given a reward (*e.g.*, candies, cookies, permission to watch television) when they perform a 15-minute motor task without disruption will tend to display less acting-out behavior during task performance than nonrewarded peers. Both of these propositions can be put to a test in the real world. If the hypotheses are confirmed, the theory will be supported and we can place more confidence in it. Thus, hypotheses offer the possibility of linking abstractions with concrete, observable phenomena.

Not all hypotheses are derived from theory. Even in the absence of a theoretical framework, however, the researcher who proceeds to collect data without having made predictions about the outcome jeopardizes the contribution that the findings can make to human knowledge. Well-conceived hypotheses offer direction and suggest explanations.

Perhaps an example will clarify this point. Suppose we were to hypothesize that nurses who have received a baccalaureate education are more likely to experience stress in their first nursing job than nurses with diploma-school education. We could justify our speculation on the grounds of theory (role conflict, cognitive dissonance theory, reality shock theory), on the basis of earlier studies, as a result of personal observations, on the basis of logic, or on the basis of some combination of these. *The need to develop justification in and of itself forces the researcher to think logically, to exercise critical judgment, and to tie together earlier research findings.* Now let us suppose the above hypothesis is not confirmed by the evidence collected; that is, we find that baccalaureate and diploma nurses demonstrate an equal amount of stress in their first nursing assignment. *The failure of data to support a prediction forces the investigator to critically analyze theory or previous research, to carefully review the limitations of the study's methods, and to explore alternative explanations for the findings.* The use of hypotheses, in other words, induces critical thinking and, hence, promotes understanding.

Characteristics of Workable Hypotheses

An essential characteristic of a usable research hypothesis is that it states the relationship between two or more variables. The variables that are related to one another through the hypothesis are the independent variable (the presumed cause or antecedent) and the dependent variable (the presumed effect or phenomenon of primary interest). One of the most common flaws of the predictions of beginning researchers is the failure to make a relational statement. The following prediction is not a scientifically acceptable hypothesis: Pregnant women who receive prenatal training will have favorable reactions to the labor and delivery experience. This statement expresses no anticipated relationship; in fact, there is only one variable (the woman's reactions to the labor and delivery experience), and a relationship by definition requires at least two variables. This prediction can, however, be altered to make it a suitable hypothesis with an independent and dependent variable: Pregnant women who receive prenatal training will have *more* favorable reactions (the dependent variable) to the labor and delivery experience *than* pregnant women with no prenatal training. Here the second variable (the independent variable) is the woman's status with respect to prenatal training—some will have received it and others will not have received it.

The relational aspect of the prediction is embodied in the phrase "more than." If a hypothesis lacks a phrase such as "more than," "less than," "greater than," "different from," "related to," or something similar, it is not amenable to scientific testing. As an example of why this is so, consider the original prediction: Pregnant women who receive prenatal training will have favorable reactions to the labor and delivery experience. How would we know whether the women's reactions are favorable? That is, what absolute standard could be used for deciding whether the women's reactions to their labor and delivery experiences were favorable or not? Perhaps this point will be clearer if we illustrate it more specifically. Suppose that we ask a group of women who have taken an 8-week prenatal training course to respond to the following question*:

On the whole, how would you describe your labor and delivery experience?

1. Very favorably
2. Rather favorably
3. Neither favorably nor unfavorably
4. Rather unfavorably
5. Very unfavorably

Based on this question, how could we compare the actual outcome with the predicted outcome that the women would have favorable responses? Would all of the women questioned have to respond "very favorably?" Would our prediction be supported if half the women say "very favorably" or "favorably"? There is simply no adequate way of testing the accuracy of the prediction. If we modify the prediction, as suggested above, to "Pregnant women who receive prenatal training will have more favorable reactions to the labor and delivery experience than pregnant women with no prenatal training," a test is quite simple. We could simply ask two groups of women with different prenatal training experiences to respond to the question and then compare the responses of the two groups. The absolute degree of favorability of either group would not be at issue.

Hypotheses, ideally, should be based on a sound, justifiable rationale. The most defensible hypotheses follow from previous research findings or are deduced from a theory. When a new area is being investigated, the

---

*This rather simple question is provided primarily for the sake of illustrating the need to have a relational statement in a hypothesis. Normally, a measure of a dependent variable would be somewhat more complex than this example suggests.

researcher may have to turn to logical reasoning or personal experience in order to justify the predictions. There are, however, very few topics for which research evidence is totally lacking.

Wording the Hypothesis

Hypotheses state the expected relationship between the independent and dependent variables. When there is a single independent and dependent variable, the hypothesis is referred to as a *simple* (or univariate) *hypothesis*. A *complex* (or multivariate) *hypothesis* is one that predicts a relationship between two (or more) independent variables or two or more dependent variables. Complex hypotheses offer the advantage of allowing researchers to mirror the complexity of the real world in their research designs. It is not always possible, of course, to design a study with complex hypotheses. A number of practical considerations, including the research-er's technical skills, resources, and time, may render the testing of com-plex hypotheses impossible or inadvisable. It should be understood, how-ever, that an important goal of research is to explain the dependent variable as thoroughly as possible and that two or more independent vari-ables are typically more successful than one alone.

Table 5-2 presents ten specific examples of simple and complex hypotheses. Most of these hypotheses would need further elaboration in terms of the specification of operational definitions, but each of these hypotheses is potentially testable and each delineates a predicted relation-ship. Beginning research students would probably profit from a careful scrutiny of this table in order to familiarize themselves with the language and style of scientific hypotheses. The first column specifies the hypotheses themselves, while the last three columns indicate the inde-pendent and dependent variables for each hypothesis and designate whether it is simple or complex.

It should be pointed out that, while researchers typically adopt a cer-tain style in the phrasing of hypotheses, there is, nevertheless, some degree of flexibility. The same hypothesis can generally be stated in a vari-ety of ways, so long as the researcher specifies (or implies) the relation-ship that will be tested. As an example of how a hypothesis can be reworded while maintaining its integrity and usefulness, consider the third hypothesis from Table 5-2:

1. Older nurses are less likely to express approval of the expanding role of nurses than younger nurses.
This hypothesis can be stated in several alternative ways:

2. There is a relationship between the age of a nurse and approval of the nurse's expanding role.

3. The older the nurse, the less likely it is that she or he will approve of the nurse's expanding role.

Table 5-2. Examples of Hypotheses

HYPOTHESIS	INDEPENDENT VARIABLE	DEPENDENT VARIABLE	SIMPLE OR COMPLEX
1. The infants born to heroin-addicted mothers have lower birthweights than infants of nonaddicted mothers.	Addiction or nonaddiction of infant's mother	Birthweight	Simple
2. There is a relationship between tactile and auditory stimulation and heart rate response in premature infants.	Tactile stimulation; auditory stimulation	Heart rate response	Complex
3. Older nurses are less likely to express approval of the expanding role of nurses than younger nurses.	Age of nurses	Approval of nurses' expanding role	Simple
4. Structured preoperative support is more effective in reducing surgical patients' perceptions of pain and requests for analgesics than structured postoperative support.	Timing of nursing intervention	Surgical patients' pain perceptions; requests for analgesics	Complex
5. Teenage girls are better informed about the risks of venereal disease than teenage boys.	Gender of teenager	Knowledge about venereal disease	Simple
6. Nurses who are scheduled by the block-rotation method will have a lower number of reported sick days and express a higher level of job satisfaction than nurses scheduled by a random-rotation method.	Schedule method	Absenteeism; level of job satisfaction	Complex

4. Older nurses will differ from younger nurses with respect to approval of the nurse's expanding role.

5. Younger nurses will tend to be more approving of the nurse's expanding role than will older nurses.

6. Approval of the nurse's expanding role decreases with the age of the nurse.

Other variations are also possible. The important point to remember is that the statement should specify the independent and dependent variables and the anticipated relationship between them.

Table 5-2. (*Continued*)

HYPOTHESIS	INDEPENDENT VARIABLE	DEPENDENT VARIABLE	SIMPLE OR COMPLEX
7. Nursing students who have been with a patient who has died will be more likely to report a physical complaint within 72 hours than students who have not had this experience.	Experiencing death of patient	Physical complaint	Simple
8. Patients who have a primary nurse assigned to them on admission report a more favorable impression of their nursing care than patients who do not have a primary nurse assigned on admission.	Assignment of primary nurse	Impression of nursing care	Simple
9. Patients who receive a copy of the "Patient's Bill of Rights" ask more questions about their treatment and diagnosis than those who do not receive this document.	Receipt of "Patient's Bill of Rights"	Number of questions	Simple
10. Physicians spend less time explaining treatment plans to patients than do nurse practitioners.	Medical role (physician vs. nurse practitioner)	Time spent explaining treatment plans to patients	Simple

Sometimes hypotheses are described as being either directional or nondirectional. A *directional hypothesis* is one that specifies the expected direction of the relationship between variables. That is, the researcher predicts not only the existence of a relationship, but also the nature of the relationship. In the six versions of the same hypothesis above, versions 1, 3, 5, and 6 are all directional because there is an explicit expectation that older nurses will be less approving of the expanding role of nurses than younger nurses.

A *nondirectional hypothesis,* by contrast, does not stipulate the direction of the relationship. Such a hypothesis predicts that two or more variables are related but makes no projections about the exact nature of the association. The second and fourth variations in the example illustrate the wording of nondirectional hypotheses. These hypotheses state the prediction that a nurse's age and the degree of approval of the nurse's expanding role are related; they do not stipulate, however, whether the researcher thinks that older nurses or younger nurses will be more approving.

Hypotheses derived from theory will almost always be directional, because theories attempt to explain phenomena and, hence, provide a rationale for expecting variables to behave in certain ways. Existing studies also typically supply a basis for specific expectations and, hence, for directional hypotheses. When there is no theory or related research, when the findings of related studies are contradictory, or when the researcher's own experience results in ambivalent expectations, the investigator may use nondirectional hypotheses. Some people argue, in fact, that nondirectional hypotheses are generally preferable because they connote a degree of impartiality or objectivity. Directional hypotheses, it is said, carry the implication that the researcher is intellectually committed to a certain outcome, and such a commitment might lead to bias. This argument fails to recognize that researchers typically do have specific expectations or hunches about the outcomes, whether they state those expectations explicitly or not. Directional hypotheses have three distinct advantages: (1) they demonstrate that the researcher has thought critically and carefully about the phenomena under investigation; (2) they make clear to the readers of a research report the framework within which the study was conducted; and (3) they may permit a more sensitive statistical test of the hypothesis. This last point, which refers to whether the researcher chooses a one-tailed or two-tailed statistical test, is a rather fine point that is discussed in most statistical texts.

One further distinction should be noted, and that is the difference between research and statistical hypotheses. *Research hypotheses* (also referred to as substantive, declarative, or scientific hypotheses) are statements of expected relationships between variables. All of the hypotheses in Table 5-2 are research hypotheses. Such hypotheses indicate what the researcher expects to find as a result of conducting a study.

The logic of statistical inference operates on principles that are somewhat confusing to many beginning students. This logic requires that hypotheses be expressed such that no relationship is expected. *Statistical hypotheses*, or *null hypotheses*, state that there is no relationship between the independent and dependent variables. The null form of hypothesis 1 in Table 5-2 would be "Infants born to heroin-addicted mothers have the same birthweight as infants born to nonaddicted mothers." As another illustration, the null hypothesis for example 2 in the table would read "There is no relationship between tactile and auditory stimulation and heart rate response in premature infants." The null hypothesis might be compared to the assumption of innocence of an accused criminal in our system of justice: the variables are assumed to be "innocent" of any relationship until they can be shown "guilty" through appropriate statistical procedures. The null hypothesis represents the formal statement of this assumption of innocence.

In designing a study, the researcher is typically concerned only with the research hypotheses. While some research reports express the hypotheses in null form, it is more common (and more desirable) to state the researcher's actual expectations. When statistical tests are performed, the underlying null hypothesis is usually assumed without being explicitly stated.

Hypothesis Testing and Scientific Research

The testing of hypotheses constitutes the heart of empirical investigations. After the hypotheses are formulated, the researcher must select a research design, identify the appropriate population and sample, develop or choose data-collection instruments, gather the data, and analyze the results. Strictly speaking, the statistical analysis performs the test of the hypothesis, but the steps leading up to the analysis are such an integral part of the research process that they may also be considered as operations designed to test the hypotheses.

It must again be emphasized, however, that neither theories nor hypotheses are ever proven in an ultimate sense through hypothesis testing. It is inappropriate to say that the data proved the validity of the hypothesis, or that the conclusions proved the worthiness of the theory. Findings are always considered tentative. Certainly, if the same results are repeatedly produced in a large number of investigations, then greater confidence can be placed in the conclusions. Hypotheses, then, come to be increasingly accepted or believed with mounting evidence, but ultimate proof is never possible.

At this point, the reader may be wondering whether a hypothesis is always necessary. Most research that can be classified as descriptive proceeds without an explicit hypothesis. Descriptive research (i.e., research that predominantly aims to describe phenomena rather than explain them) is very common in the emerging field of nursing research. Examples of descriptive investigations include surveys of the health needs of elderly citizens, studies of the coping patterns of mothers of handicapped children, and surveys of the nutritional status of low-income preschool children. This kind of study is often extremely important in laying a foundation for later research. When a field is new, it may be difficult to provide adequate justification for the development of explanatory hypotheses because of a dearth of facts or previous findings. Thus, there are some studies of a descriptive nature for which hypotheses may not be required.

However, initial efforts to investigate phenomena are usually strengthened by the formulation of hypotheses. Even when related literature on a topic is lacking, a nurse's experience is an extremely valuable source of ideas for predicting outcomes. Most research problems are concerned with relationships between variables. Where there is a relationship, there is a potential hypothesis. Researchers have nothing to lose and stand to gain important knowledge and guidance by developing predictions before collecting data.

Research Example

McKenzie was interested in studying nonverbal communication between nurses and patients.* After some preliminary reading and discussions with colleagues, she decided to focus on touch as the medium of communication. She described her research problem as follows: Does the amount of touching nurses give to patients speed the patients' recovery? Based on McKenzie's readings regarding the effects of touch as a therapeutic device, she formulated the following hypotheses:

Without specific instruction regarding touching as a therapeutic form of communication, nurses do not engage in much touching behavior.

The more nurses touch their patients, the higher the patients' morale.

The greater the amount of physical contact between nurses and patients, the greater the likelihood of the patients' compliance with nurses' instructions, and the fewer the number of days of hospitalization.

This example illustrates how the researcher narrowed and refined a broad topic of interest—nonverbal communication—and developed several research hypotheses in a series of steps. Those steps involved reviewing the literature, consulting with other nurses, identifying a specific area of interest for investigation, preparing a problem statement, considering how to operationalize key variables, and, finally, formulating the research hypotheses.

---

*This example is fictitious.

Using the criteria presented in this chapter, we can evaluate Nurse McKenzie's problem statement and hypotheses. The research problem appears to meet the criterion of significance: there are some tangible and important applications that can be made of the findings for the nursing profession. The question does not deal with a moral/ethical issue and meets the criterion of researchability. Without a further description of the study, we cannot judge the feasibility of the study, but presumably the study could be readily accomplished without undue constraints.

The researcher chose to state the problem in the interrogatory form, which is the preferred form. However, it should be noted that the leap between the problem statement and the hypotheses is a great one. The first hypothesis, though thematically related to the research problem, does not address the issue of patient recovery at all. The second hypothesis is also tenuously connected to the problem statement; improved patient morale is undoubtedly a desirable outcome, but it is not really an acceptable way to operationalize speed of recovery. The final hypothesis (a complex hypothesis) is an appropriate translation of the problem statement into hypothesis form. Here the researcher is defining patient recovery in terms of compliance with instructions and days spent in the hospital.

Besides the gap between the problem statement and hypotheses, there are additional problems with the hypotheses. The first hypothesis is untestable because it fails to state a predicted relationship between two variables. What criterion can we use to decide what "much touching" is? This hypothesis could be tested if rephrased, such as "Nurses who receive instruction on the therapeutic value of touching will engage in more touching of patients than those who do not receive instruction." A second criticism is that the variables have not been adequately defined (operationalized).

In summary, there are many laudable features of McKenzie's efforts. She has identified a significant, researchable topic and formulated some testable hypotheses. However, several modifications to the problem statement or hypotheses are in order.

Summary

The process of developing a research problem is not a smooth and direct one. The researcher usually starts with the identification of several topics of broad interest. After a topic has been tentatively selected, the researcher must begin the task of successively narrowing the scope of the problem.

A number of criteria should be considered in making the final selection of the problem. First, the problem should be a significant one. That is, the research question should contribute to nursing practice or nursing theory in a meaningful way. Second, the problem should be researchable. Questions of a moral or ethical nature are inappropriate, and concepts that defy precise definition and measurement should be avoided. Third, a problem may have to be abandoned if the investigation is not feasible. Feasibility involves the issues of time and timing, availability of subjects, cooperation of other people, availability of facilities and equipment, monetary requirements, experience and competency of the researcher, and ethical considerations. Finally, the research question should be one that is of interest to the researcher.

The selected problem should be stated formally (in writing) before proceeding to the design of the study. The problem may be stated in either declarative or interrogative form; the latter is preferred because it is simpler and more concise and because it leads more directly to a solution. The problem statement should be accompanied by a set of clear definitions of the concepts involved.

The successful progression from initial problem statement to the final collection and analysis of data is often intimately associated with the development of one or more clear, workable hypotheses. A hypothesis is a statement of predicted relationships between two or more variables. A workable hypothesis states the anticipated association between the independent and dependent variables. A hypothesis that projects a result for only one variable is essentially untestable because there is typically no criterion for assessing absolute, as opposed to relative, outcomes. The testability of a hypothesis also depends on the ability of the researcher to observe or measure the variables and the absence of any value-laden, moral, or ethical questions. Finally, a good hypothesis should be justifiable. In other words, it should be consistent with existing theory or knowledge (or with the researcher's own experiences) and with logical reasoning.

Hypotheses can be classified according to various characteristics. *Simple hypotheses* express a predicted relationship between one independent and one dependent variable, while *complex hypotheses* state an anticipated relationship between two or more independent and two or more dependent variables. Complex hypotheses are powerful because they offer the possibility of mirroring the complexity of the real world in research designs. A *directional hypothesis* specifies the expected direction or nature of a hypothesized relationship. *Nondirectional hypotheses* denote a relationship but do not stipulate the precise form that the relationship will take. Directional hypotheses are generally preferable. Sometimes a distinction between research and statistical hypotheses is made. *Research hypotheses* predict the existence of relationships; *statistical* or *null hypotheses* express the absence of any relationships.

After hypotheses are developed and refined, they are subjected to an empirical test through the collection, analysis, and interpretation of data.

It must be stressed, however, that hypotheses are never proved or disproved in an ultimate sense. Scientists say that hypotheses are "accepted" or "rejected," "supported" or "not supported." Through replication of studies, hypotheses and theories can gain increasing acceptance, but scientists, who are essentially skeptics, avoid the use of the word "proof."

Study Suggestions

1. Examine the following five problem statements. Are they researchable problems as stated? Why or why not? If a problem statement is not researchable, modify it in such a way that the problem could be studied scientifically.

   a. What are the factors affecting the attrition rate of nursing students?

   b. What is the relationship between humidity and heart rate in humans?

   c. Should licensure examinations for nurses be discontinued?

   d. How effective are walk-in clinics?

   e. What is the best approach for conducting patient interviews?

2. Below are three general topics that could be investigated. Develop at least one problem statement for each. Assess the adequacy of the problems in terms of their researchability and feasibility.

   a. Nurse–patient interaction

   b. Sleep disturbances

   c. Preoperative anxiety

3. Below are five problem statements. Develop a hypothesis based on each one. Try to state each hypothesis in more than one way.

   a. Are the scores on nurses' licensure examinations related to the type of curriculum they have experienced for their basic education?

   b. Is the clinical specialty of nurses related to their attitudes toward alcoholism?

   c. Are nutritional habits related to a person's age and sex?

   d. Is there a relationship between the prematurity of an infant and the mother's smoking behavior?

   e. Do nurse practitioners perform triage functions as well as a physician?

4. Below are five hypotheses. For each hypothesis, give a possible problem statement from which the hypothesis might have been developed.

   a. Absenteeism is higher among nurses in intensive care units than among nurses on other wards.

   b. Patients who are not told their diagnosis report more subjective feelings of stress than do patients who are told their diagnosis.

c. The educational preparation of a nurse (associate's degree, diploma, or baccalaureate degree) will affect her or his ability to conduct thorough patient interviews.

d. Patients with roommates will call for a nurse less often than patients without roommates.

e. Women who have participated in Lamaze classes will request pain medication less often than will women who have not attended these classes.

5. For each of the five hypotheses in suggestion 4, indicate whether the hypothesis is simple or complex, and directional or nondirectional; then state the independent and dependent variables.

PART III
Designs for
Nursing Research

Chapter 6
Experimental Versus Nonexperimental Research

The choice of a research approach is one of the major decisions that must be made in conducting a research study. This section of the text examines some of the basic kinds of research strategies that have been used in nursing research. In this chapter we will examine various research designs that differ primarily according to the degree of control the researcher has over the variables under investigation. Since research control has important implications for the interpretability and validity of results, the distinctions made in this chapter deserve particular attention. We begin with a discussion of the strongest kind of research designs— experimental studies.

Experimental Research

Experiments differ from nonexperiments in one very important respect: the researcher is an active agent in experimental work rather than a passive observer. Early physical scientists learned that while observation of natural phenomena is valuable and instructive, the complexity of the events occurring in the natural state often obscures the understanding of important relationships. This problem was handled by isolating the phenomenon of interest in a laboratory setting and controlling the conditions under which it occurred. The procedures developed by physical scientists were profitably adopted by biologists during the 19th century, resulting in many achievements in physiology and medicine. The 20th century has witnessed the utilization of experimental methods by scholars and researchers interested in human behavior and psychological states.

Characteristics of True Experiments

The term "experiment" is often used loosely in everyday speech to connote the idea of trying something out or of using something tentatively. Thus, we might say that we are experimenting with a new method of preparing for exams or a new brand of cough syrup. In scientific parlance an experiment has a very precise and unambiguous meaning. A *true experiment* is characterized by the following properties:

> *Manipulation:* The experimenter does something to at least some of the subjects in the study.
>
> *Control:* The experimenter introduces one or more controls over the experimental situation, including the use of a control group.
>
> *Randomization:* The experimenter assigns subjects to a control or experimental group on a random basis.

Manipulation. In experimental research, the investigator manipulates the independent variable by administering an *experimental treatment* (or *experimental intervention*) to some subjects while withholding it from others (or by administering some other treatment, such as a placebo). The experimenter, in other words, consciously varies the independent variable and observes the effect that the manipulation has on the dependent variable of interest. Let us illustrate the concept of manipulation with an example.

Suppose that we are interested in investigating the effect of being physically restrained by Posey belt on heart rate. We might choose to begin our experimentation with some subhuman species, such as the rat. One possible experimental design for addressing the research problem is a before–after design (also known as a pretest–posttest design), as shown in Figure 6-1. This scheme involves the observation of the dependent variable—heart rate—at two points in time, before and after the administra-

	Experimental Group	Control Group
Before (Pretest)		
After (Posttest)		

Figure 6-1. Classical experimental design

tion of the experimental treatment. Each of the rats in the experimental group is restrained with a Posey belt, while those in the control group are not. This scheme permits us to examine what changes in heart rate were produced as a result of being physically restrained (the independent variable), since only half of the rats were exposed to it. In this example, we have manipulated whether the rat would be exposed to restraint by Posey belt, thus meeting the first criterion of a true experiment.

Control. This example also meets the second requirement for experimental research, the use of a *control group*. Campbell and Stanley (1963), in a classic monograph on research design, observed that obtaining scientific evidence requires making at least one comparison. But not all comparisons provide equally persuasive evidence. Let us look at an example. If we were to supplement the diet of a group of premature neonates with a particular combination of vitamins and other nutrients every day for 2 weeks, the weight of these infants at the end of the 2-week period would give us absolutely no information about the effectiveness of the treatment. At a bare minimum, we would need to compare their posttreatment weight with their pretreatment weight to determine if, at least, their weight had increased. But let us assume for the moment that we find an average weight gain of half a pound. Does this finding support the conclusion that there is a causative relationship between the nutritional supplements (the independent variable) and weight gain (the dependent variable)? No, it does not. Babies will normally gain weight as they mature. Without a control group—a group that does not receive the supplements—it is impossible to separate the effects of maturation from those of the treatment. The term "control group," in other words, refers to a group of subjects whose performance on a dependent variable is used as a basis for evaluating the performance of the experimental group (the group that receives the treatment of interest to the researcher) on the same dependent variable.

Randomization. It must be stressed that the presence of a control group and the introduction of an experimental intervention are not in themselves sufficient conditions for a true experiment. To qualify as an experiment, the design must also involve randomization, or the assignment of subjects to groups on a random basis. The term *random* essentially means that every subject has an equal chance of being assigned to any group. If subjects are recruited to groups randomly, there is no *systematic bias* in the groups with respect to attributes that may affect the dependent variable under investigation.

Before going on to discuss the mechanics of random assignment, we should pause to consider the function of randomization. Suppose a researcher wishes to study the effectiveness of a hospital-based contraceptive counseling program for a group of multiparous women who have just given birth. Two groups of subjects are established, one of which will be counseled and the other of which will receive no counseling. The women as a whole may be expected to differ on a number of characteristics, such as age, marital status, financial situation, attitude toward the parent role, and the like. Any of these characteristics could have an effect on the diligence with which a woman practices contraception, quite independent of whether or not she receives counseling. The researcher naturally wants to have the counsel and no-counsel groups equal with respect to these characteristics in order to adequately assess the impact of the counseling. The random assignment of subjects to one group or the other is designed to perform this equalization function. One method might be to flip a coin for each woman (more elaborate procedures are discussed later). If the coin is "heads" the woman would be assigned to one group and if the coin is "tails" she would be assigned to the other group.

The reader must be warned, however, that while randomization is the preferred scientific method for equalizing groups, there is no guarantee that they will, in fact, be equal. Let us take as an extreme example the case in which only ten women, all of whom have given birth to at least four children, have volunteered to participate in a contraceptive counseling program. Five of the ten women are aged 35 or older and the remaining five are under 35. One would anticipate that a random assignment of women to a control and experimental group would result in approximately two or three women from the two age ranges in each group. But let us suppose that by chance alone the older five women ended up in the experimental group. Since these women are nearing the end of their childbearing years, it might be expected that the likelihood of their conceiving is diminished. Thus, follow-ups on their reproductive behavior (the dependent variable) might suggest that the counseling program was successful for the experimental group, while a higher birthrate for the control group may only reflect the age and, hence, a fertility difference and not the lack of exposure to counseling.

Despite this possibility, randomization remains the most trustworthy and acceptable method of equalizing groups. Unusual or deviant assignments such as this one are rare, and the likelihood of obtaining grossly unequal groups is reduced as the number of subjects increases.

To demonstrate how random assignment is actually performed, we will turn to another example. Suppose we have 15 people who are interested in losing weight. We would like to try one method of weight reduction that is based on caloric intake with one group of five subjects, a second method based on a protein-enriched diet with another group of five subjects, while the third group maintains its previous eating habits. We decide to use an experimental approach to test the effectiveness of the two special diets, and this approach requires that the subjects be assigned to the groups randomly. Since there are three groups, we can no longer use the flip of a coin to decide the group to which a person will be assigned.

Researchers typically use a table of random numbers to perform the randomization process. A portion of such a table is reproduced in Table 6-1. A random-number table is set up by using the digits from zero to nine in such a way that each number is equally likely to follow any other. These tables are often generated by computers. Going in any direction from any point in the table produces a random sequence.

To return to the example at hand, we would number the 15 people from 1 to 15 as shown in the second column of Table 6-2 and then draw numbers between 1 and 15 from Table 6-1. A simple procedure for finding a starting point is to close your eyes and let your finger fall at some point on the table. For the sake of following the example, let us assume that we have done this and that the starting point is at number 52, as circled on Table 6-1. We can now move from that point in any direction on the table. Our task is to select the first five numbers that fall between 01 and 15. Let us move from the starting point to the right, looking at two-digit combinations to be sure to get numbers from 01 to 15. The next number to the right of 52 is 06. The person whose number is 06, that is, Gary S., is assigned to the first group. Moving along in the table, we find that the next number within the range of 01 to 15 is 11. Jane N., whose number is 11, is also assigned to Group I. When we get to the end of the row, we move down to the next row, and so forth. To find numbers in the required range, we may have to bypass a good many numbers. The next three numbers we find are 01, 15, and 14. Thus Sharon M., Rick S., and Jim M. are all put in the first group. The next five numbers between 01 and 15 that emerge in the random-number table are used to assign five people to the second group in the same fashion, as shown in the third column of Table 6-2. The remaining five people are put into the third group. It should be noted that numbers that have already been used often reappear in the table before our randomization task is completed. For example, the number 15 appeared four times before the assignment procedure was completed. This is perfectly normal since the numbers are random. After the first time a number appears and is used, subsequent appearances can be ignored.

It might be useful to look at the three groups to see if they are approximately equal with respect to one readily discernible characteristic, that is, the sex of the person. We started out with eight females and seven males in the total group. The breakdown of the three groups by sex is presented in Table 6-3. As this table shows, the randomization procedure did a good job of allocating the two sexes approximately equally across the three groups. We must accept on faith the probability that other characteristics are fairly well distributed in the randomized groups as well.

We now have fulfilled all three requirements for a true experiment: we have manipulated the situation by devising distinct treatments (the three diets), we have a control group, and we have randomly assigned subjects to the treatments. If any one of these elements had been missing, we would not have had a true experimental design.

Table 6-1. Small Table of Random Digits

46	85	05	23	26	34	67	75	83	00	74	91	06	43	45
69	24	89	34	60	45	30	50	75	21	61	31	83	18	55
14	01	33	17	92	59	74	76	72	77	76	50	33	45	13
56	30	38	73	15	16	⑤②	06	96	76	11	65	49	98	93
81	30	44	85	85	68	65	22	73	76	92	85	25	58	66
70	28	42	43	26	79	37	59	52	20	01	15	96	32	67
90	41	59	36	14	33	52	12	66	65	55	82	34	76	41
39	90	40	21	15	59	58	94	90	67	66	82	14	15	75
88	15	20	00	80	20	55	49	14	09	96	27	74	8̲2̲	57
45	13	46	35	45	59	40	47	20	59	43	94	75	16	80
70	01	41	50	21	41	29	06	73	12	71	85	71	59	57
37	23	93	32	95	05	87	00	11	19	92	78	42	63	40
18	63	73	75	09	82	44	49	90	05	04	92	17	37	01
05	32	78	21	62	20	24	78	17	59	45	19	72	53	32
95	09	66	79	46	48	46	08	55	58	15	19	11	87	82
43	25	38	41	45	60	83	32	59	83	01	29	14	13	49
80	85	40	92	79	43	52	90	63	18	38	38	47	47	61
80	08	87	70	74	88	72	25	67	36	66	16	44	94	31
80	89	01	80	02	94	81	33	19	00	54	15	58	34	36
93	12	81	84	64	74	45	79	05	61	72	84	81	18	34
82	47	42	55	93	48	54	53	52	47	18	61	91	36	74
53	34	24	42	76	75	12	21	17	24	74	62	77	37	07
82	64	12	28	20	92	90	41	31	41	32	39	21	97	63
13	57	41	72	00	69	90	26	37	42	78	46	42	25	01
29	59	38	86	27	94	97	21	15	98	62	09	53	67	87
86	88	75	50	87	19	15	20	00	23	12	30	28	07	83
44	98	91	68	22	36	02	40	08	67	76	37	84	16	05
93	39	94	55	47	94	45	87	42	84	05	04	14	98	07
52	16	29	02	86	54	15	83	42	43	46	97	83	54	82
04	73	72	10	31	75	05	19	30	29	47	66	56	43	82

Experimental Designs

The most basic experimental design involves the random assignment of subjects to two groups and the subsequent collection of data. A more refined design, illustrated in Figure 6-1, involves the collection of pretest data prior to any experimental manipulation.

Solomon Four-Group Design. Sometimes the pretest may have the potential to distort the results. That is, the posttest measures may be affected not only by the treatment but also by exposure to the pretest. For example, if our intervention was a workshop to improve nurses' attitudes

Table 6-2. Example of Random-Assignment Procedure

NAME OF SUBJECT	NUMBER	GROUP ASSIGNMENT
Sharon M.	1	I
Fred F.	2	III
Sheryl W.	3	III
Pam W.	4	II
Gretchen E.	5	II
Gary S.	6	I
Polly O.	7	III
Barrett T.	8	III
Mike H.	9	II
Sherry B.	10	III
Jane N.	11	I
Paula S.	12	II
Chip C.	13	II
Jim M.	14	I
Rick S.	15	I

Table 6-3. Breakdown of the Sex Composition of the Three Groups

	GROUP I	GROUP II	GROUP III
Male	3	2	2
Female	2	3	3

toward the mentally ill, a pretest attitudinal measure may in itself constitute a sensitizing "treatment" and could obscure an analysis of the workshop's effect. Such a situation might call for the *Solomon four-group design.* In this design there are two experimental groups and two control groups. One experimental group and one control group would be administered the pretest and the other groups would not, thereby allowing the effects of the pretest measure and intervention to be segregated.

Factorial Design. We have to this point considered designs in which the experimenter systematically varies or manipulates only one independent variable at a time. Modern statistical and research design procedures have made it possible to manipulate two or more variables at a time. As usual, we will look at a hypothetical example to illustrate this point. Suppose that we are interested in comparing two therapeutic strategies for premature infants: one method involves tactile stimulation and the second approach involves auditory stimulation. At the same time, however, we are interested in learning if the daily amount of stimulation is related to the progress of the infant. The dependent variables for this study will be various measures of infant development, such as weight gain, cardiac responsiveness, and so forth. Figure 6-2 illustrates the structure of this experiment.

This type of study, which is known as a *factorial experiment,* offers a number of advantages to the researcher. In effect, factorial designs permit the testing of three hypotheses in a single experiment. In the present example the three research questions being addressed are as follows:

1. Does auditory stimulation have a more beneficial effect on the development of premature infants than tactile stimulation?

2. Is the duration of stimulation (independent of modality) related to infant development?

3. Is auditory stimulation most effective when linked to a certain "dose" and tactile stimulation most effective when coupled with a different dose?

This third question demonstrates a major strength of factorial designs: they permit us to evaluate not only *main effects* (effects resulting from experimentally manipulated variables, as exemplified in questions 1 and 2) but also *interaction effects* (effects resulting from combining the treatment methods). We may feel that it is not sufficient to say that auditory stimulation is preferable to tactile stimulation (or vice versa) and that 45 minutes of stimulation per day is more effective than 15 minutes per day. Rather, it is how these two variables interact (how they behave in combination) that is of interest. Our results may indicate that 15 minutes of tactile stimulation and 45 minutes of auditory stimulation are the most

	TYPE OF STIMULATION	
	Auditory A1	Tactile A2
15 min. B1	A1 B1	A2 B1
DAILY EXPOSURE 30 min. B2	A1 B2	A2 B2
45 min. B3	A1 B3	A2 B3

Figure 6-2. Schematic diagram of a factorial experiment

beneficial treatments. We could not have obtained these results by conducting two separate experiments that manipulated only one independent variable and held the second one constant.

In factorial experiments such as the ones being discussed here, subjects would be assigned at random to a combination of conditions. In the example that Figure 6-2 illustrates, the premature infants would be assigned randomly to one of the six cells. The term *cell* is used in experimental research to refer to a treatment condition; it is represented in a schematic diagram as a box (cell) in the design.

Figure 6-2 can also be used to define some design terminology frequently encountered in the research literature. The two independent variables in a factorial design are referred to as the *factors*. The "type of stimulation" variable is factor A and the "amount of daily exposure" variable is factor B. Each factor must have two or more *levels* (if there were only one level, the factor would not be a variable). Level one of factor A is "auditory" and level two of factor A is tactile. When describing the dimensions of the design, researchers refer to the number of levels. The design in Figure 6-2 would be described as a 2 × 3 design: two levels in factor A times three levels in factor B. If a third source of stimulation, such as visual stimulation, were added, and if a daily dosage of 60 minutes were also added, the design would be referred to as a 3 × 4 design.

Factorial experiments can be performed with three or more independent variables (factors). However, designs with more than four factors are rare, because the analysis becomes complex and because the number of subjects required would be prohibitive.

Advantages and Disadvantages of True Experiments

Advantages. True experiments are the most powerful method available to scientists for testing hypotheses of cause-and-effect relationships between variables. Because of its special controlling properties, the scientific experiment offers greater corroboration than any other research approach that, if the independent variable (e.g., diet, drug dosage, teaching approach) is manipulated in a certain way, then certain consequences in the dependent variable (weight loss, recovery of health, learning) may be expected to ensue. The great strength of experiments, then, lies in the confidence with which causal relationships can be inferred.

Paul Lazarsfeld, a sociologist, has identified three criteria for causality (1955). The first criterion is temporal: a cause must precede an effect in time. If we were testing the hypothesis that saccharin causes bladder cancer, it would obviously be necessary to demonstrate that the subjects had not developed cancer prior to exposure to saccharin. The second requirement is that there be an empirical relationship between the presumed cause and the presumed effect. In the saccharin/cancer example, the researchers would have to demonstrate an association between the inges-tion of saccharin and the presence of a carcinoma. The final criterion in a causal relationship is that the relationship cannot be explained as being due to the influence of a third variable. Suppose, for instance, that people who use saccharin tend also to drink more coffee than nonusers. There is, thus, a possibility that any empirical relationship between saccharin use and bladder cancer in humans reflects an underlying causal relation-ship between a substance in coffee and bladder cancer. It is particularly because of this third criterion that the experimental approach is so strong. Through the controls imposed by manipulation, comparison, and ran-domization, alternative explanations to a causal interpretation can often be ruled out or discredited.

Disadvantages. Despite the overwhelming advantages of experimen-tal research, this approach has several limitations. First of all, there are a number of interesting variables that are simply not amenable to experi-mental manipulation. A large number of human characteristics, such as sex, height, or intelligence, or environmental characteristics, such as weather, cannot be experimentally controlled.

A second, but related, limitation is that there are many variables that could technically be manipulated except that ethical considerations pro-hibit such manipulation. For example, to date there have not been any experiments using human subjects to study the effect of cigarette smoking on lung cancer. Such an experiment would require us to randomly assign people to a smoking or nonsmoking group. Experimentation with humans, therefore, is subject to a number of ethical constraints.

In many situations experimentation may not be feasible simply because it is impractical. This often will be the case in hospital settings. It may, for instance, be impossible in the real world to secure the necessary cooperation to conduct an experiment from administrators or other key people. Cooperation may be withheld for many reasons, from a desire to avoid disruptions to a basic suspicion and uneasiness about the concept of experimentation.

Another problem with experiments is the so-called Hawthorne effect, which is a kind of placebo effect. The term is derived from a series of experiments conducted at the Hawthorne plant of the Western Electric Corporation in which various environmental conditions, such as light and working hours, were varied to determine their effect on worker produc-tivity. Regardless of what change was introduced, that is, whether the light was made better or worse, productivity increased. Thus, it seems that the knowledge of being included in a study may be sufficient to cause people to change their behavior, thereby obscuring the effect of the vari-able of interest.

In a hospital situation the researcher might have to contend with a double Hawthorne effect. For example, if an experiment to investigate the effect of a new postoperative patient routine were conducted, nurses and hospital staff, as well as patients, might be aware of their participation in a study, and both groups could alter their actions accordingly. It is precisely for this reason that *double-blind experiments*, in which neither the subjects nor those who administer the treatment know who is in the experimental or control group, are so powerful. Unfortunately, the double-blind approach is not feasible for some kinds of nursing research since nursing interventions are harder to disguise than medications.

In sum, despite the clear-cut superiority of experiments for testing causal hypotheses, they are subject to a number of limitations that make them difficult to apply to many real-world problems. Nevertheless, the fact that experimental conditions are difficult to establish does not mean that all attempts to achieve them should be abandoned. True experiments probably are possible in many situations in which nonexperimental methods are used.

Quasi-experimental Research

Research that uses a *quasi-experimental design* often looks very much like an experiment. *Quasi-experiments*, however, lack at least one of the three properties that, as we have seen, characterize an experiment. The missing ingredient is either the randomization or control-group component (or both). Quasi-experiments do involve the manipulation of an independent variable, that is, the institution of a treatment. The basic difficulty with the quasi-experimental approach is its weakness, relative to experiments, in allowing us to make causal inferences. We want to know if an intervention does, in fact, cause the effect we observe in the dependent variable. Experimental evidence for cause-and-effect relationships is more convincing than findings from quasi-experiments.

Perhaps the problems inherent in quasi-experiments will become clear if we present a few hypothetical examples. Before doing this, however, it will be useful to introduce some notation that will facilitate our discussion.* Figure 6-3 presents a symbolic representation of a pretest–posttest experimental design, identical to the design shown in Figure 6-1. According to the notation used in Figure 6-3, R means that there has been a random assignment to separate treatment groups. An O represents the collection of data on the dependent variable, and the X stands for the exposure of a group to an experimental treatment. Thus the top line in Figure 6-3 represents the experimental group that has had subjects randomly assigned to it (R), has had both a pretreatment test (O_1) and a posttreatment

---

*The notation, as well as most of the concepts in this section, are derived from Campbell and Stanley's classic monograph (1963).

| R = randomization | R | O₁ | X | O₂ |

R = randomization

O = observation or measurement

X = treatment or intervention

R   O₁   X   O₂

R   O₁   O₂

Figure 6-3. Symbolic representation of a pretest–posttest experimental design

test (O_2), and has been exposed to the experimental treatment of interest (X). The second row in the figure represents the control group, which differs from the experimental group only by the absence of exposure to the experimental treatment. We are now equipped to examine a few quasi-experimental designs.

Quasi-experimental Designs

Nonequivalent Control-Group Design. Suppose that we wished to study the effect of introducing the problem-oriented method of charting on nursing staff morale. The system is to be implemented in a 600-bed hospital in a large metropolitan area. Since we anticipate that there might be staff-dissatisfaction problems, at least initially, we arrange to conduct a study. There are a number of alternative strategies available in designing the investigation. Suppose, however, that a true experiment is not feasible because the new system is being implemented throughout the hospital, making randomization impossible. Therefore, we decide to find another hospital with similar characteristics (size, geographic location, and the like) that is not instituting the problem-oriented method of charting. We also decide to collect baseline data by administering a staff morale questionnaire in both hospitals (the pretest). Data are again collected after the system is installed in the first hospital (the posttest). This is called a *non-equivalent control-group design.*

Figure 6-4 depicts this hypothetical study symbolically. The top row is our experimental (problem-oriented charting) hospital and the second row is the hospital using traditional methods. A comparison of this diagram with the one in Figure 6-3 shows their close resemblance to one another. They are, in fact, identical except that subjects have not been randomly assigned to treatment groups in the second diagram. The design in Figure 6-4 is the weaker of the two because *it can no longer be assumed that the experimental and comparison groups are equal.** Because of the inability to randomize subjects, our study is quasi-experimental rather than truly experimental. The design is, nevertheless, a very strong one

---

*In quasi-experiments, the term "comparison group" is generally used in lieu of "control group" to refer to the group against which outcomes in the treatment group- will be evaluated.

$$O_1 \qquad X \qquad O_2$$

$$O_1 \qquad\qquad O_2$$

Figure 6-4. Nonequivalent control-group pretest–posttest design (quasi-experimental)

because the collection of pretest data allows us to determine whether the groups were initially similar in terms of their morale. If the comparison and experimental groups responded similarly, on the average, on their pretest questionnaire, we could be relatively confident that any posttest difference in self-reported morale was the result of the experimental treatment.

Let us pursue this same example a bit further. Suppose we had not thought to or had been unable to collect pretest data before the new method of charting was introduced. The resulting study could be diagramed to show the scheme in Figure 6-5. This design, which is not uncommon, has a flaw that is difficult to remedy. We have no basis on which to judge the initial equivalence of the two nursing staffs. If we find that the morale of the experimental hospital staff is much lower than that of the control hospital staff, can we conclude that the new method of charting caused a decline in staff morale? There could be several alternative explanations for the posttest differences. Campbell and Stanley (1963), in fact, would call the design shown in Figure 6-5 *preexperimental* rather than quasi-experimental because of its essentially unreconcilable weaknesses. Thus, while quasi-experiments lack some of the controlling properties inherent in true experiments, the hallmark of the quasi-experimental approach is the effort to introduce other controls to compensate for the absence of either the randomization or control-group component.

Time-Series Design. The designs reviewed above illustrate studies in which a clearly identified control group was used but randomization was not. The designs we examine below have neither a control group nor randomization. In some cases where both characteristics are absent there are inherent weaknesses that seriously jeopardize the validity of the findings. However, there are several designs that offer the researcher some measure of protection against these problems.

Let us suppose that a hospital decides to adopt a requirement that all its nurses accrue a certain number of continuing-education units before being considered for a promotion or raise. The nurse administrators want to assess some of the positive and negative consequences of this mandate. Some of the indicators they might examine include turnover rate, absen-

$$X \qquad O$$
$$O$$

Figure 6-5. Nonequivalent control-group (posttest only) design (pre-experimental)

$$O_1 \qquad X \qquad O_2$$

Figure 6-6. One-group pretest–posttest design (pre-experimental)

tee rate, qualifications of employment applicants, number of raises and promotions awarded, and so on. For the purposes of this example, let us assume that there is no other comparable hospital that could reasonably serve as a comparison for this study. In such a case, the only kind of comparison that could be made is a before–after contrast. If the requirement were inaugurated in January, one could compare the turnover rate, for example, for the 3-month period prior to the new rule with the turnover rate for the subsequent 3-month period. The schematic representation for such a study is shown in Figure 6-6.

While this design seems logical and straightforward, there actually are a number of problems with it. What if either of the 3-month periods is atypical, apart from any regulation? What about the effects of any other hospital rules inaugurated during the same period? What about the effects of external factors, such as parking facilities, employee benefits at other nearby hospitals, changes in the economy, and the like? The design in question offers no way of controlling any of these factors. This design again falls into the group that has been called preexperimental by Campbell and Stanley (1963) because it fails to control for so many possible extraneous variables.

The inability to obtain a meaningful control group, however, does not eliminate the possibility of conducting research with integrity. The design presented in Figure 6-6 could be modified in such a way that at least some of the alternative explanations for any change in the turnover rate of nurses could be ruled out. Remember that what we want to assess is the effect of the continuing-education requirement on the turnover rate. If there are plausible alternative ways to explain an increase or decrease in nurses' resignations, then we cannot solve our research problem.

A design that can come to our assistance in this case is known as the *time-series design* and is diagramed in Figure 6-7. The basic notion underlying the time-series design is the collection of information over an extended time period and the introduction of an experimental treatment during the course of the data-collection period. In the figure, O_1 through O_4 represent four separate instances of observation or data collection on a dependent variable prior to treatment; X represents the treatment (the introduction of the independent variable); and O_5 through O_8 represent four posttreatment observations. In our present example, O_1 might be the number of nurses who left the hospital in January through March in the year prior to the new continuing-education rule, O_2 the number of resig-

$$O_1 \qquad O_2 \qquad O_3 \qquad O_4 \qquad X \qquad O_5 \qquad O_6 \qquad O_7 \qquad O_8$$

Figure 6-7. Time-series design (quasi-experimental)

nations in April through June, and so forth. After the rule is implemented, data on turnover are similarly collected for four consecutive 3-month periods, giving us observations O_5 through O_8.

While the time-series design does not eliminate all of the problems of interpreting changes in turnover rate, the extended time perspective immensely strengthens our ability to attribute any change to our experimental manipulation. Figure 6-8 attempts to demonstrate why this is so. The two diagrams (A and B) in this figure show two possible outcome patterns for the eight measures of nurse turnover. The dotted line in the center represents the time at which the continuing-education rule was implemented. Both A and B reflect a feature that is common to most time-series studies, and this is the fluctuation from one observation or measurement to another. These fluctuations are, of course, perfectly normal. One would not expect resignations to be spaced evenly during the course of the year with exactly the same number of resignations per month. It is precisely because of these fluctuations that the design shown in Figure 6-6, with only one observation before and after the experimental treatment, is so weak.

Let us compare the kind of interpretations that can be made for the outcomes reflected in A and B of Figure 6-8. In both cases, the number of

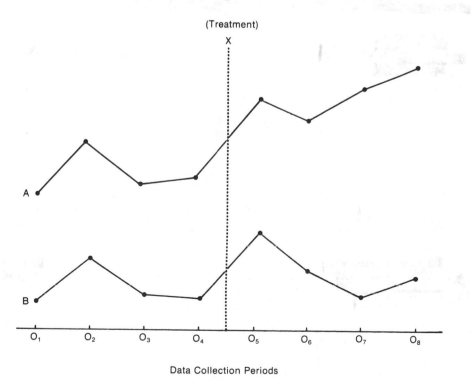

Data Collection Periods

Figure 6-8. Two possible time-series outcome patterns

resignations increases between O_4 and O_5, that is, immediately after the introduction of the continuing-education requirement. For pattern B, however, the number of resignations falls at O_6 and continues to decrease at O_7. The increase at O_5 looks very similar to other apparently haphazard fluctuations in the turnover rate at other periods. Therefore, it probably would be erroneous to conclude that the treatment had had an effect on resignations. In A, on the other hand, the number of resignations increases at O_5 and remains relatively high for all subsequent periods of data collection. It is true, of course, that there may be other explanations for a change in turnover rate from 1 year to the next. The time-series design, however, does permit us to rule out the possibility that the data reflect an unstable measurement of resignations made at only two points in time. If we had used the design in Figure 6-6 to study this problem, it would have been analogous to obtaining the measurements at O_4 and O_5 of Figure 6-8 only. The outcomes in both A and B of this figure look quite similar at these two points in time. Yet, as we have seen, the use of a broader time perspective leads us to draw very different conclusions about the nature of the changes from one pattern of outcomes to the next.

Advantages and Disadvantages of Quasi-experiments

Advantages. The great strength of quasi-experiments lies in their practicality, feasibility, and, to a certain extent, their generalizability. In the "real world" it is often quite impractical, if not impossible, to conduct true experiments. A good deal of the research that is of interest to nurses occurs in natural settings. Frequently, it is difficult to deliver an innovative treatment to only half of a group, and randomization may be even more unmanageable. The inability to randomize, or even to secure a control group, need not force a researcher to abandon all hopes of conducting an investigation. Quasi-experimental designs are research plans that introduce some controls when full experimental rigor is lacking.

Disadvantages. It is precisely because the control inherent in true experiments is absent in quasi-experiments that the researcher needs to be acquainted with the weaknesses of the quasi-experimental approach. The major disadvantage of quasi-experiments is that the kinds of cause-and-effect inferences that we typically seek in conducting research cannot be made as easily as with true experiments. With quasi-experiments there are generally several "rival hypotheses" that compete with the experimental manipulation as explanations for observed results. Take as an example the case in which we administer certain medications to a group of babies whose mothers are heroin addicts. Suppose we are interested in determining whether this treatment will result in a weight gain in these typically low-weight babies. If we use no comparison group or we utilize a nonequivalent control group and then observe a weight gain, we must ask ourselves the following questions: Is it plausible that some other external factor caused or influenced the gain? Is it plausible that pretreatment differences resulted in differential posttreatment weight gains? Is it plausible that the changes would have occurred in the absence of any intervention? If we answer "yes" to any of these questions, then the inferences we can make about the effect of the experimental treatment are weakened considerably. With quasi-experiments there is typically at least one plausible rival explanation. We hasten to add that the quality of a study is not necessarily a function of its design. There are many excellent quasi-experimental investigations, as well as very poor experiments.

Nonexperimental Research

When a researcher is in a position to introduce a "treatment," the effects of which he or she is interested in assessing, we say that the independent variable is being controlled or manipulated by the investigator. We noted above that manipulation is a key element in true experiments, and in quasi- and pre-experimental designs as well. When experimentation or quasi-experimentation is possible, these approaches are generally the most highly effective methods for testing hypotheses about the relationships among variables.

There are, nevertheless, a number of research problems that, for one or more reasons, do not lend themselves to an experimental or even quasi-experimental design. Let us say, for example, that we are interested in studying the effect of widowhood on physical and psychological functioning. We could use as our dependent variables an existing psychological diagnostic instrument, such as the Minnesota Multiphasic Personality Inventory, as well as physiological and medical measures, such as blood pressure, number of medications consumed, and self-reports on eating and sleeping patterns. Our independent variable is widowhood versus nonwidowhood. Clearly, researchers would be unable to manipulate widowhood. Spouses of hospitalized patients become widows or widowers by a process that is neither random nor subject to research control. Thus, the investigator must proceed by taking the two groups as they naturally occur and comparing them in terms of psychological and physical well-being.

Many of the research studies in which human beings are involved are nonexperimental in nature. This is certainly true of a large number of nursing research investigations. There are essentially four reasons for doing nonexperimental research. First, there are many situations in which the independent variable is inherently nonmanipulable. For instance, sex, blood type, personality, medical diagnosis, and age are examples of characteristics that people bring with them to the research situation. The effects of these characteristics on some phenomenon of interest cannot be studied experimentally. We simply cannot, for example, randomly confer upon incoming hospital patients various diagnoses in order to study the effect of the diagnosis upon preoperative anxiety. Nevertheless, the relationship between these variables and a whole range of criterion variables is often of considerable theoretical or practical interest. Does the size of a hospital affect a patient's perception of the quality of nursing care? Does a patient's age affect the incidence of decubitus ulcers? Such questions cannot be answered using experimental procedures.

Second, there are numerous variables that could technically be manipulated but that should not be manipulated for ethical reasons. One example we have already discussed is the number of cigarettes smoked per day by humans. If the nature of the independent variable is such that its manipulation could cause physical or mental harm to subjects, then that variable should not be controlled experimentally.

Third, there are many research situations in which it is simply not practical or even desirable to conduct a true experiment. Such constraints might involve insufficient time, inconvenience, lack of cooperation, or lack of adequate funds. For instance, let us suppose that we were interested in studying the effect of hospital noise levels on patient well-being and recovery. Certain areas of the hospital might be particularly noisy while other areas might be much quieter. Let us say that we have categorized all the rooms as either above average or below average in terms of noise intensity. Technically, it might be possible to randomly assign incoming patients to rooms, but this would typically be rather impractical. We must be content in this situation to perform a nonexperimental study. That is, we would collect information on patient well-being—number of hours slept, blood pressure, need for medications, and so on—and compare groups exposed to the two different noise conditions.

A fourth situation that calls for a nonexperimental approach involves research in which the investigator observes the manifestation of some event or situation and tries to determine what factors have caused it. In other words, it is research in which the consequences (the dependent variables) are in evidence, and the task is to determine the antecedents. In such a case the investigator must take the relationships among variables as they are without being able to control any of the presumed determinants.

In sum, there are many situations in which the researcher cannot control or manipulate the independent variable. When this is the case, the researcher has no choice but to conduct a nonexperimental study.

Types of Nonexperimental Research

Ex Post Facto Research.   There are two broad classes of nonexperimental research. One is referred to as *ex post facto research*. The literal translation of the Latin term *ex post facto* is "from after the fact." This expression is meant to indicate that the research in question has been conducted after the variations in the independent variable have occurred in the natural course of events.

The basic purpose of ex post facto research (or *correlational research*, as it is sometimes called) is essentially the same as experimental research—to determine the relationships among variables. The most important distinction between the two is the difficulty of inferring causal relationships in ex post facto studies because of the lack of manipulative control of the independent variables. In experiments, the investigator makes a prediction that a deliberate variation in X, the independent variable, will result in the occurrence of some event or behavior, Y (the dependent variable). For example, the prediction is made that if some medication is administered, then patient improvement will ensue. The experimenter has direct control over the X: the experimental treatment can be administered to some and withheld from others.

In ex post facto research, on the other hand, the investigator does not have control of the independent variables because they have already occurred. The examination of independent variables—the presumed causative factors—is done retrospectively. Because of this, attempts to draw any cause-and-effect conclusions may be totally unwarranted. There is a famous research dictum that is relevant: correlation does not prove causation. That is, the mere existence of a relationship—even a strong one—between two variables is not enough to warrant the conclusion that one variable has caused the other. Thus, ex post facto research can demonstrate functional but not causal relationships among variables. Of course, even experimentation is not sufficient to prove a causal relationship, but the experimenters can place considerably more confidence in their inferences than can researchers using an ex post facto approach.

Descriptive Research. The second broad class of nonexperimental research is pure *descriptive research*. Descriptive studies are not concerned with relationships among variables. Their purpose is to observe, describe, and document aspects of a situation. For example, an investigator may wish to determine the percentage of teenage mothers who received no prenatal care. Or a researcher might be interested in the incidence of fetal abnormalities among women who discontinued use of birth-control pills. Because the intent of such research is not to explain or to understand the underlying causes of the variables of interest, experimental designs are not required.

Pure descriptive research is relatively uncommon. Most studies present opportunities for looking at how phenomena are interrelated, and, therefore, most nonexperimental research is correlational. On the other hand, most studies have a component that is purely descriptive.

Two types of studies that often have a primarily descriptive intent are field studies and trend studies. *Field studies* are investigations that are done in real social settings, such as hospitals, clinics, intensive care units, nursing homes, and the like. The purpose of field studies is to systematically examine the practices, behaviors, attitudes, and characteristics of individuals or groups as they normally function in life. Typically, the investigator focuses on a single social setting, and in this manner the ongoing processes and structure can be studied in depth.

Trend studies document changes (or absence of changes) of various phenomena over time. For example, an investigator may wish to describe changes in the life expectancy for patients on dialysis over time. As another example, a researcher may be interested in documenting trends in the use of midwives. Trend studies, like all descriptive research, are designed to describe the status of some condition, but in such studies the dimension of time is added.

Advantages and Disadvantages of Nonexperimental Research

Disadvantages. Relative to experimental and quasi-experimental research, nonexperimental research is weak in its ability to reveal causal relationships. Descriptive research, of course, does not focus on relationships. The major limitation of pure descriptive research, in fact, is its inability to provide insight into why the phenomena of interest are occurring or behaving the way they are. Descriptive research may give us "facts," but it offers neither explanations nor any possibility of prediction or control.

Ex post facto studies suffer from problems of ambiguity that leave open the possibility of faulty interpretation. This situation stems in large part from the fact that in ex post facto studies the researcher works with preexisting groups that have not formed by a random process but, rather, by what might be termed a self-selecting process. Kerlinger (1973) has offered the following description of self-selection.

Self-selection occurs when the members of the groups being studied are in the groups, in part, because they differentially possess traits or characteristics extraneous to the research problem, characteristics that possibly influence or are otherwise related to the variables of the research problem. (p. 381)

In correlational research the researchers cannot assume that the groups being studied were similar at the beginning of the investigation. Because of this fact, preexisting differences may be a plausible alternative explanation for any observed differences on the dependent variable of interest.

As an illustration of this problem, let us take a hypothetical study in which the researcher is interested in examining the relationship between type of nursing program (the independent variable) and job satisfaction after graduation. If the investigator finds that diploma-school graduates are more satisfied with their work than baccalaureate graduates 1 year after graduation, the conclusion that the diploma-school program provides better preparation for actual work situations and, hence, leads to increased satisfaction may or may not be accurate. The students in the two programs were undoubtedly different to begin with in terms of a number of important characteristics, such as social class, personality, career goals, and so forth. In other words, students self-selected themselves into one of the two programs, and it may be the selection traits themselves that have resulted in different job expectations and satisfactions.

A large part of the difficulty of interpreting correlational findings stems from the fact that behaviors, states, attitudes, and characteristics are interrelated (correlated) in complex ways. An example might help to make this clear. Let us suppose we were interested in studying the differences between the postoperative convalescence behavior of patients who had undergone surgery for two different medical problems—hernia and ulcers. Our independent variable in this hypothetical study is the type of medical problem. We might use as our measure of the dependent variable (postoperative convalescent behavior) one or more of the following: ratings of nurses on the degree of cooperativeness of the patient, number of times the patient calls the nurse for help, the patients' self-ratings of distress, and the number of medications required to induce sleep or alleviate pain. Let us say that we find that the hernia patients receive a significantly lower rating by the nurses on degree of cooperation than the ulcer patients. We could interpret this finding to mean that particular medical problems and their accompanying surgical treatment produce different patterns of cooperative behavior in individuals. This relationship is diagramed in Figure 6-9 A. Note that, even with this interpretation, it is essen-

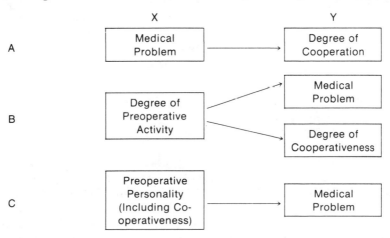

Figure 6-9. Three possible explanations for the relationship between medical diagnosis and degree of cooperativeness in patients. Arrows show the direction of influence; variable X is presumed to "cause" variable Y.

tially impossible to separate the effects of (1) the type of medical problem and (2) the type of surgical procedure on cooperativeness, since one necessarily follows the other.

For the sake of this discussion, let us examine some alternative explanations for the findings. Perhaps there is a third variable that influences both the degree of convalescent cooperativeness and the type of medical ailment, such as the degree of physical activity to which a person is accustomed. That is, it may be possible that hernia patients are usually engaged in a greater degree of physical activity than are ulcer patients, and this fact may be one of the causes of both the diagnosis and the inability to cope properly with the sedentary hospital routine. This set of relationships is diagramed in Figure 6-9 B.

A third possibility may be reversed causality, as shown in Figure 6-9 C. Willingness to cooperate in general may be thought of as one aspect of a person's personality, and it is possible that the dynamics of a person's psychological makeup will result in the manifestation of different medical problems. In this interpretation, it is the person's disposition that causes the diagnosis, and not the other way around. Undoubtedly, the reader will be able to invent other alternatives. The point is that interpretations of ex post facto results should generally be considered tentative, particularly if the research has no theoretical basis.

Advantages. Despite the limitations of ex post facto studies, they will undoubtedly continue to play a crucial role in nursing, medical, and social-science research because many of the interesting problems to be solved in those fields are not amenable to experimentation. Correlational research is often an efficient and effective means of collecting a large amount of data about a problem area. For example, it would be possible to collect extensive information about the health histories and eating habits of a large number of people. Researchers could then examine which health problems are correlated with which diets. By doing this, a large number of interrelationships could be discovered in a relatively short amount of time. By contrast, an experimenter usually looks at only a few variables at a time. For example, one experiment might be devoted to manipulating foods high in cholesterol to observe the effects on certain medical symptoms, while another experiment could manipulate saccharin consumption, and so forth.

One final advantage is that ex post facto research, particularly those investigations referred to as field studies, is very realistic and, therefore, has an intrinsic appeal for the solution of many practical problems. Unlike many experimental studies, ex post facto research can seldom be criticized for its artificiality. In general, the results of studies in realistic settings are more likely to be generalizable to other settings than are the results from laboratory research.

Research Example

> Branch (1984) tested the hypothesis that food additives result in hyperactivity in children.* A sample of 30 hyperactive children from Callaway and 30 hyperactive children from Columbia were selected to participate in the study. All 60 children were age 7 to 10. The children from Callaway constituted the experimental group. With the cooperation of parents and school personnel, these children were put on a strict additive-free diet for a 3-month period. The children from Columbia (the comparison group) were allowed to continue their normal diets, which included foods with artificial colors and flavors. At the end of 3 months, Branch collected data regarding the children's hyperactivity. Each child was observed for a 1-hour session by an independent observer who did not know to which group each child belonged. The observer rated each child for the amount and intensity of hyperactive behavior. The investigator found that the children from Callaway were rated as significantly less hyperactive than those from Columbia, on average. Branch concluded that food additives cause hyperactivity among school-age children.

This study used a preexperimental design. Its major strength is that the investigator had the opportunity to manipulate the independent variable, the children's diet. Assuming that cheating was minimal, the investigator could be reasonably confident that the two groups were, in fact, distinct. She did not have to rely on retrospective accounts of what children had consumed in the previous 3 months, as would be the case if she had used an ex post facto design.

There are, nevertheless, some serious design problems. Although Branch has included a comparison group, there is no way to know if the two groups were really equivalent prior to the intervention. Were the two groups equally hyperactive to begin with? Are the two groups comparable in terms of sex, age distribution, or other characteristics that could affect hyperactive behavior? Are there differences in the way the school systems are handling the hyperactivity? These questions suggest that there may be rival explanations for the observed relationship between the children's diets and their hyperactive behavior.

It was noted earlier that three conditions are necessary to infer causality. First, a cause must precede an effect in time. In this case the diets were instituted for 3 months and then the children's behaviors were observed. Second, an empirical relationship must exist. Again, this requirement was satisfied: children from Columbia were rated as more hyperactive than those from Callaway. Third, the relationship cannot be

---

*This example is fictitious.

explained in terms of the influence of a third variable. This is where Branch's design is weak. Because the two groups of children might have been different in many important respects prior to the study, there is no way to rule out the possibility that some other factor caused the posttreatment differences in hyperactivity.

Perhaps a true experiment would not have been feasible for this researcher, though certainly an experimental design could be used to test the hypothesis. The investigator could have strengthened the research considerably by the inclusion of a pretreatment observation of the children's behavior.

Summary

In this chapter we discussed research designs that vary in their capacity to reveal causal relationships. Experimental designs are especially strong in this regard. *True experiments* are characterized by three fundamental properties. *Manipulation* involves doing something to or acting upon at least some of the subjects in a research study. The experimenter manipulates, or varies, the independent variable (often referred to as the *experimental treatment*) to see if the manipulation has an effect on the dependent variable or variables of interest. True experiments always require the utilization of a *control group*, whose performance on the criterion or dependent measures is used as a basis for assessing the performance of the experimental group on the same measure. The third requirement for an experiment is that subjects be assigned to control the experimental groups by a process known as *randomization*. The random-assignment procedure can be accomplished by any method that allows every subject an equal chance of being included in any group. Randomization does not guarantee that all groups will be equal, but this technique is the most reliable method for equating groups on all possible characteristics that could affect the outcome of the study.

Various experimental designs exist for testing research hypotheses, including a pretest–posttest design when a measure of the dependent variable before the intervention is desirable. If pretest sensitization might obscure the effect of the treatment, a *Solomon four-group design* might be needed. When a researcher manipulates more than one variable at a time, the design is known as a *factorial experiment*. Such a design is efficient in that it permits two simultaneous experiments with one pool of subjects. Furthermore, with factorial designs we can test both *main effects* (effects resulting from the experimentally manipulated variables) and *interaction effects* (effects resulting from combining the treatments). In factorial designs each independent variable is referred to as a *factor* and each factor consists of two or more *levels* of the treatment.

While experiments are the most rigorous scientific approach to studying cause-and-effect relationships, there are many situations in which an experimental design is either not ethical or not feasible. *Quasi-experiments* involve a manipulative component but lack a comparison group or randomization. Quasi-experimental designs are designs in which efforts are made to introduce controls into the study in order to compensate in part for the absence of one or both of these important characteristics. By contrast, *preexperimental designs* have no such safeguards and, therefore, are subject to ambiguity and multiple interpretations of results.

A number of specific quasi-experimental designs were presented. The *nonequivalent control-group design* involves the use of a control group that was not designated by a randomization procedure. Since the problem with the use of such a comparison group is the possibility that the groups are initially different in ways that will affect the research outcomes, the collection of pretreatment data becomes an important means of assessing their initial equivalence. In studies in which there is no control group, a method for overcoming some of the difficulties in the interpretation of results is the collection of information over a period of time before and after the treatment is instituted. Such a study is known as the *time-series design*. Despite some of the problems inherent in quasi-experimental designs, they are often more practical in the nursing field than the more rigorous experimental designs and, therefore, merit increased attention by nursing researchers.

Nonexperimental research includes two broad categories: descriptive research and ex post facto/correlational research. *Descriptive research* is designed to summarize the status of some phenomena of interest as they currently exist. *Ex post facto* or *correlational studies* are research investigations designed to examine the relationships among variables. Unlike experimental or quasi-experimental studies, however, ex post facto research lacks active manipulation of the independent variable. Since the investigation of the independent variables is done retrospectively, that is, after they have occurred in the natural course of events, it becomes very difficult to draw cause-and-effect conclusions. It is for this reason that, methodologically speaking, experimental studies are considered more rigorous. On the other hand, since experimentation is often impractical or impossible, nonexperimental research remains a common approach to studying problems in the field of nursing.

Study Suggestions

1. Assume that you have ten people—Z, Y, X, W, V, U, T, S, R, and Q—who are going to participate in an experiment you are conducting. Using a table of random numbers, assign five people to group I and five to group II.

2. Suppose that you were interested in testing the hypothesis that systematic relaxation procedures taught by nurses to presurgical patients would reduce stress. Describe what you might do to test this hypothesis on an experimental and quasi-experimental basis. Compare the kinds of conclusions you could make with each approach.

3. In the hypothetical example of the hospital administration that wanted to study the effect of a new continuing-education requirement on its nursing staff, preexperimental and quasi-experimental designs were discussed. What might some of the problems be in trying to study this problem experimentally?

3. A nurse researcher is interested in studying the success of several different approaches to feeding patients with dysphagia. Can the researcher use an ex post facto design to examine this problem? Why or why not? Could an experimental or quasi-experimental approach be used? How?

5. A nurse researcher is planning to investigate the relationship between the social class of hospitalized children and the frequency and content of children-initiated communications with the nursing staff. Which is the independent variable and which is the dependent variable? Would you classify this research as basically experimental or correlational, or could both approaches be used?

6. Classify the following list of potential independent variables in terms of whether it would be impossible, unethical, or impractical to manipulate the variable and, hence, to conduct an experiment: psychiatric disorder, method of contraception, body weight, preoperative anxiety in patients, body temperature, method of asthma therapy, white blood cell count, heroin addiction, membership in a professional nursing association, and marital status.

Chapter 7
Nursing Research Approaches

Although there are many different kinds of nursing investigations, there does not exist any neat and orderly typology of nursing research studies. One way to categorize scientific investigations is according to research design, that is, the degree of control the researcher exercises over the independent variable. Various research designs were discussed in the previous chapter. Another distinction concerns the purpose of the study, while yet another relates to the nature or the timing of the data collection. We do not attempt here to categorize nursing research according to any of these dimensions, because the boundaries are often not clear-cut. The purpose of this chapter is to introduce various research approaches in order to acquaint the reader with commonly used terms and to demonstrate the breadth of study possibilities for nurse researchers.

Survey Research Studies

A *survey* is designed to obtain information regarding the prevalence, distribution, and interrelations of variables within a population. In a survey there is no experimental intervention; surveys are inherently nonexperimental. The dicennial census of the U.S. population is one example of a survey. Political opinion polls, such as those conducted by Gallup or Harris, are other examples. When surveys obtain data from samples, as they usually do, they are often referred to as *sample surveys* (as opposed to a *census*, which covers the entire population).

Generally, surveys obtain information from a sample of people by means of self-report; that is, the people in the sample respond to a series of questions posed by the investigator. Self-report instruments are used to collect data in other types of research studies besides surveys, but refinements to the "art of asking questions" have generally come from survey research.

The content of a self-report survey is essentially limited only by the extent to which respondents are willing to report on the topic. Any information that can reliably be obtained by directly asking a person for that information is acceptable for inclusion in a survey. Often, a survey focuses on what people do: how or what they eat, how they care for their health needs, their compliance in taking medications, what kinds of family-planning behaviors they engage in, what their sleeping patterns are, and so forth. In some instances, particularly in political surveys, the emphasis is on what people plan to do—how they plan to vote, for example. Surveys also collect information on people's knowledge, opinions, attitudes, and values. For example, we might be interested in learning about the public's knowledge of and attitude toward health-maintenance organizations. Another example would be a survey of nurses' opinions about proposed legislation to limit the activities of nurse practitioners.

Almost invariably, survey researchers ask respondents for information about their personal background or situation. Most surveys secure data on many of the following characteristics: age, sex, nationality (or ethnicity), marital status, education, religion, political preference, occupation, income, father's and mother's education, race, and family size. Demographic characteristics such as those mentioned are rarely the focus of any survey except in the case of a national census. There are, however, two important reasons for collecting background data. First of all, personal characteristics such as age, education, and sex have been shown time and again to be related to a person's behavior and attitudes. These variables, in other words, often play a valuable explanatory role. The second reason for collecting this information is to enable the researcher to compare characteristics of the sample with those of the population. If it is known, for instance, that the population under examination was comprised of about 50% men and 50% women, one might have reason to question the validity of conclusions based on the survey of a sample in which 85% of the respondents were women.

Personal Interviews. Survey data can be collected in a number of ways. The most powerful method of securing survey information is through *personal interviews*, the method in which interviewers meet with people face-to-face and secure information from them. In most cases the interviewer will use a carefully developed set of questions, referred to as an *interview schedule*. Generally, personal interviews are rather costly. They require considerable planning and interviewer training in order to be successful; they also tend to involve a lot of personnel time. Nevertheless, personal interviews are regarded as the most useful method of collecting survey data because of the depth and quality of the information they yield. Furthermore, personal interviews usually result in a high number of "returns"; that is, relatively few people refuse to be interviewed in person.

Telephone Interviews. Interviewing persons over the telephone is a less costly, but less effective, method of gathering survey information. Whenever detailed information is needed from respondents, the researcher would be well advised not to use this approach. When the interviewer is unknown, respondents may be uncooperative and unresponsive in a telephone situation. *Telephone interviews* inherently lack the ability to build the rapport that is a feature of face-to-face interviews. However, telephoning can be a convenient method of collecting a lot of information quickly if the interview is short, specific, and not too personal.

Written Questionnaires. Questionnaires differ from interviews primarily in that they are self-administered. That is, the respondent reads the questions on the schedule and gives an answer in writing. The most common way of distributing questionnaires is through the mail. Compared with personal interviews, the cost of a mailed questionnaire is quite low, especially if the population is spread over a wide geographical area. The most serious drawback of a mailed questionnaire, however, is the generally low response rate. Questionnaires mailed to the general public, to people who have no particular interest in the topic under investigation, may yield a response rate of as low as 10% to 20%.

There are a number of alternatives to using the postal services for the distribution of questionnaires. When the population of interest is students, the questionnaires usually can be administered in classrooms. Other face-to-face situations, such as with hospitalized patients, at employee meetings, or at gatherings of social or professional organizations, also lend themselves to greater ease of administration and cooperation of the respondents.

Survey research is noteworthy for its flexibility and a broadness of scope. It can be applied to many populations, it can focus on a wide range of topics, and its information can be used for many purposes. However, it should be noted that the information obtained in most surveys tends to be relatively superficial. Interviews and questionnaires rarely probe very deeply into such complexities as contradictions of human behavior and feelings. This lack of depth is not necessarily a weakness. The fact is that survey research is better suited to extensive analysis rather than intensive analysis.

Evaluation Research

Evaluation research is inherently an "applied" form of research. The purpose of evaluation research is to find out how well a program, practice, or policy is working.* In clinical nursing, nursing administration, and nursing education, there is often a great need to sit back and pose such questions as "How are we doing?" or "Are we accomplishing our goals?" For example, a clinical nurse may want to evaluate the effectiveness of structured observations, as opposed to informal observations, of patients in the development of nursing-care plans. A nursing administrator may want to assess the effect of a new hospital policy on nurses' performance and job satisfaction. A nursing educator may want information about the effectiveness of an autotutorial approach in teaching nursing students how to administer subcutaneous injections.

In each of these examples, the research objective is utilitarian. The purpose of the evaluation is to answer the practical questions of people who must make decisions: Should the practice be continued? Do current policies need to be modified or should they be abandoned altogether? When practices are found to be only partially effective, evaluation research can often provide direction for making improvements.

The traditional strategy for the conduct of evaluation research consists of four broad phases: (1) determining the objectives of the program; (2) developing a means of measuring the attainment of those objectives; (3) collecting the data; and (4) interpreting the data vis-à-vis the objectives. The most difficult task is to spell out in detail the goals of a program or practice. Typically, there are numerous objectives of a program, and these objectives are vague and not clearly articulated. For example, the principal goal of many nursing practices is the improvement of patient care. This aim, though laudable, is so general as to be almost meaningless in terms of evaluating its realization. What exactly do we mean by improving patient care? How will we know if we have succeeded?

The term *behavioral objective*, frequently referred to in the evaluation research literature, is a concept that has evolved as a means of coping with the broadness and fuzziness of program goals. A behavioral objective is the intended outcome of a program stated in terms of the behavior of the persons at whom the program is aimed. Thus, the goal of "improved patient care" might in one instance translate as "the patient will walk the length of the corridor within 5 days after surgery." Note that behavioral objectives always focus on the behavior of the beneficiaries, rather than the agents, of the program. In the example above, the objective was worded to reflect the intended behavioral outcome of the patient—not the behavior of the nurse or other medical personnel. It would be inappropriate, for example, to use the objective "the nurse will teach the patient to measure his heart rate by counting his radial pulse for a full minute" since the main concern is the activity of the patient rather than of the

---

*We will, for the most part, use the term "program" throughout our discussion, but the reader should be aware that this term is meant to include practices and policies as well.

nurse. Once the program goals have been delineated, the evaluation using a traditional approach can be designed much like other research studies. Evaluations can employ an experimental, quasi-experimental, or nonexperimental design and can collect research data by the full range of methods to be described in Chapter 10.

Needs Assessments

Like evaluation research, a *needs assessment* represents an effort to provide a decision-maker with information for action. A needs assessment is a nonexperimental study in which a researcher collects data for estimating the needs of a group, community, or organization.

Nursing educators may wish to assess the needs of their clients (students), hospital staff members may wish to learn the needs of those they serve (patients), or a mental-health outreach clinic may wish to gather information on the needs of some target population (*e.g.*, adolescents in the community). Thus, while an evaluation might seek to ascertain if a program is attaining its objectives, the aim of needs assessments is to determine (1) if the objectives of a program are meeting the needs of the people who are supposed to benefit from it; or (2) whether a new program needs to be instituted.

Key-Informant Approach. Several approaches can be used to conduct a needs assessment. The *key-informant approach*, as the name implies, collects information about the needs of a group from key individuals who are presumed to be in a position to know those needs. These key informants could be community leaders, prominent health-care workers, agency directors, or other knowledgeable persons. Questionnaires or interviews would generally be used to collect the data.

Survey Approach. A second method is the *survey approach* in which data are collected from a sample from the target group whose needs are being assessed. In a survey there would be no attempt to question only persons who are in positions of authority or who are knowledgeable. Any member of the group or community could be asked to give his or her viewpoint.

Indicators Approach. Another alternative is to use an *indicators approach*, which relies on inferences made from statistics available in existing reports or records. For example, a school of nursing that is interested in analyzing the needs of its students could examine over a 5-year period the drop-out rate of its students, performance on licensure examinations, job placement rates 6 months after graduation, financial-aid patterns, utilization of library materials, and so forth. The indicators approach is very flexible and is usually economical since the data are generally available but need organization and interpretation.

The final phase of a needs assessment almost always involves the development of recommendations. These recommendations for action typically involve the delineation of priorities as revealed by the findings. The role of the researcher conducting a needs assessment is often that of making judgments about priorities in light of considerations such as costs and feasibility and in advising on means by which the most highly prioritized needs can be serviced.

Retrospective Studies

Retrospective studies are ex post facto investigations in which the manifestation of some phenomenon existing in the present is linked to other phenomena occurring in the past. That is, the investigator is interested in some outcome and attempts to shed light upon the antecedent factors that have caused it. Many epidemiological studies are retrospective in nature, and this approach has been used by medical researchers for over a century. For example, most lung cancer research with humans has been retrospective in nature. In retrospective lung cancer research, the investigator begins with those who have already developed the disease and, usually, with a sample of those who have not. Then the researcher looks for differences between the two groups in antecedent behaviors or conditions, such as smoking habits.

In nursing research, as in medical research, retrospective studies are quite prevalent. Patient well-being, recovery, or satisfaction are phenomena that have been linked retrospectively to different nursing interventions or modes of treatment. Many studies in the field of nursing education have also been of this type. As another illustration of a retrospective study, let us take as an example the case of a nursing school staff that is trying to understand the factors that cause certain students to drop out of its baccalaureate program while other students continue until graduation. The researcher's problem is to try to identify and disentangle the independent variables (such as motivation, academic ability, financial problems, personality traits, and so on) that have caused some students to leave the program before completion.

In a sense, this kind of ex post facto study can be viewed as the converse of true experiments. In experiments the researcher creates the "cause" by directly manipulating the independent variable and then observes the effect of the manipulation on some dependent variable. In contrast, in a retrospective study the investigator begins with a description of some situation and attempts a retrospective search to identify the causative factors. Retrospective studies are considerably weaker than experiments in their ability to shed light on causal relationships. Findings from a single retrospective study are rarely convincing and, thus, often require confirmatory research efforts.

Prospective Studies

Another nonexperimental type of research that focuses on causal relations is the *prospective study,* which starts with an examination of presumed causes and then goes forward in time to the presumed effect. For example, a researcher might want to test the hypothesis that the incidence of rubella during pregnancy is related to malformations in the offspring. To test this hypothesis prospectively, the investigator would begin with a sample of pregnant women, some of whom have contracted the disease during their pregnancy while others have not. The subsequent occurrence of congenital anomalies would be observed. The researcher would then be in a position to test whether women who had contracted the disease during pregnancy were more likely to bear malformed babies than women who did not have rubella.

Prospective studies are often more costly than retrospective studies and perhaps are less common for this reason. Prospective research often requires large samples, particularly if the dependent variable of interest is rare. For example, in prospective studies of the antecedents of heroin addiction, a very large sample would be required initially in order to yield a sufficient number of heroin addicts for the purposes of generalization. Another difficulty with prospective studies is that a substantial follow-up period may be necessary before the phenomenon or effect under investigation manifests itself, as is the case in prospective studies of cigarette smoking/lung cancer.

Despite these problems, prospective studies are considerably stronger than retrospective studies. For one thing, any ambiguity concerning the temporal sequence of phenomena usually is resolved in prospective research. In addition, samples are more likely to be representative, and investigators may be in a position to impose numerous controls to rule out competing explanations for observed effects. Despite these advantages, causal inferences cannot be made with the same degree of confidence in prospective studies as in the case of experiments. Without the ability to manipulate the independent variable and randomly assign people to different conditions, there is no way to equate groups on all relevant factors. Because of this fact, alternative causes or antecedents may compete with those that the researcher has hypothesized.

Case Studies

Case studies are in-depth investigations of a person, group, institution, or other social unit. The researcher conducting a case study attempts to analyze and understand the variables that are important to the history, development, or care of the subject or the subject's problems. As befits an intensive analysis, case studies typically focus on *why* the subject of the investigation thinks, behaves, or develops in a particular manner, rather than *what* his or her status, progress, actions, or thoughts are. It is not unusual for probing research of this kind to require a detailed study over a considerable time period. Data are often collected relating not only to the subject's present state, but also on past experiences and situational and environmental factors relevant to the problem being examined.

. In most case studies, the researcher is a passive observer, gathering information about the subject's behaviors and characteristics as they naturally occur. However, some case studies involve the administration of a treatment and an analysis of ensuing consequences on the person. An accurate, scientific examination of the effects of a treatment would call for an experimental design in which subjects are randomly assigned to either a control or experimental group. However, steps can be taken to introduce some of the rigor of scientific logic into case studies that involve an intervention. Let us say that we are interested in examining the effect of a certain therapeutic approach on the behavior of an autistic child. We would begin by isolating one or more kinds of specific behavior as a measure of the child's status, as for example, the child's ability to play quietly without becoming violent, or the child's willingness to take medications. Before instituting any treatment (therapy), the researcher would record the child's behavior on the criterion measures for a short period of time. These data generally are referred to as *baseline data*. Once therapy begins, the criterion measures are carefully monitored and recorded either until the sought-for behavior patterns are obtained or for a specified period of time.

The appearance of desirable behavior (or the disappearance of undesirable behavior) after the institution of a therapeutic treatment is not in and of itself sufficient evidence that the treatment was effective. In this particular example, other events or circumstances in the child's life may be responsible for improved behavior, less acting-out, and so forth. For this reason, two additional phases of data collection are highly recommended. The *reversal phase* is the period in which the treatment is withheld. If there is subsequent deterioration in the subject's behavior pattern, the researcher will have more confidence that it is the treatment, rather than extraneous factors, that is producing the desired effect. Finally, treatment is *reinstituted*, and further measurements of the criterion variable are made. Figure 7-1 presents some ideal hypothetical data for the example of the autistic child's play behavior. These data are ideal in the sense that they provide rather clear-cut evidence of the treatment's efficacy. Most actual data would probably be less conclusive.

Unquestionably the greatest advantage of case studies is the depth that is possible when a limited number of people, institutions, or groups is

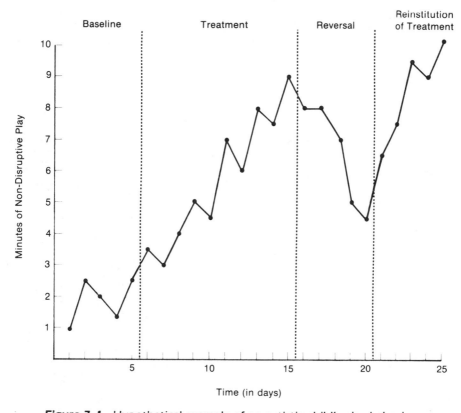

Figure 7-1. Hypothetical example of an autistic child's play behavior

being investigated. A common complaint leveled at other types of research is that the data tend to be rather superficial. Case studies provide the researcher with the opportunity of having an intimate knowledge of the subject's condition, thoughts, feelings, actions (past and present), intentions, and environment.

On the other hand, this same strength is a potential weakness, because the familiarity of the researcher with the subject makes objectivity more difficult. Objectivity may be particularly problematic if the data are collected by observational techniques for which the researcher is the main (or only) observer. The other major drawback of the case-study approach is its questionable adequacy as a basis for generalization. The dynamics of one person's physiological or psychological functioning may bear little resemblance to those of other persons. That is, if the researcher reveals the existence of important relationships, it would be difficult to argue that the same relationships would manifest themselves in other subjects. Inasmuch as case studies cannot be counted on to produce valid generalizations, their usefulness as an approach to testing hypotheses is severely limited. However, the information obtained in case studies can be extremely useful in the production of hypotheses to be tested more rigorously in subsequent research. The intensive probing that characterizes case studies often leads to insights about previously unsuspected relationships.

Historical Research

Historical research is the systematic collection and critical evaluation of data relating to past occurrences. Generally, historical research is undertaken in order to test hypotheses or to answer questions about causes, effects, or trends relating to past events that may shed light on present behaviors or practices. An understanding of contemporary nursing theories, practices, or issues can often be enhanced by an investigation of a defined segment of the past. Particularly today, when nurses are working to define and extend their professional roles, a knowledge of the roots of nursing has the capacity to put nursing theories and procedures into an appropriate context.

The student should be careful not to confuse historical research with a review of the literature, although a literature review is typically an early step in the research process. The purpose of historical research is to explain the present or to anticipate future events; it is not merely to find out what is already known about an issue and to paraphrase it. Like other types of research, historical inquiry has as its goal the discovery of new knowledge.

One important difference between historical research and a literature review is that a historical researcher is often guided in the collection of information by the formulation of specific hypotheses or questions. The hypotheses represent attempts at explaining and interpreting the conditions, events, or phenomena under investigation. Hypotheses in historical research are not usually tested in a statistical sense. They are, generally, broadly stated conjectures about relationships among historical events, trends, and phenomena. For example, it might be hypothesized that a relationship exists between the presence or absence of war on the one hand and the amount of scientific nursing knowledge generated on the other. This hypothesis could be tested by analyzing research trends in nursing during the 20th century.

Data for historical research are usually in the form of written records of the past: periodicals, diaries, books, letters, newspapers, minutes of meetings, legal documents, reports, and so forth. However, a number of nonwritten materials may also be of interest. For example, physical remains and objects are potential sources of information. Visual materials such as photographs, films, and drawings are forms of data, as are audio materials such as records, tapes, and so forth.

Historical evidence usually is subjected to two types of evaluation, which historians refer to as external and internal criticism. *External criticism* is concerned basically with the authenticity and genuineness of the data. For example, a nursing historian might have a diary presumed to be written by Dorothea Dix. External criticism would involve asking questions such as the following: Is this the handwriting of Ms. Dix? Is the paper on which the diary is written of the right age? Are the writing style and ideas expressed consistent with her other writings?

Internal criticism of historical data refers to the evaluation of the worth of the evidence. The focus of internal criticism is not so much on the physical aspects of the materials, but rather on their content. An important issue here is the accuracy or truth of the data. For example, the historian must question whether a writer's representations of historical events are unbiased. It may also be appropriate to ask if the author of a document was in a position to make a valid report of an event or occurrence, or whether the writer was competent as a recorder of fact. After evaluating the authenticity and accuracy of historical data, the researcher must begin to pull the materials together, to analyze them, and to test the research hypotheses. The historian must, to a greater degree than other researchers, be cautious in generalizing the results of the research. Since events can never be duplicated exactly, there is reason to question the validity of generalizations from historical data. Nevertheless, the same can be said of virtually all research that involves human beings in social settings, as is the case with many nursing research studies. Indeed, it is precisely when a situation or event is unlikely to be duplicated that historical research represents the only feasible type of investigation.

Research Example: A Retrospective Study

Wright (1985) hypothesized that teenage girls exposed to a sex-education course in high school are less likely to become pregnant during their teen years than those with no sex education.* To test this hypothesis, she interviewed 200 girls aged 15 to 18 and asked them about the type and amount of instruction they had received in school regarding sexual responsibility, pregnancy, and contraception. One hundred of these girls were young mothers who had just delivered babies at two county hospitals. The remaining 100 were girls attending high schools in the same two counties. According to their self-reports, the girls in this second group had had no prior pregnancies. The two groups of girls were then compared with respect to their exposure to a school course on sex education. According to Wright's findings, the girls in both groups were equally likely

---

*This example is fictitious.

to have had a sex-education course. She concluded that a school-based sex-education program has no effect on reducing the risk of teenage pregnancy.

Wright conducted a retrospective study of the effects of sex education. She chose to test her hypothesis by beginning with the effect of interest (pregnancy versus no pregnancy) and then looking backward for a presumed determinant (exposure to a sex-education course).

Given the cause-and-effect nature of her hypothesis (*if* sex education, *then* reduced risk of pregnancy), Wright chose a relatively weak testing method. Several problems deserve special mention. The most serious flaw of Wright's study is that virtually no steps were taken to control extraneous variables. The two groups of girls were known to differ in one respect—their pregnancy history. (Note that even this depends on the girls' truthfulness in reporting prior pregnancies.) But the two groups could differ systematically in a number of ways, independent of their exposure to sex education. Perhaps the groups were different with regard to socioeconomic status, religious beliefs, educational aspirations, relationship with their parents, and so on; any of these variables might be related to the girls' sexual behavior or contraceptive practices. Such differences could mask a true relationship between sex education and the rate of teenage pregnancy.

A second problem with Wright's study is its dependence on the subjects' recall. The teens were expected to provide information about the nature of their previous sex-education training. Wright might have been able to obtain more accurate information directly from the schools.

Several things could be done to improve Wright's study. Clearly, a true experiment would have been the best approach, and the research problem lends itself to an experimental design. The investigator would have had to work within a school setting, randomly assigning some students to a sex-education course and others to a control group with no sex education. The two groups would then have to be followed up to see if pregnancy rates were higher in one group than in the other. A quasi-experimental approach could also be implemented, using a nonequivalent comparison-group design. Even if active interventions (*i.e.*, controlling the sex-education program) were not possible, a prospective design would have been better than a retrospective design. A prospective study would follow-up students who either did or did not have sex education to see if they eventually became pregnant. Even if all these alternatives had to be ruled out, Wright could have taken steps within the retrospective design to rule out competing explanations for the teens' pregnancy status. For example, she could have controlled social class by ensuring that an equal number of working-class and middle-class teens were in both the pregnant and nonpregnant groups. This and other techniques for controlling extraneous variables are discussed in the next chapter.

Summary

This chapter described several types of research that are used to study nursing research problems. It should be noted that these are not exhaustive (*i.e.*, there are many studies that do not fall under one of the categories presented); neither are they mutually exclusive (*e.g.*, a retrospective study could involve a survey). The purpose of presenting these various categories of research is to familiarize students with some research terminology and to illustrate different uses to which research can be put in nursing. It should also be noted that the types of research described here are not necessarily linked to a specific kind of research design, as shown in Table 7-1.

Survey research is that branch of research that examines the characteristics, behaviors, attitudes, and intentions of a group of people by asking people belonging to that group (typically only a subset) to answer a series of questions. Survey research is an extremely flexible research approach and, therefore, is quite diversified with respect to populations studied, scope, content, and purpose. Various approaches are used to collect survey information. The most powerful method is the *personal interview* in which interviewers meet with participants face-to-face and question them directly. This method has the advantage of encouraging cooperation, which results in higher response rates and a better quality of data. *Telephone interviews* have grown in popularity in recent years but, while this approach is convenient and economical, it is not recommended when the interview is long or detailed or when the questions are sensitive or highly personal. *Written questionnaires* are probably the most common means of collecting survey data. Questionnaires are not oral; that is, questions are read by the respondent, who then gives a written response. Questionnaires are often distributed through the mail, but, because of the generally low response rates of mailed surveys, some type of personal contact generally is recommended.

Evaluation research is the process of collecting and analyzing infor-

Table 7-1. Designs Possible for Various Types of Research

RESEARCH APPROACH	RESEARCH DESIGN		
	Experimental	Quasi-experimental	Nonexperimental
Survey			X
Evaluation	X	X	X
Needs assessment			X
Retrospective study			X
Prospective study			X
Case study		X	X
Historical research			X

mation relating to the functioning of a program, policy, or procedure in order to assist decision-makers in choosing a course of action. Evaluations are undertaken with the aim of providing answers to questions about the effectiveness of the program under consideration. The traditional evaluation approach begins with a determination of the goals of the program. Goals are typically phrased in the form of *behavioral objectives*, which delineate the intended outcomes of a program in terms of the behaviors of the program's beneficiaries. The research task is then one of establishing the degree of congruence between program objective and actual outcomes.

A *needs assessment* is another type of applied research approach aimed at providing useful information for planners and decision-makers. A needs assessment is an investigation of the needs of a group, community, or organization for certain types of services or policies. Since organizations and groups are almost constantly in transition, and since their needs may change over time, needs assessments can serve a useful purpose both before and after a service program is in operation. Several techniques or approaches are used in the conduct of needs assessments, notably the *key-informant, survey,* or *indicator approaches.*

Retrospective studies are investigations in which the researcher observes the manifestation of some phenomenon (the dependent variable) and tries to identify its antecedents or causes (the independent variable). *Prospective studies* start with an observation of presumed causes and then go forward in time to observe the consequences. Prospective research is typically initiated after evidence of important relationships are suggested by retrospective investigations. Both retrospective and prospective studies are nonexperimental approaches that attempt to shed light on hypothesized cause-and-effect relationships; both are less powerful than true experiments or quasi-experiments because the researcher has no control over the independent variable.

Case studies are intensive investigations of a single entity or a small number of entities. Typically, that entity is a human being, but groups, organizations, families, or institutions may sometimes be the focus of concern. In a case study the investigator examines the person in depth by probing into the history or development of the subject with respect to the characteristics or behaviors of interest. Case studies can be quite valuable in the production of hypotheses or the demonstration of some clinical approach that could be subjected to more rigorous testing. When an intervention is being demonstrated or assessed, it is quite useful to collect data over an extended time period and, when possible, to subdivide the time frame into *baseline, treatment, reversal,* and *reinstitution* phases. The case study offers the potential of great depth but runs the risk of subjectivity and severely limited generalizability.

Historical research is the systematic attempt to establish facts and relationships about past events. The historical researcher utilizes the scientific method insofar as possible to answer questions or test hypotheses by objectively evaluating and interpreting available historical evidence. Historical data are usually in the form of written records from the past (such as letters, diaries, or legal documents), but physical artifacts and audio or visual materials represent another source of information. Historical data are normally subjected to two forms of evaluation: *external criticism*, which is concerned with the authenticity of the source, and *internal criticism*, which assesses the worth of the evidence. Historical research is extremely valuable in nursing at this time because the profession is striving to understand and conceptualize the practice and process of nursing.

Study Suggestions

1. Suppose you were interested in studying the attitude of nurses toward abortion. Would you use a personal interview, telephone interview, or questionnaire to collect your data? Why?

2. A nurse researcher is interested in studying the attitude of nursing students toward working with the elderly. Suggest at least five personal background characteristics about which you would recommend gathering information from the respondents. Justify why you feel such variables would enhance the study.

3. A nurse researcher is developing a study to evaluate the effectiveness of a program that uses nurse practitioners to manage common respiratory infections. Suggest a design for the evaluation.

4. For each of the following practices or procedures derive one or more hypothetical objectives and state them as behavioral objectives:

   a. A crisis-intervention program for drug abusers

   b. Procedures to educate primiparas with respect to breast-feeding of their infants

   c. A program to interest nursing students in working with elderly people

   d. An instructional unit to teach student nurses how to administer subcutaneous injections

5. Explain how you would use the key informant, survey, and indicator approaches to assess the need to teach Spanish to nurses in a given community.

6. In the section on prospective studies, an example relating to rubella and congenital anomalies was cited. How could such a problem be studied retrospectively? Would an experimental approach with humans be possible? Why or why not?

7. Suppose you are interested in conducting a case study on sleep promotion. What kinds of baseline data would you need to collect? What

might your treatment be? What ethical considerations are involved in withdrawing the treatment?

8. Identify a problem for study using the historical-research approach. Formulate hypotheses. What might serve as primary sources for the data? How would you check the data for internal criticism?

Chapter 8
Principles of Research Design

The preceding chapter introduced the reader to a variety of research approaches, but little attention was paid to the actual conduct of the study. Designing a research study involves the development of a plan or strategy that will guide the collection and analysis of data. Research designs that are well-conceived and properly executed have the greatest potential of adding information to the store of human knowledge. The principle aim of this chapter is to introduce design techniques that strengthen the quality of scientific studies and the interpretability of their findings. Most of these techniques are applicable to experimental, quasi-experimental, and nonexperimental research.

Techniques of Research Control

Basically, the central purpose of research design is to maximize the amount of control that an investigator has over the research situation and variables. As discussed in Chapter 2, the researcher needs to control extraneous variables in order to determine the true nature of the relationships between the independent and dependent variables under investigation. Extraneous variables, it will be recalled, are variables that have an irrelevant association with the dependent variable and that can confound the testing of the research hypothesis. There are two basic types of extraneous variables: (1) those that are intrinsic to the subjects of the study and (2) those that are external factors stemming from the research situation.

Controlling External Factors

In high-quality research, steps usually are taken to minimize situational contaminants. The researcher should seek to make the conditions under which the data are collected as similar as possible for every participant in the study. The control that a researcher imposes on a study by attempting to maintain constancy in the research conditions probably represents one of the earliest forms of scientific control.

The environment has been found to exert a powerful influence on people's emotions and behavior. In designing research, therefore, the investigator needs to pay attention to the environmental context within which the study is to be conducted. Control over the environment is most easily achieved in *laboratory experiments* in which all subjects are brought into an environment that the experimenter is in a position to arrange.* Researchers have much less freedom in controlling the environment in studies that occur in natural settings, which are sometimes referred to as *field studies*. This does not mean that the researcher should abandon all efforts to make the environments as similar as possible. For example, in conducting a survey in which the information is to be gathered by means of an interview, the researcher should attempt to conduct all interviews in basically the same kind of environment. That is, it would not be desirable to interview some of the respondents in their own homes, some in their place of work, some in the researcher's office, and so forth. In each of these settings the participant normally assumes different roles (wife, husband, parent; employee; client or patient; and so forth) and responses to questions may be influenced to some degree by the role in which the respondent is operating.

One of the advantages of conducting a study in an artificial setting such as a laboratory is that the researcher has greater confidence of having control over the independent and extraneous variables. In real-life settings, even when there are randomly assigned groups, the differentiation between groups may be difficult to control. Let us look at another example to see why this is so. Suppose we are planning to teach nursing students a unit on dyspnea, and we have used a lecture-type approach in the past. If we are interested in trying an individualized, autotutorial approach to cover the same material and want to evaluate the effectiveness of this method before adopting it for all students, we might randomly assign students to one of the two methods. Scores on a test covering the content of the unit could be used as the dependent or criterion variable. But now, suppose the students in the two groups talk to one another about their learning experiences. Some of the lecture-group students might go through parts of the programmed text. Perhaps some of the students in the autotutorial group will sit in on some of the lectures. In short, field experiments are often subject to the problem of *contamination of treatments*. In the same study, it would also be difficult to control other vari-

---

*The term "laboratory" typically connotes a setting in which scientific equipment is installed. Here, the term is used in a general sense to refer to a physical location apart from the routine of daily living, which is used by the researcher as the site for the collection of data and where subjects report to participate in the research project.

ables, such as the time or place in which the learning takes place for the individualized group.

A second external factor that should be controlled is the time factor. Depending on the topic of the study, the criterion variable may be influenced by the time of day or time of year in which the data are collected, or both. It would, in such cases, be important for the researcher to ensure that constancy of time is maintained. If an investigator were studying fatigue or perceptions of physical well-being, it would probably matter a great deal whether the data were gathered in the morning, afternoon, or evening, or in the summer as opposed to the winter. While time constancy is not always critical, it is often relatively easy for the researcher to control and should, therefore, be sought whenever possible.

Another aspect of maintaining constancy of conditions concerns constancy in the communications to the subjects and in the treatment itself in the case of experiments or quasi-experiments. In most research efforts, participants are informed about the purpose of the study, what use will be made of the data, under whose auspices the study is being conducted, and so forth. This information should be prepared ahead of time and the same message should be delivered to all subjects. To ensure constancy of communication, there should generally be as little ad libbing as possible. Surveys, for example, almost always make use of a structured interview schedule rather than having the interviewer develop questions in the course of the interview situation.

In studies involving the implementation of a treatment, care should be taken to adhere to the specifications (often referred to as *research protocols*) for that treatment. For example, in experiments to test the effectiveness of a new drug to cure a medical problem, great care would have to be taken to ensure that the subjects in the experimental group received the same chemical substance and the same dosage, that the substance was administered in the same way, and so forth. Some treatments are much "fuzzier" than in the case of administering a drug, as is the case for most nursing interventions. In such a situation, the investigator should spell out in detail the exact behaviors required of the personnel responsible for delivering or administering the treatment.

One of the features that distinguishes nonexperimental research from experimental and quasi-experimental studies is that if the researcher has not manipulated the independent variable, there is no means of ensuring constancy of conditions. Let us take as an example an ex post facto study that attempts to determine if there is a relationship between a person's knowledge of nutrition and his or her own eating habits. Suppose the investigator finds no relationship between nutritional knowledge and eating patterns. That is, the investigator finds that persons who are well-informed about nutrition are just as likely as uninformed persons to maintain inadequate diets. In this case, however, the researcher has had no control over the source of a person's nutritional knowledge (the independent variable). This knowledge was measured after the fact (post facto), and the conditions under which the information was obtained cannot be assumed to be constant or even similar. The researcher may conclude from the study that it is useless to teach nutrition to people since knowledge has no impact on their eating behavior. It may be, however, that different methods of providing nutritional information vary in their ability to motivate people to alter their nutritional habits. Thus, the ability of the investigator to control or manipulate the independent variable of interest may be extremely important in understanding what the relationships between variables really mean.

Controlling Intrinsic Factors

Characteristics of the participants in the study almost always need to be controlled. For example, in a study of the effects of a physical training program on physical fitness, such variables as age, sex, and occupation of the subjects might be considered extraneous variables. Each of these characteristics might be related to the outcome of interest (physical fitness) independently of the physical training program. In other words, the effects that these variables have on the dependent variable are extraneous to the research topic.

Randomization. We have already discussed the most effective method of controlling such extraneous variables, and that is randomization. The primary function of randomization is to secure comparable groups, that is, to equalize the groups with respect to the extraneous variables. A distinct advantage of random assignment, compared with other methods of controlling extraneous variables, is that randomization controls *all* possible sources of extraneous variation, without any conscious decision on the researcher's part about which variables need to be controlled.

Homogeneity. When randomization is not feasible, there are several other methods of controlling intrinsic subject characteristics that could contaminate the relationships under investigation. The first alternative is to use only subjects who are homogeneous with respect to those variables that are considered extraneous. The extraneous variables, in this case, are not allowed to vary. In the example of the physical training program cited above, if sex were considered to be an important confounding variable, the researcher might wish to use only men (or only women) as subjects. Similarly, if the researcher were concerned about the effects of the subjects' age on physical fitness, participation in the study could be limited to those within a specified age range. This method of utilizing a homogeneous subject pool is fairly easy and offers considerable control. However, the limitation of this approach lies in the fact that the research findings can only be generalized to the type of subjects who participated in the study. If the physical training program was found to have beneficial effects on the physical fitness of a sample of men aged 40 to 45, its usefulness for improving the physical fitness of women in their 60s would be strictly a matter of conjecture.

Blocking. Another approach to controlling extraneous variables is to include them in the design of a study as independent variables. To pursue our example of the physical training program, if sex was thought to be a confounding variable, it could be built into the study design, as shown in Figure 8-1. This procedure would allow us to make an assessment of the impact of our training program on physical fitness for both men and women.

Let us consider this approach in greater detail. We will refer to the design shown in Figure 8-1 as a *randomized block design*. The variable sex, which cannot be manipulated by the researcher, is known as a *blocking variable*. In an experiment to test the effectiveness of the physical training program, the experimenter obviously could not randomly assign subjects to one of four cells: the sex of the subjects is a "given." But the experimenter can and should randomly assign men and women separately to the experimental and control conditions. Let us say there are 40 men and 40 women available for the study. The researcher should not take the 80 subjects and assign half to the physical training program group and the other half to the no-program group if gender is believed to be an extraneous variable. Rather, the randomization procedure should be performed separately for the two sexes, thereby guaranteeing 20 subjects in each cell of the four-cell design.

Strictly speaking, the type of design we have discussed is appropriate only in experimental studies, but in reality it is used quite commonly in

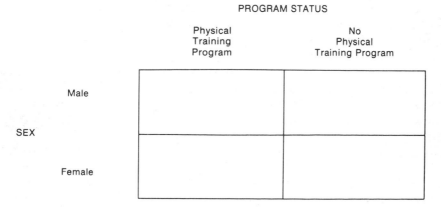

Figure 8-1. Schematic diagram of a randomized block design

quasi-experimental and ex post facto studies as well. If an investigator were studying the effects of a physical training program on physical fitness after the fact (*i.e.*, subjects self-selected themselves into one of the two groups and the researcher had no control over who was included in each group), he or she might want to set up the analysis in such a way that differential effects for men and women would be analyzed. The design structure would look the same as the one presented in Figure 8-1, although the implications and conclusions that could be drawn from the results would be different than if the researcher had been in control of the manipulation and randomization procedures.

Matching. The third alternative method of dealing with extraneous variables is known as *matching*. Matching involves using knowledge of subject characteristics to form comparison groups. If a matching procedure were to be adopted for our physical training program example, and age and sex were the extraneous variables of concern, we would need to match two subjects with respect to age and sex. That is, the researcher would begin with a sample of subjects participating in the training program and would then create a comparison group by matching, one by one, people in terms of age and sex of the experimental subjects.

There are a number of reasons why matching should be avoided if possible. First, in order to match effectively, the researcher must know in advance what the relevant extraneous variables are. This knowledge is not always available, or may be imperfect. Second, after two or three variables, it often becomes impossible to match adequately. Let us say we are interested in controlling for the age, sex, race, and type of work of the subjects. Thus, if subject number one in the physical training program is a black woman, aged 30, who is a physical therapist, the researcher must seek another woman with these same or similar characteristics as a control. With more than three variables, the matching procedure becomes extremely cumbersome, if not impossible. For these reasons, matching as a technique for controlling extraneous variables should, in general, be used only when other, more powerful procedures are not feasible, as might be the case for some ex post facto studies.

Analysis of Covariance. Yet another method of controlling unwanted variables is through statistical procedures. It is recognized that at this point many readers are unfamiliar with basic statistical procedures, let alone sophisticated techniques such as are being referred to here. Therefore, a detailed description of a powerful statistical control mechanism, known as *analysis of covariance*, will not be attempted. The interested reader with a background in statistics should consult a textbook on advanced statistics for fuller coverage of this topic. However, since the possibility of statistical control may mystify readers, we will attempt to explain the underlying principle with a simple illustration.

Returning to the example used throughout this section, suppose we have a group that is undergoing a physical training program and we have another group that is not. The groups represent intact groups (*e.g.,* employees of two companies), and, therefore, randomization is not possible. As our measure of physical fitness, let us say we have devised a test that involves ratings on a number of activities (running, throwing, weight lifting, and so forth), and each participant receives a total physical-fitness score. As with most things in life, our test undoubtedly will reveal individual differences. Some people will do quite well on the test and others will perform poorly. The research question is "Can some of the individual differences be attributed to a person's participation in the physical training program?" Unfortunately, the individual differences in physical fitness are also related to other, extraneous characteristics of the subjects, such as age. The large circles in Figure 8-2 may be taken to represent the total variability (extent of individual differences) in scores for both groups on the physical-fitness measure. A certain amount of that total variability can be explained simply by virtue of the subject's age, which is schematized in the figure as the small circle on the left in part A of Figure 8-2. Another part of the variability can be explained by the subject's participation or nonparticipation in the physical training program, represented here as the small circle on the right. In part A, the fact that the two small circles (age and program participation) overlap tells us that there is a relationship between those two variables. In other words, subjects in the group receiving the physical training program are, on average, either

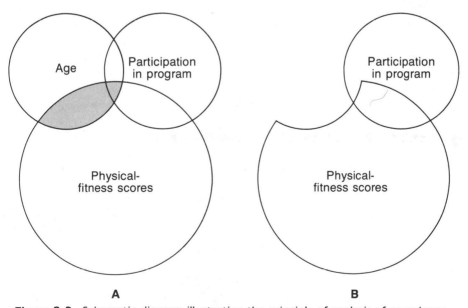

A   **B**

Figure 8-2. Schematic diagram illustrating the principle of analysis of covariance

older or younger than members of the comparison group. Therefore, age should be controlled.

Analysis of covariance can accomplish this control function by statistically removing the effect of the extraneous variable on the dependent variable. In our illustration, that portion of the physical-fitness variability that is attributable to age could be removed through the analysis of covariance technique. This is designated in part A of Figure 8-2 by the darkened area in the large circle. Part B illustrates that the final analysis would examine the effect of program participation on fitness scores after removing the effect of age on those scores. With the variability of physical-fitness scores resulting from age controlled, we can have a much more precise estimate of the effect of the training program on physical fitness. Note that even after removing the variability resulting from age, there is still individual variability not associated with the program treatment (the bottom half of the large circle). This means that the precision of the study could probably be further enhanced by controlling additional extraneous variables, such as sex, type of occupation, and so forth. The analysis of covariance procedure can accommodate multiple extraneous variables.

The four alternatives to randomization described here have one characteristic in common: the researcher must know or predict in advance what the relevant extraneous variables are. In order to select homogeneous samples, develop a randomized block design, match, or perform an analysis of covariance, the researcher must make a decision about what variable or variables need to be controlled. This constraint may pose severe limitations on the degree of control that is possible, particularly since the researcher can seldom deal explicitly with more than two or three extraneous variables at a time. It cannot be emphasized too strongly that the random assignment of subjects to groups is the most effective approach, overall, of managing extraneous variables, because randomization tends to produce a "cancelling out" of individual variation on all possible extraneous variables.

Evaluating Research Designs: Internal Validity

Campbell and Stanley (1963) have provided us with a useful framework with which to evaluate various research designs. These authors use the term *internal validity* to refer to the extent to which it is possible to make an inference that the independent variable is truly related to the dependent variable. True experiments possess a high degree of internal validity because the use of control procedures (comparison groups and randomization) enables the researcher to control extraneous variables, thereby ruling out most alternative explanations for the results. With quasi-experiments and ex post facto studies the investigator must always contend with competing explanations for the obtained results. These competing explanations, referred to as *threats to internal validity*, have been grouped into several classes, a few of which will be examined here.

History

The threat of *history* refers to the occurrence of events that take place concurrently with the introduction of the independent variable that can affect the dependent variables of interest. For example, suppose we were studying the effect of a hospital requirement for continuing education on the nurse turnover rate. Now let us further suppose that at about the same time the continuing-education rule was put into effect, a nurse in the hospital was sued for malpractice. The lawsuit might bring to the nurses' attention a host of problems concerning their legal liability and the method used by the hospital in handling these problems. Our dependent variable in this case, turnover rate, is now subject to the influence of (at least) two forces, and it becomes impossible for us to "unconfound" the two effects. In a true experiment, history generally is not a threat to the internal validity of a study because we can assume that external events are as likely to affect one group as another.

Selection

The term *selection* encompasses biases resulting from pretreatment differences between experimental and comparison groups. When people are not assigned randomly to groups, we must always be aware of the possibility that the groups are not equivalent. They may differ, in fact, in ways that are quite subtle and difficult to detect. If the groups are non-equivalent, the researcher is faced with the possibility that any posttreatment differences are due to initial differences rather than to the effect of the experimental treatment. The problem of selection is clearly reduced when, in quasi-experimental designs, pretreatment data are collected, but the problem does not disappear altogether. In ex post facto studies, the collection of data prior to the introduction of the independent variable is rarely possible. Selection biases are among the most problematic threats to the internal validity of studies not using an experimental design.

Maturation

In a research context, *maturation* refers to processes occurring within the subjects during the course of the study as a result of time rather than as a result of the independent variable, such as developmental growth, fatigue, and the like. To take an example, if we wanted to evaluate the

effects of a special sensorimotor-development program for develop-
mentally retarded children, we would have to take into account the fact
that progress does take place in these children even without special
assistance.

There are many areas of nursing research in which maturation
would be a relevant consideration. Remember that the term here does not
refer to aging or developmental changes exclusively, but, rather, to any
kind of change that occurs as a function of time. Thus, wound healing,
postoperative recovery, and many other bodily changes that can occur
with little or no nursing intervention must be considered as an explanation that rivals the independent variable.

Mortality

Mortality refers to the differential loss of subjects from comparison
groups. The loss of subjects during the course of a study, often referred to
as *attrition*, may differ from one group to another because of initial differences in interest, motivation, and the like. For example, suppose we used
a nonequivalent control-group design to assess the morale of the nursing
personnel from two different hospitals, one of which was initiating the
problem-oriented method of charting. The dependent variable, nursing
staff satisfaction, is measured before and after the intervention. The comparison group, which may have no particular commitment to the study,
may be reluctant to complete a posttest questionnaire. Those who do fill
it out may be totally unrepresentative of the group as a whole; they may
be those who are highly enthusiastic about their work environment, for
example. Thus, on the average, it might appear that the morale of the control hospital improved, but this improvement might only be an artifact of
the "mortality" of a biased segment of this group.

Internal Validity and Research Design

Quasi-experimental and ex post facto studies are especially susceptible to threats to internal validity. The four threats described above (and
others, which were too technical to review here) represent alternative
explanations that compete with the independent variable as a cause of the
dependent variable. The aim of a good research design is to rule out these
competing explanations.

A good experimental design will normally control for these factors,
but it must not be assumed that in a true experiment the researcher need
not worry about them. For example, if constancy of conditions is not
maintained for experimental and control groups, then history might be a

rival explanation for obtained results. Experimental mortality is, in particular, a salient threat in true experiments. If the experimenter does something differently with two or more groups, then subjects may drop out of the study differentially among the comparison groups. This is particularly apt to happen if the experimental treatment is painful, inconvenient, or time-consuming or if the control condition is boring to the subjects. When this happens, the subjects remaining in the study may differ from those who left in important ways, thereby nullifying the initial equivalence of the groups.

Researchers engaged in nonexperimental studies should, in particular, consider the various competing explanations for the results they obtain. When the investigator does not have control over the numerous extraneous variables that can interfere with a straightforward understanding of relationships, great caution should be exercised in interpreting the results and in drawing conclusions from them.

External Validity

The term *external validity* refers to the generalizability of the research findings to other settings or samples. Research is almost never conducted with the intention of discovering relationships among variables for one group of people at one point in time. For example, if a nursing intervention under study is found to be successful, others will want to adopt the procedure. Therefore, an important question is whether the intervention will work in another setting or with different patients.

One aspect of a study's external validity concerns the adequacy of the sampling design. If the characteristics of the sample are representative of those of the population, then the generalizability of the results is enhanced. Sampling designs are described at length in the next chapter.

In addition to subject characteristics, there are various characteristics of the environment or research situation that affect the study's external validity. For example, when a treatment is new (e.g., a new curriculum for nursing students), subjects and research agents alike might alter their behaviors in a variety of ways. People may be either enthusiastic or skeptical about new methods of doing things. The results may, thus, reflect reactions to the novelty rather than to the intrinsic qualities of the treatment.

Sometimes the demands for internal and external validity conflict. If a researcher exercises tight control over a study to maximize internal validity, the setting may become too artificial to generalize to a more naturalistic environment. Thus, a compromise must sometimes be reached. The need for replication of studies in different settings with new subjects cannot be overemphasized.

Characteristics of a Good Design

A consideration of the threats to the internal and external validity of a study represents one frame of reference for evaluating the study's research design. In this section we examine other criteria for assessing the worth of a research design.

Appropriateness for Research Question

The requirement that the research design should be appropriate for the questions being asked seems so obvious that it may be overlooked. Generally, a given research problem can be handled adequately with a number of different designs, so that the researcher typically has some flexibility in selecting a design. Yet many designs will be completely unsuitable for dealing with the research problem.

A misconception that frequently leads to inappropriate designs arises from the belief that the researcher can only have two groups—an experimental group and a control group. This misunderstanding probably stems from the fact that many studies, particularly older ones, use a two-group design and because textbooks often illustrate the concept of an experiment with the most basic design possible. If the investigator is interested in comparing four treatments, then a design that includes four groups is clearly indicated. A related error is the belief that the investigator can or should manipulate only one variable at a time.

Lack of Bias

A second characteristic of good research design is that it results in data that are not biased. Bias can operate in a variety of ways, some of which are very subtle. The most obvious source of bias is in the allocation of subjects to groups. When groups are formed on a nonrandom basis, the risk of bias is always present. Note that we do not mean that the investigator is necessarily responsible for the bias. In ex post facto studies in which subjects "self-select" themselves into groups, the biases are generally beyond the researcher's control.

In studies in which the data are collected by means of observation, the researcher's preconceptions might unconsciously bias the objective collection of data. In such a case, the researcher should take a number of steps to minimize this risk. Whenever possible, *double-blind* procedures are highly recommended. This technique removes observer biases by virtue of the fact that neither the subject nor the observer (or the person collecting the data) knows in which group a given subject is. When this approach is not feasible, it is a good practice to have two or more observers so that at least an estimation of the biases can be made.

Bias can enter the data whenever there is an opportunity for human subjectivity. There will always be a need for human judgment and sensitivity in the design of studies but, whenever it is possible to use an objective procedure such as randomization, the researcher should pursue this course. A general scientific principle is to *randomize whenever possible*. The reader may have the impression that randomization is irrelevant in nonexperimental research, but this is not the case. Although in quasi-experiments and ex post facto studies subjects are not randomly assigned to treatments, other aspects of the research design are subject to control through randomization. For example, in a study of nurses' attitudes toward death, the investigator might present subjects with 20 or so statements relating to death and dying with which respondents would be asked to agree or disagree. The order of these statements should ideally be randomized to avoid any ordering that might lead the respondents to express certain attitudes. In general, then, the researcher should utilize every possible opportunity for randomization that does not conflict with either theoretical, ethical, or practical considerations.

Precision

The term *precision* as used in the present context refers to the appropriateness of the statistical procedures used to analyze the data. This concept will be discussed more extensively in subsequent chapters. However, the idea will be treated here briefly in a simple form since statistical analyses often depend on research design.

The first section of this chapter dealt with the notion of control over extraneous variables. What this control is actually all about is *control over variability in the dependent measures.* In an example used repeatedly, we talked about the variability from one person to another on a measure of physical fitness. The various control mechanisms discussed represent attempts to isolate that portion of the variability in physical fitness that could be attributable to participation in a physical training program. Let us express what the researcher is attempting to do in the form of a ratio:

$$\frac{\text{Variability in physical fitness}}{\text{Variability in physical fitness due to age, sex,}}$$
$$\frac{\text{due to training program}}{\text{occupation, initial level of fitness, etc.}}$$

This ratio, though greatly simplified here, captures the essence of many statistical procedures. The researcher wants to make the variability in the numerator (the upper half) as large as possible relative to the variability in the denominator (the lower half) in order to demonstrate most clearly the relationship between program participation and physical fitness. The smaller the variability caused by extraneous variables, such as age and sex, the easier it will be for the researcher to detect differences in physical fitness between those who did and those who did not participate in the physical training program. Designs that enable the researcher to reduce the variability caused by the extraneous variables are said to increase the precision of the research. As a purely hypothetical illustration of why this is so, we will attach some numerical values to the ratio above*:

$$\frac{\text{Variability due to training program}}{\text{Variability due to extraneous variables}} = \frac{10}{4}$$

Now, if we can make the bottom number smaller, say from four to two, we will have a purer and more precise estimate of the effect of program participation on physical fitness. How can a research design help to reduce the variability caused by extraneous variables?

A randomized block design is one example of a design that increases the precision of an analysis. Let us say we performed the physical-fitness study as a true experiment, using age group (persons aged 20 to 35 vs. those aged 36 to 50) as the blocking variable. The total variability in scores on the physical-fitness measure (*i.e.*, the extent to which persons obtained different scores) can be conceptualized as having three components:

Total variability = Variability due to program + Variability due to age
+ Variability due to other extraneous variables

This equation can be taken to mean that part of the reason why some people did well and others did less well on the physical-fitness test is that (1) some participated in the training program and others did not; (2) some people are older and some younger; and (3) other factors, such as sex, occupation, and so forth, had an effect.

The randomized block procedure allows us to segregate the variability that is due to age and remove it from the variability resulting from all other extraneous variables. By doing this, the training program becomes greater relative to the extraneous variability. Thus, we can say that the randomized block design has enabled us to get a more precise estimate of the effect of having participated in the training program. Research designs

---

*The reader should not be concerned at this point with how these numbers can be obtained in a real analysis. The procedure will be explained in Chapter 16.

differ considerably in the sensitivity with which the effects of the independent variable can be detected with statistical tools.

The Time Dimension

Certain research problems are concerned with phenomena that evolve over time: healing, learning, growth, recidivism, physical development, and so on, are all variables that involve a time dimension. There are various designs available to researchers interested in such phenomena. These designs fall into two broad categories: cross-sectional and longitudinal.

Cross-sectional Designs

Cross-sectional studies involve the collection of data at one point in time. The phenomena under investigation are captured, as they manifest themselves, during the one static time period of data collection. Suppose, for example, we are interested in studying the changes in nursing students' attitude toward professionalism as they progress through a 4-year baccalaureate program. One way to investigate this issue would be to survey students when they are freshmen and resurvey them every year until they graduate. On the other hand, we could use a *cross-sectional design* by surveying members of the four classes at one point in time and then comparing the responses of the four groups. If seniors manifested more positive attitudes toward nursing professionalism than freshmen, it might be inferred that nursing students become increasingly socialized professionally by their educational experiences. In order to make this kind of inference, the researcher must assume that the senior students would have responded as the freshmen responded had they been questioned 3 years earlier, or, conversely, that freshmen students would demonstrate increased favorability toward professionalism if they were surveyed 3 years later.

The main advantage of cross-sectional designs is that they are practical. They are relatively easy to manage and economical. There are, however, a number of problems in inferring changes and trends over time using a cross-sectional design. The overwhelming amount of social and technological change that characterizes our society frequently makes it questionable to assume that differences in the behaviors, attitudes, or characteristics of different age groups are the result of the passage through time rather than to cohort or "generational" differences. In the above example, seniors and freshmen may have different attitudes toward the nursing profession, independent of any experiences they had during their 4 years of education. In cross-sectional studies there are frequently several rival hypotheses for any observed differences. Furthermore, ex post facto studies aimed at shedding light on causal relationships are handicapped when a cross-sectional design is adopted because the doubtful temporal ordering of phenomena mitigates against drawing causal conclusions.

Longitudinal Designs

Research projects that are designed to collect data at more than one point in time are referred to as *longitudinal studies*. As the preceding discussion suggested, the main value of a longitudinal design lies in its ability to clearly demonstrate (1) trends or changes over time and (2) the temporal sequencing of phenomena, which is an essential criterion for establishing causality.

Four types of longitudinal studies deserve special mention—trend, cohort, panel, and follow-up studies. *Trend studies* are investigations in which samples from a general population are studied over time with respect to some phenomenon. Different samples are selected at repeated intervals, but the samples are always drawn from the same population. Trend studies permit researchers to examine patterns and rates of change over time and to make predictions about future directions. For example, trend studies have been initiated to analyze the number of students entering nursing programs and to forecast future supplies of nursing personnel.

Cohort studies are a particular kind of trend study in which specific subpopulations are examined over time. Once again, different samples are selected at different points in time, but the samples are drawn from specific subgroups that are often age-related. For example, the cohort of women born during the 1946–1950 period may be periodically surveyed to determine their employment/unemployment patterns. A sophisticated design known as the *cross-sequential design* combines the features of cohort studies with a cross-sectional approach. In cross-sequential studies, two or more different age cohorts are studied longitudinally so that both changes over time and generational or cohort differences can be detected.

Panel studies differ from trend and cohort studies in that the same subjects are used to supply the data at two or more points in time. The term "panel," which is used almost exclusively in the context of longitudinal survey projects, refers to the sample of subjects involved in the study. Panel studies typically yield more information than trend studies because the investigator can usually reveal patterns of change and reasons for the changes. Since the same people are contacted at two or more points in time, the researcher can identify the subjects who did and did not change and then isolate the characteristics of the subgroups in which changes occurred. As an example, a panel study could be designed to explore over time the nutritional habits of a sample of adults. Panel studies are intuitively appealing as an approach to studying change but are extremely difficult and expensive to manage. The most serious problem is the loss of participants at different points in the study. Attrition is problematic for the researcher because those who drop out of the study may differ in important respects from the people who continue to participate; hence, the generalizability of the findings may be impaired.

Follow-up studies are similar in design to panel studies except that follow-up studies are usually associated with experiments or other types of nonsurvey research. Follow-up investigations are generally undertaken to determine the subsequent development of subjects with a specified condition or who have received a specified intervention. For example, patients who have received a particular nursing intervention or clinical treatment may be followed up to ascertain the long-term effects of the treatment. To take a nonexperimental example, samples of premature and normal babies may be followed up to assess their later perceptual and motor development.

In sum, longitudinal designs are useful for studying the dynamics of a variable or phenomenon over time. The number of data-collection periods and the time intervals in between the data-collection points depend on the nature of the study. When change or development is rapid, numerous time points at short intervals may be required to document the pattern and to make accurate forecasts.

Research Example

Casteel (1985) hypothosized that nursing effectiveness is higher in primary nursing than in team nursing.* To test this hypothesis she obtained data from 100 patients in two medical–surgical units at the Laclede Hospital (which used primary nursing) and from a similar sample hospitalized at Osage Hospital (which used team nursing). Casteel used three measures of nursing effectiveness: patients' length of stay in hospital, ratings of effectiveness by an objective expert observer, and total number of errors of omission and commission by the nursing staff.

Casteel realized that numerous factors influence nursing effectiveness and that these factors needed to be controlled in order to test the research hypothesis. However, random assignment of nurses to the two types of nursing and random assignment of patients to hospitals was not possible. Therefore, Casteel took other steps to

*This example is fictitious.

enhance the internal validity of the study. First, she designed her study in such a way that the conditions in the two hospitals were as comparable as possible. For example, she selected two private hospitals that were similar in size, modernity, reputation, and proximity to an urban center. She focused on two medical–surgical units that were similar with respect to staff–patient ratio, number of beds, type of medical problems, and number of private and semiprivate rooms. Casteel also recognized that staff characteristics were important. Therefore, a group of 15 nurses in each hospital who provided the care were matched with respect to number of years of experience in nursing (more than 5 or less than 5 years) and educational credentials (baccalaureate degree, associate degree, and diploma). Finally, the 100 patients in each hospital were matched in terms of their sex, age (in 5-year age groupings), and medical diagnosis. The data were collected by two objective observers who had no affiliation with either of the two hospitals and no personal acquaintance with any of the nursing staff. The data supported Casteel's hypothesis that primary nursing is more effective than team nursing.

Casteel's study is nonexperimental; she had no control over the implementation of either the primary or team nursing. She tested her hypothesis using intact, preestablished groups of nursing staff and their patients. Although an experimental design might technically be possible for this problem, it would probably not be feasible from a practical point of view.

Given that Casteel had to work with existing conditions, she nevertheless was careful in designing a study that controlled for numerous external and intrinsic extraneous variables. She maintained constancy over numerous external conditions, such as the environmental context and the data-collection procedures. One possible uncontrolled source of bias is the observers' values with respect to primary versus team nursing. If the observers prefer primary nursing, then their ratings of nursing effectiveness could have been colored by their opinions. However, this potential flaw would surface even with an experimental design. Double-blind procedures for this situation seem unmanageable. Perhaps the best approach would have been to ask observers to rate the nurses without telling the observers what the research problem was.

Casteel controlled several important intrinsic characteristics (of both nurses and patients) through matching. Although this procedure has numerous shortcomings, the use of matching in this case was preferable to totally ignoring the problem of extraneous variables. One alternative would have been to use homogeneous groups of nurses (e.g., all baccalaureate nurses) or patients (e.g., all with the same medical diagnosis), but this would have severely limited the generalizability of the results. The problem with matching, as noted earlier, is that only two or three matching variables can be used, and there may be far more than two or three extraneous variables. For example, such factors as age, amount of continuing education, level of empathy, and number of years of experience could affect nursing effectiveness. If systematic differences on these variables exist between nurses in the two hospitals, then these differences represent rival explanations, competing with the type of nursing approach as causes of the differences in nursing effectiveness. Thus, selection is a primary threat to the internal validity of the study. If some event external to the study occurred in only one hospital during the data-collection period, then history might also have been a threat.

In sum, the researcher took many commendable steps in controlling extraneous variables in this study. Given the constraints of not being able to manipulate the independent variable or to randomize nurses to groups, the matching procedure was one of the best alternatives. The only more rigorous approach would have been to gather data on any other extraneous variables (e.g., amount of continuing education, age, etc.) and to control these variables statistically using analysis of covariance.

Summary

The purpose of research design is to guide the collection and analysis of data in such a way that the results it yields are interpretable and generalizable. We plan and design studies, rather than simply rush out to collect information, because research that is carefully designed increases our confidence in the conclusions. The researcher must design a study that controls *extraneous variables*, that is, the unwanted or irrelevant variables in the research setting, or irrelevant characteristics of the participants, that could influence the results of the study.

One important type of control relates to the constancy of conditions under which a study is performed. A number of aspects of the study, such as the environment, timing, communications, and the implementation of treatment, should be held constant or kept as similar as possible for each participant.

The most problematic and pervasive extraneous variables are intrinsic characteristics of the subjects. Several techniques are available to control such characteristics. First, a homogeneous sample of subjects can be used such that there is no variability relating to characteristics that could affect the outcome of a study. Second, the extraneous variables can be built into the design of a study so that a direct assessment of their impact can be made. One such design that accomplishes this is the *randomized block design*, in which the extraneous variable is referred to as the *blocking variable*. The third approach, *matching*, is essentially an after-the-fact attempt to approximate a randomized block design. This procedure matches subjects on the basis of one or more extraneous variables in an attempt to secure comparable groups. A fourth technique is to control extraneous variables by means of a statistical procedure known as an *analysis of covariance*. All four procedures for controlling extraneous individual characteristics share one disadvantage, and that is that the researcher must know which variables need to be controlled. The fifth procedure, randomization, effectively controls for all possible extraneous variables because it tends to produce groups in which individual variation is cancelled out.

The control mechanisms reviewed here help to improve the *internal validity* of studies. Internal validity is concerned with the question of whether or not the results of a project are attributable to the independent variable(s) of interest or to other extraneous factors. A number of plausible rival explanations, known as threats to the internal validity of a study, were discussed. These threats include *history, selection, maturation,* and *mortality* (or *attrition*). These threats are least likely to emerge in experimental designs. *External validity* refers to the generalizability of study findings to other samples and settings.

In addition to being internally valid, a good research design is one that is appropriate for the question being asked, free from bias, and capable of enhancing statistical *precision*. Precision refers to the sensitivity with which treatment effects, relative to the effects of extraneous variables, can be detected.

Research designers need to consider what time frame is best suited to their problem. *Cross-sectional studies* involve the collection of data at one point in time, whereas *longitudinal studies* collect data at two or more points in time. Research problems that involve trends, changes, or development over time are best addressed through longitudinal designs. *Trend studies* investigate a particular phenomenon over time by repeatedly drawing different samples from the same general population. *Cohort studies* represent a type of trend study in which a particular subpopulation is studied over time with respect to some phenomenon. Longitudinal survey studies in which the same sample of subjects is questioned twice (or more often) are known as *panel studies. Follow-up studies* similarly deal with the same subjects studied at two or more points in time, and they generally refer to those investigations in which subjects who have received a treatment or who have a particular characteristic of interest are followed up in order to study their subsequent development. Longitudinal studies are typically expensive, time-consuming, and plagued with such difficulties as attrition but are often extremely valuable with respect to the information they produce.

Study Suggestions

1. How do you suppose the use of identical twins in a research study can enhance control?

2. Suppose you were planning to conduct a nonexperimental study concerning the effects of three types of nursing preparation (baccalaureate program, associate-degree program, and diploma school) on membership in professional organizations. What types of extraneous variables relating to characteristics of the subjects would be important to consider and, if possible, control?

3. With respect to the preceding question, how would you go about controlling for the extraneous variables you have identified?

4. Suppose that you are studying the effects of range-of-motion exercises on radical mastectomy patients. You start your experiment with 50 experimental subjects who come for daily sessions over a 2-week period, while control subjects come only once at the end of 2 weeks. Your final group sizes are 40 for the experimental group and 49 for the control group. The results of your study indicate that the experimental group did better in raising the arm of the affected side above head level. What effects, if any, do you think the subject attrition would have on the internal validity of your study?

5. A nurse researcher wants to study how nurses' attitudes toward death change as a function of years of nursing experience. Design a cross-sectional study to research this question, specifying the samples that you want to include. Then design a longitudinal study to research the same problem. Identify the problems and strengths of each approach.

6. For each of the examples below, indicate (1) the types of research designs that could be used to study the problem (experimental, quasi-experimental etc.); (2) the design you would recommend using; and (3) how you would go about obtaining a sample, collecting data, and establishing control procedures.

   a. What effect does the presence of the newborn's father in the delivery room have on the mother's subjective report of pain?

   b. What is the effect of different types of bowel-evacuation regimens on quadriplegics?

   c. Does the reinforcement of intensive care unit nonsmoking behavior in smokers affect postintensive care unit smoking behaviors?

   d. Is the degree of change in body image of surgical patients related to their need for touch?

Chapter 9
Sampling Designs

Sampling is a familiar process to all of us. In the course of our daily activities we gather knowledge, make decisions, and formulate predictions through sampling procedures. A nursing student may decide on an elective course for a semester by sampling two or three classes on the first day of the semester. Patients may generalize about the quality of nursing care as a result of their exposure to a sample of nurses during a 1-week hospital stay. We all come to conclusions about phenomena on the basis of contact with a limited portion of those phenomena.

The scientist, too, must derive knowledge from samples. In testing the efficacy of a medication for asthma victims, a scientific researcher must reach a conclusion without administering the drug to every asthmatic. Nevertheless, the scientist cannot afford the luxury that we experience in our private lives of coming to conclusions based on a sample size of three or four subjects. The consequences of making erroneous generalizations are typically much more severe in scientific investigations than in private decision making. Therefore, research methodologists have devoted considerable attention to the development of sampling plans that produce accurate and meaningful information. In this chapter we review some of these plans.

Basic Sampling Concepts

Sampling is an indispensable step in the research process, and a step to which too little attention is typically paid. To understand the importance of sampling, the reader must first become familiar with the terms associated with sampling. Much of this terminology has been introduced in earlier chapters but will be explained in more detail here to avoid any possible confusion in subsequent discussions.

Populations

A *population* is the entire aggregation of cases that meets a designated set of criteria. For instance, if a nurse researcher were studying American nurses with doctorates, the population could be defined as all United States citizens who are RNs and who have acquired a PhD, DScN, DEd, or other doctoral-level degree. Other possible populations might be (1) all the male patients who had undergone surgery in hospital X during the year 1978; (2) all women over 60 years old who are under psychiatric care; or (3) all the children in the United States with cystic fibrosis. As this list illustrates, a population may be broadly defined, involving millions of people, or may be narrowly specified to include only several hundred people.

Populations are not restricted to human subjects. A population might consist of all of the hospital records on file in the Belleville Hospital, or all of the blood samples taken from clients of a health-maintenance organization, or all of the correspondence of Florence Nightingale. Populations may be defined in terms of actions, words, organizations, animals, or days in the year. Whatever the basic unit, the population is always comprised of a specific aggregate of elements in which the researcher is interested.

A distinction is sometimes made between target and accessible populations. The *accessible population* is the aggregate of cases that conform to the designated criteria *and* that are accessible to the researcher as a pool of subjects for a study. The *target population* is the entire aggregate of cases about which the researcher would like to make generalizations. A target population might consist of all RNs currently employed in the United States, but the more modest accessible population might be restricted to employed RNs working in San Francisco. The utility of identifying both the target and accessible populations will be discussed in a later section of this chapter.

Samples and Sampling

Sampling refers to the process of selecting a portion of the population to represent the entire population. A *sample*, then, consists of a subset of the entities that comprise the population. The entities that make up the samples and populations are usually referred to as *elements*. The element is the most basic unit about which information is collected. As we have seen, the most common element in nursing research is people, but other entities can form the basis of a sample or population.

Samples and sampling plans vary in their adequacy. The overriding consideration in assessing a sample is its representativeness. Unfortunately, there is no method for really being sure that a sample is representative without obtaining the information from the entire population. Certain sampling procedures are less likely to result in biased samples than others, but there is never any guarantee of a representative sample. This may sound somewhat discouraging, but it must be remembered that the scientist always operates under conditions in which error is possible. An important role of the scientist is to minimize or control those errors, or at least to estimate the magnitude of their effects.

Sampling plans can essentially be grouped into two categories: *probability sampling* and *nonprobability sampling*. Probability samples utilize some form of random selection in choosing the sampling units. The hallmark of a probability sample is that a researcher is in a position to specify the probability that each element of the population will be included in the sample. Probability sampling is the more respected of the two types of sampling plans because greater confidence can be placed in the representativeness of probability samples. In nonprobability samples, elements are selected by nonrandom methods. There is no way of estimating the probability that each element has of being included in a nonprobability sample, and there is no assurance that every element has a chance for inclusion.

Strata

Sometimes it is useful to think of populations as consisting of two or more subpopulations or strata. A *stratum* refers to a mutually exclusive segment of a population established by one or more specifications. For instance, suppose our population consisted of all RNs currently employed in the United States. This population could be divided into two strata based on the gender of the nurse. Alternatively, we could specify three strata consisting of nurses younger than 30, nurses aged 30 to 45, and nurses 46 or older. Within a sampling context, strata are often identified and used in the sample-selection process to enhance the representativeness of the sample.

Sampling Rationale

Scientists work with samples rather than with populations because it is more economical and efficient to work with a small group of elements than with an entire set of elements. The typical researcher has neither the time nor the resources required to study all possible members of a population. The need for data in a specified time period usually makes it imperative for the researcher to sample. Furthermore, it is usually unnecessary to gather information about some phenomenon from an entire population. It is almost always possible to obtain a reasonably accurate understanding of the phenomena under investigation by securing information from a sample. Samples, thus, are practical and efficient means of collecting data.

Still, despite all of the advantages of sampling, the data obtained from samples can lead to erroneous conclusions. Finding 100 willing subjects to participate in a research project seldom poses any difficulty, even to a novice researcher. It is considerably more problematic to select 100 subjects who adequately represent the population. Bias in sampling refers to the systematic overrepresentation or underrepresentation of some segment of the population in terms of a characteristic relevant to the research question. In some cases, the biases may be conscious—that is, the result of a conscious decision on the part of the researcher to exclude certain persons who meet the sampling criteria.

Sampling bias is more likely to occur unconsciously than consciously, however. If a researcher studying student nurses systematically interviews every tenth student who enters the nursing school library, the sample of students will be strongly biased in favor of students who go to the library, even though the researcher may exert a conscientious effort to include every tenth entrant irrespective of their appearance, sex, or other characteristics.

The extent to which sampling bias is likely to give cause for concern is a function of the homogeneity of the population. If the elements in a population were all identical with respect to some critical attribute, then any sample would be as good as any other. Indeed, if the population were completely homogeneous (*i.e.*, exhibited no variability at all), then a single element would constitute a sufficient sample for drawing conclusions about the population. With regard to many physical or physiological attributes, it may be safe to assume a reasonably high degree of homogeneity and to proceed in selecting a sample on the basis of this assumption. For example, the blood in a person's veins is relatively homogeneous. A single blood sample chosen haphazardly is usually adequate for clinical purposes. For many human attributes, however, homogeneity is the exception rather than the rule. Variables, after all, derive their name from the fact that traits vary from one person to the next. Age, sex, religiosity, health condition, stress, attitudes, needs, and smoking habits are all attributes that reflect the heterogeneity of human beings. The researcher must be concerned with the problem of sampling bias to the degree that a population is heterogeneous on key variables.

Nonprobability Sampling

The nonprobability approach to selecting a sample is generally held in lower esteem than probability sampling because the latter tends to produce more accurate and representative samples. Despite this fact, the majority of samples in most disciplines, including nursing research, are nonprobability samples. There are three primary methods of nonprobability sampling: accidental, quota, and purposive.

Accidental Sampling

Accidental sampling entails the use of the most readily available persons or objects for use as subjects in a study. The faculty member who distributes questionnaires to the students in her or his class is using an accidental sample, or a *sample of convenience*, as it is sometimes called. The problem with accidental sampling is that available subjects might be untypical of the population with regard to the critical variables being measured.

Accidental samples are not necessarily comprised of people known to the researchers. Stopping people at a street corner to ask their opinion on some issue is sampling by convenience. Sometimes a researcher seeking persons with certain characteristics will place an advertisement in a newspaper or place signs in supermarkets, laundromats, or community centers. Both of these approaches are subject to serious problems of bias because people self-select themselves as pedestrians on certain streets or as volunteers in response to public notices.

Accidental sampling is the weakest form of sampling. It is also probably the most commonly used sampling method. In cases in which the phenomena under investigation are fairly homogeneous within the population, the risks of bias may be minimal. In heterogeneous populations, there is no other sampling approach in which the risk of bias is greater. What is worse is that there is no way to evaluate the biases that may be operating. It is advisable to avoid using accidental samples if possible and to exercise caution in interpreting the data if accidental samples have been used.

Quota Sampling

Quota sampling is a form of nonprobability sampling in which the researcher utilizes some knowledge about the population to build some representativeness into the sampling plan. The quota sample is one in which the researcher identifies strata of the population and determines the proportions of elements needed from the various segments of the population. By using information about the composition of a population, the investigator can ensure that diverse segments are represented in the sample in the proportions in which they occur in the population. Quota sampling gets its name from the procedure of establishing quotas for the various strata from which data are to be collected.

Let us use as an example a researcher interested in studying the attitudes of undergraduate nursing students toward the role of the industrial nurse. The accessible population is a single school of nursing that has an undergraduate enrollment of 1000 students. A sample size of 200 students is desired. The easiest procedure would be to use an accidental sample, by distributing questionnaires in classrooms or catching students as they enter or leave the library. The researcher may realize, however, that male students and female students will probably have different attitudes toward the industrial nurse's role, as will members of the four different classes. An accidental sample could easily oversample and undersample these diverse population sectors. Table 9-1 presents some fictitious data showing the proportions of each stratum for the population and for an accidental sample. As this table shows, the accidental sample seriously overrepresents freshmen and women while underrepresenting men and members of the sophomore, junior, and senior classes. In anticipation of a problem of this type, the researcher can guide the selection of subjects such that the final sample will include the correct number of cases from each stratum. The bottom of Table 9-1 shows the number of cases that would be required for each stratum in a quota sample for this example.

If we pursue this same example a bit further, the reader may better appreciate the dangers of inadequate representation of the various strata. Suppose that one of the key questions in this study was "Do you think you might ever consider taking a position as an industrial nurse?" The percentage of students in the population who would respond "yes" to this inquiry is shown in the first section of Table 9-2. Of course, these values would never be known by the researcher; they are displayed to illustrate a point. Within the population, males and older students are more willing

Table 9-1. Numbers and Percentages of Students in Strata of a Population—Accidental Sample and Quota Sample

		FRESHMEN	SOPHO-MORES	JUNIORS	SENIORS	TOTAL
Population	Males	25 (2.5%)	25 (2.5%)	25 (2.5%)	25 (2.5%)	100 (10%)
	Females	225 (22.5%)	225 (22.5%)	225 (22.5%)	225 (22.5%)	900 (90%)
	TOTAL	250 (25%)	250 (25%)	250 (25%)	250 (25%)	1000 (100%)
Accidental Sample	Males	2 (1%)	4 (2%)	3 (1.5%)	1 (0.5%)	10 (5%)
	Females	98 (49%)	36 (18%)	37 (18.5%)	19 (9.5%)	190 (95%)
	TOTAL	100 (50%)	40 (20%)	40 (20%)	20 (10%)	200 (100%)
Quota Sample	Males	5 (2.5%)	5 (2.5%)	5 (2.5%)	5 (2.5%)	20 (10%)
	Females	45 (22.5%)	45 (22.5%)	45 (22.5%)	45 (22.5%)	180 (90%)
	TOTAL	50 (25%)	50 (25%)	50 (25%)	50 (25%)	200 (100%)

Table 9-2. Students Willing to Consider Industrial Nurse Role

	NUMBER IN POPULATION	NUMBER IN ACCIDENTAL SAMPLE	NUMBER IN QUOTA SAMPLE
Freshmen Males	2	0	0
Sophomore Males	6	1	1
Junior Males	8	1	2
Senior Males	12	0	3
Freshmen Females	6	2	1
Sophomore Females	16	2	3
Junior Females	30	4	7
Senior Females	45	3	9
Number of Willing Students	125	13	26
Total Number of Students	1000	200	200
Percentage	12.5%	6.5%	13%

than others to consider the industrial nurse's role, yet these are the very groups that are underrepresented in the accidental sample. As a result, there is a sizable discrepancy between the population and sample values: nearly twice as many students are favorable toward the role of the industrial nurse (12.5%) than one would suspect based on the results obtained from the accidental sample (6.5%). The quota sample, on the other hand, does a reasonably good job of mirroring the viewpoint of the population.

Quota sampling requires neither sophisticated skills nor an inordinate amount of time or effort. Many researchers who claim that the use of an accidental sample is unavoidable for their projects could probably design a quota sampling plan, and it would be to their advantage to do so. The characteristics chosen to form the strata are necessarily selected according to the researcher's judgment. The basis of stratification should be some extraneous variable that, in the estimation of the investigator, would reflect important differences in the dependent variable under investigation. Such variables as age, sex, ethnicity, socioeconomic status, educational attainment, medical diagnosis, and occupational rank are likely to be important stratifying variables in nursing research investigations.

Except for the identification of the strata and the proportional representation for each, quota sampling is procedurally quite similar to accidental sampling. The subjects in any particular cell constitute, in essence, an accidental sample from that stratum of the population. Because of this fact, quota sampling shares many of the same weaknesses as accidental sampling. For instance, if a researcher is required by the quota sampling plan to interview ten men between the ages of 65 and 80, a trip to a nursing home might be the most convenient method of obtaining those subjects. Yet this approach would fail to give any representation to those many senior citizens who are living independently in the community. Despite its problems, quota sampling represents an important improvement over accidental sampling and should be considered by any researcher whose resources prevent the utilization of a probability sampling plan.

Purposive Sampling

Purposive or *judgmental sampling* proceeds on the belief that a researcher's knowledge about the population and its elements can be used to handpick the cases to be included in the sample. The researcher might decide to purposely select the widest possible variety of respondents or might choose subjects who are judged to be typical of the population in question. An underlying assumption in resorting to purposive sampling is that any errors of judgment will, in the long run, tend to balance out. However, this assumption may be unwarranted. Sampling in this subjective manner provides no external, objective method for assessing the typicalness of the selected subjects.

The question of whether purposive samples tend to produce more accurate, representative data than accidental samples is open to conjecture. In a purposive sample there is certainly a risk of conscious sample biases, but perhaps the necessity of making individual decisions minimizes the risk of unconscious biases. The same advice given earlier still pertains: (1) purposive samples, like accidental samples, should be avoided, particularly if the population is heterogeneous; and (2) if they are unavoidable, the resulting data should be treated with extreme circumspection.

Evaluation of Nonprobability Sampling

We have repeatedly stressed the disadvantages of using nonprobability samples in scientific research. Investigators who use nonprobability samples are in a poor position to argue that their research findings can be generalized to the population. The difficulty stems from the fact that not every element in the population has a chance of being included in the sample. Therefore, it is likely that some segment of the population will be systematically underrepresented. If the population is homogeneous on the critical attributes, then systematic biases will matter very little. But only a small fraction of the charactersitics in which nursing researchers are interested are sufficiently homogeneous to render sampling bias an irrelevant consideration.

Why then are nonprobability samples used at all? Clearly, the advantage of these sampling designs lies in their convenience and economy. Probability sampling, which will be discussed in the next section, requires skill, resources, and time. If a researcher is lacking one of these critical ingredients, there may be no option but to use a nonprobability approach or to abandon the project altogether. Even hard-nosed research consultants would hesitate to advocate a total abandonment of one's ideas in the absence of a random sample. The researcher using a nonprobability sample out of necessity must be cautious about the inferences and conclusions drawn from the data. With care in the selection of the sample, a conservative interpretation of the results, and replication of the study with new samples, the researcher may find that nonprobability samples work reasonably well.

Probability Sampling

The hallmark of probability sampling is the random selection of elements from the population. Random selection should not be confused with random assignment, which was described in connection with experimental research in Chapter 6. *Random assignment*, it will be recalled, refers to the process of allocating subjects to different experimental conditions on a random basis. Random assignment has no bearing on how the subjects participating in an experiment are selected in the first place. A *random selection* process is one in which each element in the population has an equal, independent chance of being selected. The four most commonly used probability sampling designs are simple random, stratified random, cluster, and systematic sampling.

Simple Random Sampling

Simple random sampling is the most basic of the probability sampling designs, although it is not particularly common in the research literature. Since the more complex probability sampling designs incorporate the features of simple random sampling, the procedures involved will be described here in some detail.

After the population has been identified and defined, it is necessary to establish what is known as a sampling frame. The term *sampling frame* is the technical name for the actual list of the sampling units from which the sample will be chosen. If nursing students attending Wayne State University constituted the accessible population, then a roster of those students would be the sampling frame. If the sampling unit was 400-bed (or larger) general hospitals in the United States, then a list of all such hospitals would be the sampling frame. In actual practice, a population may be defined in terms of an existing sampling frame rather than starting with a population and then developing a list of sampling units. For example, if a researcher wanted to use a telephone directory as a sampling frame, the population would have to be defined as the residents of a certain community who are clients of the telephone company and who have a listed number. Since all members of a community do not own a telephone and others fail to have their numbers listed, it would be inappropriate to consider a telephone directory the sampling frame for the entire community population.

Once a listing of the population elements has been developed or located, the elements must all be numbered consecutively. A table of random numbers would then be used to draw a sample of the desired size. An example of a sampling frame with 50 people is presented in Table 9-3. Let us assume that a sample of 20 people is sufficient for our purposes. As in the case of random assignment, we would find a starting place in the table of random numbers by blindly placing our finger at some point on the page. In order to include all numbers between 1 and 50, two-digit combinations would be read. Suppose, for the sake of the example, that we began the random selection with the very first number in the random-number table of Table 6-1 (in Chapter 6), which is 46. The person corresponding to this number, C. Yarrow, is the first subject selected to participate in the study. Number 05, J. Enochs, is the second selection, and number 23, L. Young, is the third. This process would continue until the 20 required subjects were chosen. The selected elements are circled in Table 9-3.

It should be clear that the sample selected randomly in this fashion is not subject to the biases of the researcher. There is no guarantee that the sample will be representative. Random selection does, however, guarantee that differences in the attributes of the sample and the population are purely a function of chance. Researchers using random selection proce-

Table 9-3. Sampling Frame for Simple Random Sampling Example

①. N. Alexander	⑭ P. Nelson	27. C. Champ	40. J. Quint
2. C. Bond	15. H. Ouellette	28. H. Dunn	41. K. Rothman
3. B. Cornet	16. K. Poland	29. G. Engquist	42. G. Stangler
4. D. Demske	⑰ H. Rosemonde	㉚ D. Fairweather	㊸ W. Trumbower
⑤. J. Enochs	⑱ S. Shields	㉛ J. Gitelman	44. L. Vernecke
⑥. F. Fallon	19. B. Toan	32. A. Hilson	㊺ M. Williams
7. J. Gueron	20. G. Unger	㉝ B. Judge	㊻ C. Yarrow
8. A. Harris	㉑ L. Vedrani	㉞ J. Kahn	47. D. Abraham
9. W. Innis	22. N. Woods	35. L. Logsdon	48. D. Bryant
10. M. Jennison	㉓ L. Young	36. S. Marcum	49. M. Carnahan
11. L. Kendrick	㉔ M. Zander	37. N. Norris	㊾ G. Drake
12. F. Lafser	25. B. Adler	㊳ P. O'Brien	
⑬ S. Mandell	㉖ J. Brimmer	39. L. Punch	

dures must be content with the fact that the probability of selecting a markedly deviant sample is normally low and that this probability decreases as the size of the sample increases.

Simple random sampling usually is an exceedingly laborious process. The development of the sampling frame, enumeration of all the elements, and selection of the sample elements are time-consuming chores, particularly if the population is large. Imagine enumerating all of the telephone subscribers listed in the New York City telephone directory. In actual practice, simple random sampling is seldom used because it is a relatively inefficient procedure. Furthermore, it is often impossible to get a complete listing of every element in the population, so that other methods may be required.

Stratified Random Sampling

Stratified random sampling is a variant of simple random sampling in which the population is first divided into two or more strata or subgroups. As in the case of quota sampling, the aim of stratified sampling is to obtain a greater degree of representativeness. Stratified sampling designs subdivide the population into homogeneous subsets from which an appropriate number of elements can be selected at random.

The stratification may be based on a wide variety of attributes, such as age, gender, occupation, and so forth. The difficulty lies in the fact that the variables of interest may not be readily discernible or available. If one is working with a telephone directory, it would be risky to make decisions about a person's gender, and certainly age, ethnicity, or other personal information is not listed. Patient listings, student rosters, or organizational directories might contain the information needed for a meaningful stratification. Quota sampling does not have the same problem because the prospective subject can be asked questions that determine his or her eligibility for a particular stratum. In stratified sampling, however, decisions about a person's status in a stratum must be made before a sample is chosen.

Various procedures for drawing a stratified sample have been used. The most common is to group together those elements that belong to a stratum and to select randomly the desired number of elements. The researcher may take the same number of elements from each stratum or may decide to select unequal numbers, for reasons that will be discussed below. To illustrate the procedure used in the simplest case, suppose that the list in Table 9-3 consisted of 25 men (numbers 1 through 25) and 25 women (numbers 26 through 50). Using gender as the stratifying variable, we could guarantee a sample of ten males and ten females by randomly sampling ten numbers from the first half of the list and ten from the second half.

In many cases the stratifying variables will divide the population into unequal subpopulations. For example, if the person's race were used to stratify the population of United States citizens, the subpopulation of white persons would be larger than that of black persons. In such a situation, the researcher might decide to select subjects in proportion to the size of the stratum in the population. This procedure is referred to as *proportional stratified sampling*. If an undergraduate population in a school of nursing consisted of 10% blacks, 5% Hispanics, and 85% whites, then a proportional stratified sample of 100 students, with racial background as the stratifying variable, would consist of 10, 5, and 85 students from the respective subpopulations.

When the researcher's prime concern is to understand differences between the strata, then proportional sampling may result in an insufficient base for making comparisons. In the previous example, would the researcher be justified in coming to conclusions about the characteristics of Hispanic nursing students based on only five cases? It would be extremely unwise to do so in most types of research. Researchers often adopt a *disproportional sampling design* whenever interstratum comparisons are sought between strata of greatly unequal membership size. In the example at hand, the sampling proportions might be altered to select 20 blacks, 20 Hispanics, and 60 whites. This design would ensure a more adequate representation of the viewpoints of the two racial minorities. When disproportional sampling is used, however, it is necessary to make an adjustment to the data in order to arrive at the best estimate of overall population values. This adjustment process, known as *weighting*, is a simple mathematic computation that is described in detail in most texts on sampling.

Stratified random sampling offers the researcher the opportunity to sharpen the precision and representativeness of the final sample. When it is desirable to obtain reliable information about subpopulations whose membership is relatively small, stratification provides a means of including a sufficient number of cases in the sample by oversampling for that stratum. Stratified sampling may, however, be impossible if information on the critical variables is unavailable. Furthermore, a stratified sample requires even more labor and effort than a simple random sampling, since the sample must be drawn from multiple enumerated listings.

Cluster Sampling

For many populations, it is simply not possible to obtain a listing of all the elements. The population consisting of all full-time nursing students in the country would be quite difficult to list and enumerate for the purpose of drawing a simple or stratified random sample. In addition, it would often be prohibitively expensive to sample nursing students in this way, since the resulting sample would result in no more than one or two students per institution. If interviews were involved, the interviewers would have to travel to people scattered throughout the country. Because of these considerations, large-scale studies almost never use simple or stratified random sampling. The most common procedure for large-scale surveys is cluster sampling.

In *cluster sampling*, there is a successive random sampling of units. The first unit to be sampled is large groupings, or "clusters." In drawing a sample of nursing students, the researcher might first draw a random sample of nursing schools. Or, if a sample of nursing supervisors were desired, a random sample of hospitals might first be obtained. Usually, the procedure for selecting a general sample of citizens is to successively sample such administrative units as states, cities, districts, blocks, and then households. Because of the successive stages of sampling, this approach is often referred to as *multi-stage sampling*.

For a specified number of cases, cluster sampling tends to contain more sampling errors than simple or stratified random sampling. Despite this disadvantage, cluster sampling is considerably more economical and practical than other types of probability sampling, particularly when the population is large and widely dispersed.

Systematic Sampling

Systematic sampling involves the selection of every *k*th case from some list or group, such as every 10th person on a patient list, or every 100th person listed in a directory of ANA members. Systematic sampling is sometimes used to sample every *k*th person entering a bookstore, or passing down the street, or leaving a hospital, and so forth. In such situations, unless the population is narrowly defined as consisting of all those people entering, passing by, or leaving, the sampling is nonprobability in nature. If college students were sampled systematically upon entering a bookstore, the resulting sample could not be called a random selection, since not every student would have a chance of being selected.

Systematic sampling designs can, however, be applied in such a way that an essentially random sample is drawn. If the researcher has a list, or sampling frame, the following procedure can be adopted. The desired sample size is established at some number (n). The size of the population must be known or estimated (N). By dividing N by n, the sampling interval width (k) is established. The *sampling interval* is the standard distance between the elements chosen for the sample. For instance, if we were seeking a sample of 200 from a population of 40,000, then our sampling interval would be as follows:

$$k = 40{,}000/200 = 200$$

In other words, every 200th element on the list would be sampled. The first element should be selected randomly, using a table of random numbers. Let us say that we randomly selected number 73 from a table. The persons corresponding to numbers 73, 273, 473, 673, and so forth would be included in the sample.

In actual practice, systematic sampling conducted in this manner is essentially identical to simple random sampling. Problems may arise if the list is arranged in such a way that a certain type of element is listed at intervals coinciding with the sampling interval. For instance, if every tenth nurse listed in a nursing personnel roster was a head nurse, and the sampling interval was ten, then head nurses would either always or never be included in the sample. Problems of this type are not too common, fortunately. In most cases, systematic sampling is preferable to simple random sampling because the same results are obtained in a more convenient and efficient manner.

Evaluation of Probability Sampling

Probability sampling is really the only viable method of obtaining representative samples. The superiority of probability sampling lies partially in its avoidance of conscious or unconscious biases. If all of the elements in the population have an equal probability of being selected, then the likelihood is high that the resulting sample will do a good job of representing the population.

A further advantage is that probability sampling allows the researcher to estimate the magnitude of sampling error. *Sampling error* refers to differences between population values (such as the average age of the population) and sample values (such as the average age of the sample). It is a very rare sample that is perfectly representative of a population and contains no sampling error on any of the attributes under investigation. Probability sampling does, however, permit estimates of the degree of expected error.

The great drawback of probability sampling is its expense and inconvenience. Unless the population is very narrowly defined, it is usually beyond the scope of small-scale research projects to sample using a probability design. A researcher adopting a nonprobability sampling design might well be able to argue that the homogeneity of the attribute under consideration makes an elaborate sampling scheme unnecessary. This justification will probably not be acceptable, however, if psychological, social, or economic attributes are being studied.

It might also be pointed out that the selection of elements that adequately represents the population does not guarantee the participation of all of those elements. Biased samples can result from probability samples if certain segments of the population systematically refuse to cooperate. In sum, probability sampling is the preferred and most respected method of obtaining sample elements but may in some cases be impracticable or unnecessary.

Sample Size

A major concern to beginning researchers is the number of subjects to be selected in a sample. When probability sampling procedures are used, it is possible to determine in advance the sample size needed to obtain a specified level of accuracy. There is no single formula that can be given, however, because sample size depends on numerous factors. This rather technical topic should be pursued in an advanced statistical test such as that of Cochran (1977) or Cohen (1977).

Although there is no simple equation that can automatically tell the researcher how large a sample is needed, we can offer a simple piece of advice: one should always use the largest sample possible. The larger the sample, the more representative of the population it is likely to be. Every time a researcher calculates a percentage or an average based on sample data, the purpose is to estimate a population value. Smaller samples will tend to produce less accurate estimates than larger samples. In other words, the larger the sample, the smaller the sampling error.

Let us illustrate this notion with a simple example of, say, annual aspirin consumption in a class of nursing students, as shown in Table 9-4. The population consists of 15 students whose aspirin consumption averages 16. Two simple random samples with sample sizes of two, three, five, and ten have been drawn from the population of 15 students. Each sample average on the right represents an estimate of the population average,

Table 9-4. Comparison of Population and Sample Values/Averages

NUMBER IN GROUP	GROUP	VALUES (ANNUAL NUMBER OF ASPIRINS CONSUMED)	AVERAGE
15	Population	2, 4, 6, 8, 10, 12, 14, 16, 18, 20, 22, 24, 26, 28, 30	16.0
2	Sample 1A	6, 14	10.0
2	Sample 1B	20, 28	24.0
3	Sample 2A	16, 18, 8	14.0
3	Sample 2B	20, 14, 26	20.0
5	Sample 3A	26, 14, 18, 2, 28	17.6
5	Sample 3B	30, 2, 26, 10, 4	14.4
10	Sample 4A	22,16, 24, 22, 2, 8, 14, 28, 20, 2	15.8
10	Sample 4B	14, 18, 12, 20, 6, 14, 28, 12, 24, 16	16.4

which we know is 16. Under ordinary circumstances, the population value would be unknown to us, and we would draw only one sample. With a sample size of two, our estimate might have been wrong by as many as eight aspirins in sample 1B. As the sample size increases, the averages not only get closer to the true population value, but the differences in the estimate between samples A and B get smaller as well. As the sample size increases, the probability of getting a markedly deviant sample diminishes. Large samples provide the opportunity to counterbalance, in the long run, atypical values. The safest procedure is to obtain data from as large a sample as is economically and practically feasible.

We hasten to add, however, that large samples are no assurance of accuracy. When nonprobability sampling methods are used, even a large sample can harbor extensive bias. The famous example illustrating this point is the 1936 presidential poll conducted by the magazine *Literary Digest*, which predicted that Alfred M. Landon would defeat Franklin D. Roosevelt by a landslide. Approximately 2½ million people participated in this poll—a rather substantial sample. Biases resulted from the fact that the sample was drawn from telephone directories and automobile registrations during a depression year when only the well-to-do had a car or telephone.

A large sample cannot correct for a faulty sampling design. The researcher should make decisions about the sample size and designs with the following in mind: the ultimate criterion for assessing a sample is its representativeness, not the quantity of data it produces.

Steps in Sampling

The first phase of the sampling process involves the identification of the target population. The *target population*, it will be recalled, is the entire group of people or objects about whom the researcher would like to draw conclusions or make generalizations. The target population could consist of all RNs currently unemployed in the United States, or all diabetics, or all women who have had a miscarriage, or all mentally retarded children under the age of 18.

Unless the researcher has a large amount of resources at his or her disposal, access to the entire target population usually is not possible. Therefore, it is useful to identify a portion of the target population that is accessible to the researcher. In essence, an accessible population is a sample from the larger target population. An accessible population might consist of unemployed RNs in the state of Ohio, or all diabetics under the care of a specific health-maintenance organization, or women who had a miscarriage in Centerville Hospital last year, or all mentally retarded children in a state school for the learning disabled.

Once the accessible population has been established, the researcher can implement a sampling plan, ask the sampled subjects for their cooperation, collect data, and interpret the results. It is at the interpretation phase that the researcher must be extremely cautious. Ideally, the sample is representative of the accessible population, and the accessible population is representative of the target population. By using an appropriate sample size and sampling plan, the researcher can have some assurance that the first part of this ideal has been realized. A much greater risk is involved in assuming that the second part of the ideal is also realized. Are the unemployed nurses of Ohio representative of all unemployed nurses in the United States? One can never be sure. The researcher must exercise judgment in assessing their degree of similarity.

There are, of course, no rules that a researcher can use as a guideline in making such judgments. The best advice is to be realistic and somewhat conservative. The researcher should interpret the findings and come to conclusions after asking the following: Is it reasonable to assume that the accessible population is representative of the target population? In what ways might they be expected to differ? How would such differences affect the conclusions? If the researcher decides that the differences in the two populations are too great, it would be prudent to identify a more restricted target population to which the findings could be meaningfully generalized.

Research Example

Vandiver (1984) designed a study to investigate nurses' attitudes toward surrogate motherhood, test-tube babies, and other nontraditional reproductive options.* She defined her target population as all registered nurses in the United States. She realized, however, that she did not have direct access to the entire population for selecting a sample. Therefore, she specified as her accessible population registered nurses in the state of Massachusetts. She contacted the directors of nursing in 12 hospitals chosen to represent both urban and rural, public and private settings, and enlisted their cooperation. She asked these directors to distribute 30 questionnaires to a random sample of RNs in the hospital. The number of completed questionnaires obtained from the ten hospitals ranged from a low of 16 to a high of 28, for a total of 238 completed questionnaires.

The sampling design used by Vandiver is a multi-stage design that combines both nonprobability and probability components. Vandiver handpicked 12 hospitals that yielded, in her judgment, a good mix in

---

*This example is fictitious.

terms of location and auspices. The first stage of the design, therefore, can be described as purposive sampling. Vandiver could have obtained a listing of all Massachusetts facilities and randomly chosen 12. However, with such a small sample of hospitals, it is conceivable that a skewed sample might have been obtained (*e.g.*, no rural hospitals). If the location and auspices of the hospital are related to nurses' opinions about nontraditional routes to parenthood, then perhaps Vandiver's approach is justifiable. The difficulty, however, is that we cannot be sure that Vandiver's selection of hospitals adequately represents hospitals (and nursing staff from those hospitals) in Massachusetts.

The second stage of the sampling plan involved a probability component. Within each hospital, the nursing directors were asked to select a simple random sample of 30 RNs and to distribute questionnaires to this group. Such a procedure presumably guaranteed that systematic biases would be minimized. Still, Vandiver cannot be sure that biases were not introduced because she herself did not control the random selection. By allowing the directors of nursing to select the sample, the investigator risked (1) the directors' misunderstanding of how to select a random sample, and (2) the directors' failing to comply with the request for random selection for some reason, such as practicality or personal considerations. For example, the director might decide to exclude Ms. Russell from the sample because of a recent death in her family. By allowing others to perform the random selection, Vandiver did not exercise as much control over the research situation as she might have. Furthermore, Vandiver risked even more serious biases stemming from low response rates in some hospitals (as low as 53% in one hospital). A personal delivery of the questionnaires, and good follow-up procedures, might have yielded a higher rate of returned questionnaires. Whenever response rates are low, there always remains the possibility of distortions, because nonrespondents are rarely a random subsample of the entire sample. They may self-select themselves out of the sample because, for example, they have not thought about the issues in the questionnaire or because they are strongly opposed to the topic being explored.

The key question that needs to be asked in evaluating a sampling design is the following: Is the sample sufficiently representative of the population that the results can be generalized to that population? In Vandiver's case it would be unwise to conclude that the opinions of the 238 nurses surveyed could be generalized to all RNs in the United States, or even to all RNs in Massachusetts. Given Vandiver's sampling plan, many nurses would never have had an opportunity to express their opinions. For example, nonemployed nurses and RNs working in schools, community health centers, colleges, or businesses were not sampled, and their opinions might differ systematically from those working in Massachusetts hospitals. Furthermore, response rates were not high, yielding a relatively small sample size for a survey of this type.

Despite the fact that Vandiver's sampling plan has some limitations, it is not without merit. She did well not to rely on a single hospital from which to collect data, as is so often the case. Furthermore, gross distortions were undoubtedly avoided by requesting nursing directors to select a random sample of nurses rather than by simply handing out questionnaires to the first 30 nurses available. Vandiver's results would have been enhanced had she exercised more control over sample selection and response rates, but they are nevertheless worthy of consideration. Part of the problem with the design is Vandiver's definition of the population. If Vandiver had specified a more modest target population (e.g., RNs currently employed in hospital settings in the northeast), then her sampling plan would have more credibility.

Summary

Sampling is the process of selecting a portion of the population to represent the entire population. A *population*, in turn, is the entire aggregate of cases that meet a designated set of criteria. In a sampling context, an *element* is the most basic unit about which information is collected.

The overriding consideration in assessing the adequacy of any sample is the degree to which it is representative of the population. Sampling plans vary in their ability to adequately reflect the population from which the sample was drawn. *Sampling bias* refers to the systematic overrepresentation or underrepresentation of some segment of the population. The greater the heterogeneity of the population with respect to the critical attributes, the greater the risk of sampling bias.

Sampling plans may be classified as either nonprobability or probability sampling. In *nonprobability sampling*, elements are selected by nonrandom methods. Accidental, quota, and purposive sampling are the principal nonprobability methods. *Accidental sampling* consists of using the most readily available or most convenient group of subjects for the sample. *Quota sampling* divides the population into homogeneous *strata* or subpopulations in order to ensure representative proportions of the various strata in the sample. Within each stratum, the researcher selects subjects by accidental sampling. In *purposive sampling*, subjects or objects are handpicked to be included in the sample based on the researcher's knowledge about the population. Nonprobability sampling designs have the advantage of being convenient and economical. The major disadvantage of nonprobability sampling designs is their potential for serious biases.

Probability sampling designs involve the random selection of elements from the population. A *simple random sample* involves the selection on a random basis of elements from a *sampling frame* that enumerates all the elements. A *stratified random sample* divides the population into homogeneous subgroups from which elements are selected at random. *Cluster sampling* involves the successive selection of random samples from larger to smaller units by either simple random or stratified random methods. *Systematic sampling* is the selection of every *k*th case from some list or group. By dividing the population size by the desired population size, the researcher is able to establish the *sampling interval*, which is the standard distance between the elements chosen for the systematic sample. Probability sampling designs are preferred to nonprobability methods because the former sampling plans tend to result in more representative samples and because they permit the researcher to estimate the magnitude of sampling error. Probability samples, however, are time-consuming, expensive, inconvenient, and, in some cases, impossible to obtain.

There is no simple equation that can be used to determine how large a sample is needed for a particular research project. One rule of thumb is to use as large a sample as possible and practicable. In general, the larger the sample, the more representative of the population it is likely to be. Even a very large sample, however, does not guarantee representativeness.

Study Suggestions

1. Draw a simple random sample of 20 people from the sampling frame of Table 9-3, using the table of random numbers that appears in Table 6-1. Begin your selection by blindly placing your finger at some point on the table.

2. Suppose you have decided to use a systematic sampling design for a research project. The known population size is 4400 and the sample size desired is 200. What is the sampling interval? If the first element selected is 23, what would be the second, third, and fourth elements to be selected?

3. Suppose a researcher is interested in studying the attitude of clinical specialists toward autonomy in the work situation. Suggest a possible target and accessible population. What strata might be identified by the researcher if quota sampling were used?

4. What type of sampling design was used to obtain the following samples?

   a. 15 people known by the researcher to have hypertension and 15 people known not to have hypertension

   b. The couples attending a particular prenatal class

   c. 100 nurses from a list of nurses registered in the state of Pennsylvania, using a table of random numbers

   d. 20 head nurses randomly selected from a random selection of ten hospitals located in one state

   e. Every fifth article published in *Nursing Research* during 1976

PART IV
Measurement and Data Collection

Chapter 10
Overview of Data-Collection Methods

The concepts in which a researcher is interested must ultimately be translated into observable, measurable phenomena. Defining and operationalizing variables is often one of the most difficult tasks in the research process; but without data-collection tools of high quality, researchers must always question the accuracy and robustness of the conclusions.

As is true in the case of a research design, a researcher often needs to choose from a number of alternatives in deciding how data are to be collected. For example, if a nurse researcher is interested in measuring patients' preoperative anxiety levels, a physiological measure such as the measurement of sweat gland activity could be adopted. Alternatively, observations could be made of the patients' behaviors. Or, a direct questioning method could be used. In this chapter and the following two chapters, we explore the major approaches to data collection used in nursing research. This chapter presents an overview of the purposes, advantages, and limitations of the major forms of data collection used in nursing research studies.

Self-report Methods

In the human sciences, a good deal of information can be gathered by direct questioning of people. If, for example, we are interested in learning about patients' perceptions of hospital care, patients' level of hunger or preoperative fears, or nursing students' attitudes toward the role of the school nurse, we are likely to try to find answers by posing our questions to a group of relevant persons. Sometimes alternatives to direct questions exist, and many of these alternatives are discussed below. However, the unique ability for humans to communicate verbally on a sophisticated level makes it unlikely that systematic questioning will ever be eliminated from the repertoire of data-collection techniques.

As we saw in Chapter 7, *self-report* information is generally gathered by means of a formal instrument constructed to be administered either by an interviewer (the interview schedule) or by the respondent directly in a paper-and-pencil format (the *questionnaire*). Self-report instruments aimed at gathering information on social–psychological phenomena often take the form of scales, which may be incorporated into an interview schedule or questionnaire.

Like a scale for the measurement of weight, *social–psychological scales* are devices aimed at making distinctions among people in terms of the degree to which they possess a trait, attitude, or emotion. Scales are measuring instruments that permit interindividual comparisons along some dimension of interest. For instance, a scale could be constructed for comparing the attitudes of men and women toward health-maintenance organizations. There is typically an enormous diversity among people with respect to their views, opinions, motivations, needs, and fears. The purpose of social–psychological scales is to measure these attributes quantitatively. Just as a thermometer is a scale that permits a quantitative differentiation between different temperatures, a scale that measures attitudes toward health-maintenance organizations attempts to distinguish between persons who are more or less favorable toward them.

Verbal report instruments are strong with respect to the directness of their approach. If we want to know how people think, feel, believe, or behave, the most direct means of gathering the information is to ask them about it. Perhaps the strongest argument that can be made about the self-report method is that it frequently yields information that would be difficult, if not impossible, to gather by any other means. Current behaviors can be directly observed, but only if the subject is willing to manifest them publicly. For example, it may be impossible for a researcher to observe such behaviors as child abuse, contraceptive practices, or drug usage. Furthermore, observers can only observe behaviors occurring at the time of the study; self-report instruments can gather *retrospective data* about activities and events occurring in the past, or projections about behaviors in which subjects plan to engage in the future. Information about feelings, values, opinions, and motives can sometimes be inferred through observation, but behaviors and feelings do not always correspond exactly. People's actions do not always tell us about their state of mind. Here again, self-report instruments are designed to measure such psychological characteristics through direct communication with the subject.

Despite these advantages, verbal report instruments share a number of weaknesses. The most serious issue is the question of the validity and accuracy of self-reports: How can we really be sure that respondents feel or act the way they say they do? How can we trust the information that respondents provide, particularly if the questions could potentially require them to reveal an unpopular position on a controversial issue? Investigators often have no alternative but to assume that the majority of their respondents have been frank. Yet we all have a tendency to want to present ourselves in the best light, and this may conflict with the truth. Researchers who find it necessary or appropriate to utilize verbal report instruments should be cognizant of the limitations of this method and should be prepared to take these shortcomings into consideration in interpreting the results. And consumers of research reports should similarly be alert to potential biases introduced when subjects are asked to describe themselves, particularly with respect to behaviors or feelings that our society judges to be wrong.

The next chapter describes in greater detail the characteristics of interviews, questionnaires, and social–psychological scales and presents an overview of how such data-collection instruments are constructed.

Observational Methods

When we witness events in our daily lives, we treat our observations as data for forming opinions, making decisions, predicting future events, and inferring the needs, emotions, and motives of others. The scientist, too, collects information by observing phenomena. Observational methods are, in fact, the methodological backbone in a number of scientific disciplines, such as in anthropology, zoology, astronomy, and so forth. Many kinds of information required by nurse researchers as evidence of nursing effectiveness or as clues to improving nursing practices can be obtained through direct observation. Suppose, for instance, that we were interested in studying nurses' willingness to interact with and listen to patients, or mental patients' methods of defending their personal territory, or children's reactions to the removal of a leg cast, or a patient's mode of emergence from anesthesia. These data could all be collected by the direct observation of the relevant behaviors.

Unlike our casual experiences with the environment, scientific observation places a great emphasis on the objective and systematic nature of observational operations. Weick (1968) has offered the following useful definition of scientific observational methods: "the selection, provocation, recording and encoding of that set of behaviors and settings concerning organisms 'in situ' which is consistent with empirical aims" (p. 360). Let us consider what this definition entails. The term "selection" underlines the importance of identifying specific behaviors or characteristics to be observed. By "provocation," Weick meant to point out that the observer need not be a passive observer in a naturalistic setting. It is often useful to provoke, in an experimental fashion, the very behaviors in which the investigator is interested. Observations must naturally be recorded, often according to some predetermined, systematic plan. Finally, the process of "encoding" refers to the simplification and reduction of the data into some manageable form. Specific procedures for the collection of observational data are presented in Chapter 12.

Within the area of nursing research, observational methods have broad applicability, particularly for clinical inquiries. The nurse is in an advantageous position to observe, relatively unobtrusively, the behaviors and activities of patients, their families, and hospital staff. Like self-reports, one of the reasons that scientists use observational methods is that for some variables there may be no suitable alternative. Self-report measures are inadequate, for example, in gathering data about activities and behaviors about which people may themselves be unaware or unable to verbalize. For certain groups of subjects (e.g., infants, mentally retarded adults, etc.), self-reports may be impossible to use.

Observational methods, like self-reports, are vulnerable to distortion and biases. With observations, distortions can be introduced by the observer as well as by the subject. Perceptual errors and subjectivity are a continuous threat to the quality of obtained information. Some techniques for minimizing observational biases are discussed in Chapter 12.

Physiological Measures

The trend in nursing research has been toward increasing numbers of clinical, patient-centered investigations, and this trend is likely to continue in years to come. As nurse researchers have begun to develop their own special body of clinical knowledge, they have made efforts to ascertain the effectiveness of nursing procedures by a direct examination of patient-outcome variables. An important class of outcome variables are *physiological and biophysical measures* that require specialized technical instruments for the collection of information and, often, specialized training for the interpretation of the results.

Hundreds of physiological measures are potentially available to nurse researchers; clearly, it is beyond the scope of this text to describe or even list such measures. However, the use of physiological measures by nurse researchers is illustrated here to demonstrate the range of possibilities for using such measures in a research context. Blood pressure measurement is an excellent example. Nurse researchers have used blood pressure measures in a study of the relationship between clinical signs and the need for tracheobronchial suctioning, in an evaluation of the effect of group versus individual relaxation therapy in essential hypertension, and in an investigation of time-cycle changes in young women. Other physiological measures that have been frequently used by nurse researchers include measures of blood volume, pulse rate, blood-test results, respiratory volume measures, body temperature readings, hormonal measurements, stool culture tests, and urinalysis results. To illustrate two very different uses of measures in the last category, nurse researchers have used measures from urine tests to evaluate the incidence of urinary tract infection after catheterization and, in another study, to examine the physiological effects of shift rotation among intensive care unit nurses.

Nurse researchers are increasingly collecting physiological data for their clinical research projects. The majority of nursing studies in which physiological measures have been adopted fall into one of two classes: (1) the use of physiological outcomes as the criteria against which nursing actions can be assessed; and (2) the exploration of ways in which nursing actions—including the measuring and recording of physiological functioning—can be improved.

Like other data-collection procedures that we will describe in subsequent chapters, physiological measures offer the researcher distinct advantages as well as several drawbacks. One of the greatest strengths of physiological measures is their objectivity. *Objectivity* refers to the degree of agreement between the final "scores" assigned by two independent observers. Nurse A and nurse B, reading from the same spirometer output, are likely to record the same or highly similar tidal-volume measurements for a patient. And, barring the possibility of equipment malfunctioning, two spirometers are likely to produce identical tidal-volume readouts. Furthermore, patients are unlikely to be able to deliberately distort measurements of physiological functioning.

Another advantage of physiological measurements is the relative precision and sensitivity that they normally offer. By "relative," we are implicitly comparing physiological instruments with devices for obtaining various psychological measurements, such as self-report measures of anxiety, pain, attitudes, and so forth. Furthermore, researchers are generally quite confident that physiological instrumentation provides measures of those variables in which they are interested: thermometers can be depended upon to measure temperature and not blood volume, and so forth. This characteristic may seem so obvious as to render its mention unnecessary. However, for nonphysiological measurements, the question of whether a measuring tool is really measuring the target concept is a continuously perplexing problem.

In comparison with other types of data-collection tools, the equipment for obtaining physiological measurements is rather costly. However, since such equipment is generally available in hospital settings, the costs to nurse researchers would typically be quite small or nonexistent.

A problem that physiological measures share with other data-collection approaches is the effect that the measuring tool itself has on the variables it is attempting to measure. The presence of a sensing device, such as a transducer, can change the variable of interest. For instance, a flow transducer located in a blood vessel partially blocks that vessel and, hence, alters the pressure-flow characteristics being measured. Some researchers have erroneously assumed that physiological measures are unobtrusive, based on the argument that the patients are unaware of the research purposes to which the measurements will be applied. From the body's point of view, however, physiological measures are rarely, if ever, unobtrusive.

Another difficulty is that there are normally interferences that create artifacts in physiological measurements. For example, "noise" generated within a measuring instrument interferes with the signal being produced. The subject may also create artifactual signals, particularly when the subject's movements result in movements of the sensing devices. Many transducers are highly sensitive to motion and may produce signal variations that confound or obscure variations from the critical variable. Another potential complication can result from the high degree of interaction among the major physiological systems. These interrelationships can result in problems in that stimulation of one system can create responses in other systems. Sometimes such responses are unpredictable and poorly understood, resulting in a confounding of effects that is difficult to unravel. Measuring devices themselves can produce interactions in other systems.

In summary, nurse researchers have used a wide range of physiological measurements as criteria against which they can assess nursing interventions and explore ways in which nursing actions can be improved. There are abundant measures of bodily functioning that can be utilized fruitfully by nurse researchers. To nurse researchers, the main advantages of physiological measures are their availability, objectivity, and validity.

Projective Techniques

Questionnaires, interview schedules, and psychological tests and scales normally depend on the respondents' capacity for self-insight or willingness to share personal information with the researcher. *Projective techniques* include a variety of methods for obtaining psychological measures with only a minimum of cooperation required of the person. Projective methods give free play to the subjects' imagination and fantasies by providing them with a task that permits an almost unlimited number and variety of responses. The rationale underlying the use of projective techniques is that the manner in which a person organizes and reacts to unstructured stimuli is a reflection of the person's needs, motives, attitudes, values, or personality characteristics. A stimulus of low structure is sufficiently ambiguous that respondents can "read in" their own interpretations and in this way provide the researcher with information about their perception of the world. In other words, people project part of themselves into their interaction with phenomena, and projective techniques represent a means of taking advantage of this fact.

Projective techniques are highly flexible, since virtually any unstructured stimuli or situation can be used to induce projective behaviors. One class of projective methods utilizes pictorial materials.

One particularly useful *pictorial device* is the Thematic Apperception Test (TAT). The TAT materials consist of 20 cards that contain pictures. The subject is requested to make up a story for each picture, inventing an explanation of what led up to the event shown, what is happening at the moment, what the characters are feeling and thinking, and what kind of outcome will result. The responses are then scored according to some scheme for the variables of interest to the researcher. The TAT and other similar instruments have been used in a variety of contexts. Variables that have been measured by TAT-type pictures are achievement motivation, need for affiliation, parent–child relations, attitude toward minority groups, creativity, religious commitment, attitude toward authority, and fear of success.

Verbal projective techniques present subjects with an ambiguous verbal stimulus rather than a pictorial one. Verbal methods can be categorized into two classes, according to the type of response elicited—association techniques and completion techniques. *Word-association methods* present subjects with a series of words, to which subjects respond with the first thing that comes to mind. The word list often combines both neutral and emotionally tinged words, which are included for the purpose of detecting impaired thought processes or internal conflicts. The word-association technique has also been used to study creativity, interests, and attitudes.

The most common completion technique is *sentence completion*. The person is supplied with a set of incomplete sentences and is asked to complete them in any desired manner. This approach is frequently used as a method of measuring attitudes or some aspect of personality. Some examples of incomplete sentences include the following:

When I think of a nurse practitioner I think . . .

The thing I most admire about nurses is . . .

A good nurse should always . . .

The sentence stems are designed to elicit responses toward some attitudinal object or event in which the investigator is interested. Responses are typically categorized or rated according to a prespecified plan.

A third class of projective measures falls into a category known as *expressive methods*. These techniques encourage self-expression, in most cases through the construction of some product out of raw materials. The major expressive methods are play techniques, drawing and painting, and role-playing. The assumption is that people express their feelings, needs, motives, and emotions by working with or manipulating various materials.

Projective measures are among the most controversial in the behavioral sciences. Critics point out that projective techniques are, by and large, incapable of being scored objectively. A high degree of inference is required in gleaning information from projective tests, and the quality of the data is heavily dependent upon the sensitivity and interpretive skill of the investigator or analyst. It has been pointed out that the interpretation of the responses by the researcher is almost as projective as the subjects' reactions to original stimuli.

Another problem with projective techniques is that there have been difficulties in demonstrating that they are, in fact, measuring the variables that they purport to measure. If a pictorial device is used to score aggressive expressions, can the researcher be confident that individual differences in aggressive responses really reflect underlying differences in aggressiveness?

Projective techniques have supporters as well as critics in the research community. People have advocated using projective devices, arguing that they probe the unconscious mind, encompass the whole personality, and provide data of a breadth and depth unattainable by more traditional methods. One useful feature of projective instruments is that they are less susceptible to faking than self-report measures. Another strength is that it is often easier to build rapport and gain the subject's interest with a projective measure than with a questionnaire or scale. Finally, some projective techniques are particularly useful with special groups, such as children, persons with speech and hearing defects, and so forth. Nevertheless, the use of projective techniques for research applications appears to be associated with more disadvantages than advantages.

Q Sorts

Q methodology is the term coined by William Stephenson to refer to a constellation of concepts relating to research on people. Q methodology utilizes a procedure known as the *Q sort*, which involves the sorting of a deck of cards according to specified criteria.

In a Q sort, the subject is presented with a set of cards on which words, phrases, statements, or other messages are written. The subject is then asked to sort the cards according to a particular dimension, such as approval/disapproval, most like me/least like me, or highest priority/lowest priority. The number of cards to be sorted is typically between 60 and 100. Usually, the subject sorts the cards into 9 or 11 piles, with the number of cards placed in each pile determined by the researcher. A common practice is to have the subjects distribute the cards such that fewer cards are placed at either of the two extremes and more cards are placed toward the middle. Table 10-1 shows a hypothetical distribution of 60 cards, with the specification of the number of cards to be placed in each of the nine piles.

The sorting instructions as well as the objects to be sorted in a Q-sort investigation vary according to the requirements of the research. Attitudes can be studied by asking subjects to sort statements in terms of agreement and disagreement or approval and disapproval. The researcher can study personality by developing cards on which personality characteristics are described. The subject can then be requested to sort items on a "very-much-like-me/not-at-all-like-me" continuum. The technique can also be

Table 10-1. Example of a Distribution of Q Sort Cards

	APPROVE OF LEAST								APPROVE OF MOST
Category	1	2	3	4	5	6	7	8	9
Number of Cards	2	4	7	10	14	10	7	4	2

used to gain information about how people see themselves, as they perceive others see them, as they believe others would like them to be, and so forth. A similar procedure could be used for different ratings of groups, such as intensive care unit nurses, nursing faculty, head nurses, and so forth. Other applications include asking patients to rate nursing behaviors on a continuum of most helpful/least helpful, asking nursing students to rate aspects of their educational preparation along a most-useful/least-useful continuum, and asking primiparas to rate various aspects of their labor and delivery experience in terms of a most-problematic/least-problematic dimension. In short, Q sorts are a versatile method of collecting data.

The number of cards in a Q sort also varies according to the research problem. However, it is unwise to use fewer than 50 or 60 items, since it is difficult to achieve stable and reliable results with a smaller number. On the other hand, 100 to 120 cards are normally considered the upper limit, inasmuch as the task becomes tedious and difficult with larger numbers.

Q methodology can be a powerful methodological tool but, like other data-collection techniques, has a number of drawbacks as well. On the plus side, we have seen that Q sorts are versatile and can be applied to a wide variety of problems. Unlike many other clinical approaches, we find in Q methodology an objective and (usually) reliable procedure for the intensive study of a person. Q sorts have been used effectively to study the progress of people during different phases of therapy, particularly psychotherapy. The requirement that people place a predetermined number of cards in each pile virtually eliminates some of the biases that often characterize responses to written scale items. Furthermore, the task of sorting cards is often more agreeable to subjects than completing a paper-and-pencil task.

On the other hand, it is difficult and time-consuming to administer Q sorts to a large sample of persons. Without a sizeable sample, it becomes problematic to generalize the results of the study to a broad population. The sampling problem is further compounded by the fact that Q sorts cannot normally be administered by the mail, thereby causing difficulties in obtaining a geographically diverse sample of subjects. Some critics have argued that the forced procedure of distributing cards according to the researcher's specifications is artificial and actually excludes information about how the subjects would ordinarily distribute their opinions.

Records and Available Data

A researcher need not collect fresh data in order to make a worthwhile scientific contribution. Existing information can be looked at in new ways, and the relationship between variables from available sources can be analyzed. Nurse researchers are particularly fortunate in the amount and quality of existing data available to them for exploration. Hospital records, nursing charts, physicians' order sheets, care-plan statements, nursing students' grades, NLN examination scores, and so forth, all constitute rich data sources to which nurse researchers may have access.

The places where a nurse researcher is likely to find useful records are too numerous to list here, but a few suggestions might be helpful. Within a hospital or other health-care setting, excellent records are kept routinely and systematically. In addition to medical records, hospitals maintain financial records, personnel records, nutritional records, and so forth. Educational institutions maintain records of varying quality. Most schools of nursing have permanent files on their students. Industries and businesses normally maintain a variety of records that might interest industrial nurse researchers, such as information on employees' absenteeism, health status, on-the-job accidents, job-performance ratings, alcoholism or drug problems, and so forth. The state and federal governments also maintain records that have been used frequently by researchers in the behavioral sciences. Census data and records on vital and health statistics are illustrations of important federal records available for use. In addition to institutional records, personal documents such as diaries and letters should be considered.

The use of information from records is advantageous to the researcher for several reasons. The most salient advantage of existing records is that they are an economical source of information. The collection of data is often the most time-consuming and costly step in the research process. The use of preexisting records also permits an examination of trends over time, if the information is of the type that is collected repeatedly. Problems of response biases may be completely absent when the researcher obtains information from records. Furthermore, the investigator does not have to be concerned with obtaining cooperation from participants.

On the other hand, since the researcher has not been responsible for the collection and recording of information, he or she may be unaware of the limitations, biases, or incompleteness of the records. Two of the major sources of biases in records are *selective deposit* and *selective survival*. If the records available for use do not constitute the entire set of all possible such records, the investigator must somehow deal with the question of how representative the existing records are. Many record keepers intend to maintain an entire universe or set of records rather than a sample but may fail to adhere to this ideal. The lapses from the ideal may be the result of some systematic biases, and the careful researcher should attempt to learn what those biases might be.

An additional problem with which researchers must contend is the increasing reluctance of institutions to make their records available for scientific studies. The Privacy Act, a federal regulation enacted to protect people against possible misuses of records, has made hospitals, agencies, schools, and industrial organizations sensitive to the possibility of lawsuits from persons who feel that their right to privacy has been violated. The major issue here is the divulgence of a person's identity. If records are maintained with an identifying number rather than a name, permission to use the records may be readily granted. However, most institutions do maintain records by their clients' names.

A number of other difficulties in the use of records for research purposes may be relevant. Sometimes the records have to be verified in terms of their authenticity, authorship, or accuracy, a task that may be difficult to execute if the records are old. The researcher using records must be prepared to deal with forms and file systems that he or she does not understand. Codes and symbols that had meaning to the record keeper may have to be "translated" in order to be usable. In using records to study trends, the researcher should always be alert to the possibility of changes in record-keeping procedures. For example, does a dramatic increase or decrease in the incidence of sudden infant death syndrome reflect changes in the causes or cures of this problem, or does it reflect a change in diagnosis or record keeping?

These considerations suggest that, while existing records may be plentiful, inexpensive, and accessible, they should not be used without paying attention to potential problems and weaknesses.

Selection of a Measurement Approach

As noted repeatedly in this chapter, every method of measuring variables has strengths and weaknesses. Sometimes the limitations involve pragmatic considerations, such as time or costs, while others involve potential problems of data quality. Barring practical constraints, the researcher should obviously attempt to use the method that yields the most unbiased, accurate information possible. There is little justification for using an approach that is creative and entertaining if the resulting data cannot be meaningfully interpreted. On the other hand, if subjects become bored with a task (e.g., completing a lengthy questionnaire), they may fail to provide honest responses, or they may not behave normally.

Biases that reduce the accuracy of the data can be introduced in many ways. As we have seen, each measurement approach has the potential for certain types of biases, usually those stemming from either the subjects or the investigator. Researchers need to be thoroughly familiar with the risks attached to each method and to take steps to minimize those risks. In addition, biases can result from environmental conditions. For example, in an interview study, biases may result if the interview takes place in a distracting setting, in a room that is too hot or cold, or under conditions in which privacy might be jeopardized. The careful researcher must take all such possibilities for distortion into consideration.

Decisions relating to the identification or development of an appropriate data-collection strategy are perhaps the most difficult of the decisions a researcher faces. Fortunately, there are some objective criteria for evaluating the quality of measuring tools (see Chap. 13), but, unfortunately, the steps required to apply such criteria are typically laborious and time-consuming. Even when a researcher takes these steps to assess the worth of a measure, the fact remains that all tools have some imperfections. Given the improbability of ever finding *the* perfect criterion measure, researchers may be well advised to employ *multiple criterion measures*, in which the measurement strengths of each complement one another.

Research Example

Hoefener (1984) investigated the effect of lactation on the nutritional patterns and status of primiparas who had just given birth.* A sample of 300 women were recruited for participation in the study during the second trimester of pregnancy. All women were instructed about the advantages of breast-feeding and were given some written materials about infant nutrition. One month after consenting to participate, prospective subjects were asked to indicate whether they intended to breast-feed or bottle-feed. All 65 bottle-feeders were then matched to 65 of the breast-feeders on the basis of prepregnancy weight (relative to height) and prepregnancy nutritional habits (rated on a 5-point scale from poor to excellent by a dietitian). Two weeks following delivery, the feeding routine of the new mothers was ascertained. Those who deviated from their original plans (*e.g.,* breast-feeders who switched to formula) were dropped from the sample, together with their matched pair. Mothers of twins or mothers with other complicating circumstances were similarly excluded. The final sample consisted of 53 matched pairs. Each subject was then requested to do a 24-hour dietary recall, recording all items consumed in a 24-hour period. For each record, total caloric intake was computed. Five-point ratings were also assigned to describe the quality of food consumed. The bottle-feeders and breast-

---

*This example is fictitious.

feeders were then compared in terms of these two measures of nutritional status. No differences between the two groups were found. The researcher concluded that lactation does not affect nutritional status.

In this example, the researcher decided to define nutritional status in terms of self-reported eating habits. We can evaluate the researcher's decision from two points of view: (1) Given that the researcher was using self-reports, were the methods employed sound? and (2) Would some alternative to self-reports have yielded more accurate and meaningful data?

With respect to the first question, a thorough critique would require an inspection of the actual instrument. Several comments based on the above summary merit comment, however. The first concerns the issue of whether or not the 24-hour period during which the information was gathered was typical for the respondents. One could argue that any "deviant" diets among the bottle-feeders would probably be compensated for by untypical diets in the breast-feeders group. Still, with only 53 subjects per group, there might be a chance that some unusual diets would be more prevalent in one or the other group. More stable estimates might have been obtained by gathering data for two 24-hour periods, ideally not on contiguous days.

A second comment concerns how the information from the dietary recalls was converted to research variables. Hoefener derived two measures based on the wealth of information provided. Caloric count, the first measure, appears to have been a good choice: it is an easily quantified measure, is readily usable in statistical operations (e.g., the average caloric intake per group can be computed), and is objective. The second measure, the evaluative ratings of the mothers' eating pattern, is less sound, particularly because of its dependence on subjective judgment. At a minimum, the researcher should have used two independent raters to assess the objectivity of the ratings. A better procedure would have been to derive from the data less judgmental indicators of a high-quality diet, such as the intake of certain nutrients (e.g., protein, iron, vitamin C) as a percentage of recommended daily allowances.

The more important question is whether the investigator could have improved the study by selecting an approach other than self-report. The main problem with the self-report method is that the respondents might—consciously or unconsciously—provide inaccurate data. The women could forget some of what they consumed, or they might be embarrassed to report eating some nonnutritious food, particularly to a nurse researcher. However, alternatives might have different problems of similar magnitude. One alternative might be to gather observational data—that is, have a person affiliated with the research observe and record what the subjects consumed. Certainly, one would expect an independent observer to record more accurate information about eating behavior than the subjects themselves, although the presence of an observer could alter the food consumed. Furthermore, unless such observation could be carried out in a structured setting, such as the postpartum unit of the hospital, there would be many practical barriers to this option, including an enormous expenditure of time and the subjects' unwillingness to cooperate in the study. Observation during hospitalization would have to be ruled out because of the timing (i.e., most women are released 2–3 days postpartum, often before a final decision about breast- or bottle-feeding is made) and because there is too little variation in hospital food (i.e., most women would be eating fairly nutritious meals). In all likelihood, the use of observational measures would not prove feasible, although it would be technically possible and methodologically desirable to do so.

Another option would be to gather information of a more physiological nature. Participants could be subjected to one or several tests that yield information about nutritional status. As one example, urinary creatinine excretion is sometimes used as an indicator of lean body mass. Physiological measures, while they are generally highly accurate, nevertheless may be problematic because they are often sensitive to conditions other than the variable of interest. Things other than yesterday's diet would affect creatinine levels, for example. Again, if it could be assumed that such influences were counterbalanced in the two groups, this would not be a problem, but with small samples this assumption might not be warranted.

In summary, a self-report approach in this example is defensible, given some of the problems with alternatives. The best method, however, would probably be to use a combination of self-report and physiological data.

Summary

A wide variety of measurement approaches is available to nurse researchers. Decisions relating to the choice of measurement tools are among the most difficult facing scientists, because each measurement approach has a number of limitations, as well as strengths. This chapter presents an overview of the major methods of data collection.

Perhaps the most commonly used method is the self-report approach, which involves direct questioning of subjects regarding the desired information. Self-report data are generally gathered by means of a formal instrument referred to as an *interview schedule* if an interviewer orally asks subjects predesignated questions, or a *questionnaire* if the subject responds in writing to questions presented in a printed format. Sometimes self-report information is gathered by means of a *social–psychological scale*, which is designed to measure the degree to which subjects are characterized by certain traits. Self-report measures are direct and take advantage of the unique verbal skills of human beings, but may suffer from deliberate or unconscious distortions.

Observational methods are techniques for acquiring information through the direct observation, recording, and interpretation of behaviors, events, or conditions. Observational techniques are versatile and have many potential applications by nurse researchers. Perhaps the greatest strength of observation is that it allows for the collection of data that would be difficult to obtain in any other way. Important descriptive information about behaviors of which subjects are unaware or about which they are reluctant to discuss can often be collected through observation. On the other hand, not all behaviors of interest to scientists are exhibited publicly. Observation can in some situations be criticized on ethical grounds with respect to invasion of privacy. In addition to problems of an ethical nature, observation is subject to a variety of biasing effects. The greater the degree of observer inference and judgment, the more likely it is that perceptual errors and distortions will occur.

Data may also be derived from *physiological or biophysical measurements*. A wide range of physiological measures have been used as criterion measures for clinical nursing studies. One of the greatest advantages in using physiological measures is their high degree of objectivity and validity. Independent researchers are apt to obtain the same results using the same measure. Disadvantages associated with the use of physiological instrumentation are malfunctioning of the equipment and artifacts that interfere with the system.

Projective techniques encompass a variety of data-collection methods that rely on the subject's projection of psychological traits or states in response to vaguely structured stimuli. *Pictorial methods* are methods in which the subject is presented with a picture or cartoon and asked to describe what is happening, what led up to the event, or what kind of action is needed. In *verbal methods*, the subject is presented with an ambiguous verbal stimulus rather than a picture. The two categories of verbal methods are *word association* and *sentence completion*. *Expressive methods* take the form of *play*, *drawing*, or *role-playing*.

Q methodology involves having the subject sort a set of statements into piles according to specified criteria. Attitudes, personality, and self-concept are some of the traits that may be measured by Q methodology. The procedure may be used to study a person in depth or to rate groups of people. Q sorts are flexible and helpful in avoiding certain biases, such as the tendency for people to present themselves in the best possible light. However, Q sorts are time-consuming and difficult to administer to large or geographically dispersed samples.

Existing *records* are often used by researchers in the conduct of scientific investigations. Such records provide an economical source of information. In using records, the researcher should try to determine how representative and accurate they are.

Researchers should strive to gather their data with measures that yield the most accurate information. However, since all measures are subject to some distortions or biases, it is often advisable to use more than one measure of key outcome variables so that the biases of one approach can be offset by the strengths of another.

Study Suggestions

1. Suppose that you were interested in studying the following variables: professionalism in nurses, fear of death in patients, achievement motivation in nursing students, job satisfaction among industrial nurses, fathers' reactions to their newborn infants, and patients' needs for affiliation. Describe at least two ways of collecting data relating to these concepts, using the following approaches:
   a. Interviews
   b. Verbal projective techniques
   c. Observational methods
   d. Records
   e. Q sorts

2. Suppose you were interested in studying each of the following research problems. Indicate for each whether you would use an observational or self-report approach. Justify your response.
   a. Does the administration of drug X to burn patients affect the patients' appetite?
   b. Are student nurses more confident about their clinical skills if they have more hours of supervised clinical instruction?
   c. Is nursing-staff morale lower in hospitals that have implemented extensive computerized systems?
   d. Are new mothers more satisfied with their childbirth experience if they have used birthing rooms rather than labor and delivery rooms?

3. Formulate a research problem in which each of the following could be used as the measurements for the dependent variable:
   a. Galvanic skin response
   b. Electromyograms
   c. Thermograms
   d. Blood-sugar levels

4. Suppose that you were interested in using a story-completion technique to study separation anxiety in young hospitalized children. Develop an introduction to the story and a set of instructions.

Chapter 11
Self-Report Techniques

The self-report approach to collecting data is a flexible and indispensable tool in scientific research with human beings. Survey research relies almost exclusively on self-reports. Other types of research—evaluations, needs assessments, retrospective and prospective studies, case studies, trend studies, and so on—also use direct questioning extensively. Self-reports can be used to collect data in experiments, quasi-experiments, and nonexperiments. In short, whenever humans can communicate accurately about the information needed to answer research questions, self-reports may be the most appropriate way to gather the data.

Self-report data are usually collected by means of a formal, written document (often referred to as an *instrument*). The instrument is generally known as an interview schedule or questionnaire. Sometimes a psychological scale is used to collect self-report data, but such scales are often incorporated into an interview schedule or questionnaire. These various types of instruments are described in greater detail below.

Questionnaires and Interview Schedules

An *interview schedule* is used in situations in which a person who represents the research team orally asks questions of the participants in the study, either in a face-to-face meeting or over the telephone. In such cases the interview schedule guides the interviewer in terms of both the phrasing of the questions and the recording of the responses. *Questionnaires*, on the other hand, are self-administered by the respondents. These two forms of self-report instruments are similar, but they are not interchangeable. An instrument designed to be used as an interview schedule should never be administered as a questionnaire. Let us examine some of the properties of self-report instruments to see why this is so.

Form of the Instrument

Self-report instruments vary in the extent to which they are structured. At one extreme, *standardized* or tightly *structured schedules* consist of a set of items in which the wording of both the question and the alternative responses is predetermined. When structured interviews or questionnaires are used, all subjects are asked to respond to exactly the same questions, in exactly the same order, and have the same set of options for their responses. The purpose of such a high degree of structure is to ensure comparability of responses.

At the other end of the continuum, information can be gathered by a totally unstructured interview in which the researcher does not specify in advance either the exact questions or the alternative responses. Questionnaires cannot fall into this category, since the investigator must make some decisions in committing the questions to a written form. Although unstructured interviews have no predetermined questions, the interviewer normally is given a set of topics to cover (sometimes called a *topic guide*). The interviewer's function is to encourage participants to talk freely about the topics of interest and to record the responses. Unstructured interviews have a number of potential difficulties, particularly in terms of making comparisons between subjects, but the flexibility of the approach is sometimes useful in exploratory research.

Most self-report instruments fall in between these two extremes by using a combination of open-ended and closed-ended questions. *Open-ended* items allow subjects to respond to the question in their own words. The question "What aspect of your professional relationship with physicians do you feel is most in need of improvement?" is an example of an open-ended question that might be used in a study investigating nurse–physician relations. In questionnaires the respondent is asked to give a written reply to open-ended items and, therefore, adequate space must be provided to allow the expression of opinions. In interviews, the interviewer is normally expected to quote the response verbatim.

Closed-ended (or *fixed-alternative*) questions offer respondents a number of alternative replies from which the subjects must choose the one that most closely approximates the "right" answer. The alternatives may range from the simple yes–no variety ("Have you smoked a cigarette within the past 24 hours?") to rather complex expressions of opinion or behavior.

Both open-ended and closed-ended questions have certain strengths and weaknesses. Closed-ended items are more difficult to construct but easier to administer and, especially, to analyze. With closed-ended questions, the researcher needs only to tabulate the number of responses to each alternative in order to gain some understanding about what the sample as a whole thinks about an issue. The analysis of open-ended items, on the other hand, is often problematic and time-consuming. The procedure that is normally followed is the development of categories and the assignment of the open-ended responses to those categories. That is, the researcher essentially transforms the open-ended responses to fixed categories in a post hoc fashion so that tabulations can be made. This classification process takes considerable time and skill. Furthermore, since the ultimate classification decision lies in the hands of the researchers rather than the respondents, there is the possibility of inappropriate categorization caused by misinterpretation of the responses or an inadequate classification system. Therefore, when the categories of interest can be developed beforehand, the researcher can facilitate the analysis of the data.

Closed-ended items are generally more efficient than open-ended questions in the sense that a respondent is normally able to complete more closed-ended items than open-ended ones in a given amount of time. This is one of the reasons that interview schedules and questionnaires are not interchangeable. Questionnaires rarely have more than a handful of open-ended questions, since most respondents are unwilling to compose lengthy written answers. A researcher who administers a questionnaire with many open-ended questions risks a high rate of refusals to participate or poor-quality data. In addition to efficiency and analytic ease, another advantage of closed-ended questions is that they can be more readily used with respondents who have difficulty in expressing themselves verbally. Furthermore, there are some types of questions that may seem less objectionable in closed form than in open form. Take the following example:

1. What was the gross annual income of your family last year?
2. In what range was your family's gross annual income last year?
   ( ) under $10,000
   ( ) $10,000 to $14,999
   ( ) $15,000 to $19,999
   ( ) $20,000 to $24,999
   ( ) $25,000 to $29,999
   ( ) $30,000 or over

The second question is more likely to be answered by respondents since the range of the options allows them a greater measure of privacy than the more blunt open-ended question.

These various advantages of the fixed-alternative question are offset by some corresponding shortcomings. The major drawback of closed-ended questions lies in the possibility of the researcher neglecting or overlooking some potentially important responses. It is often very difficult to see an issue from multiple points of view. The omission of possible alternatives can, of course, lead to inadequate understanding of the issues and to outright bias if the respondents choose an alternative that misrepresents their position.

Another objection to closed-ended items is that they are sometimes considered too superficial. Open-ended questions allow for a richer and fuller perspective on the topic of interest if the respondents are verbally expressive and cooperative. Some of this richness may be lost when the researcher later tabulates answers by developing a system of classification, but excerpts taken directly from the open-ended responses can be extremely valuable in the research report in imparting the "flavor" of the replies.

Finally, some respondents will often object to being forced into choosing from among responses that do not reflect their opinions precisely. Open-ended questions give a lot of freedom to the respondent and, therefore, offer the possibility of spontaneity unattainable when a set of responses is provided.

In conclusion, the decision about an instrument's degree of structure should be based on a number of important considerations, such as the verbal ability of the respondents, the amount of time available, and so forth. Combinations of both types are highly recommended to offset the strengths and weaknesses of each, but questionnaires will normally consist of a preponderance of fixed-alternative questions.

Question Wording and Content

Another feature that sometimes distinguishes interview schedules and questionnaires involves the actual questions themselves. One issue relates to the clarity of the wording. It seems fairly obvious that the designer of a questionnaire or interview schedule should strive for clarity and precision. A question that can be interpreted differently by different people is unlikely to produce meaningful information. Unfortunately, clarity is more easily discussed than achieved. Even seemingly simple and straightforward questions may be ambiguous or open to various interpretations to respondents who do not have the same perspective on the issues as the researcher. The question "When do you usually eat your evening meal?" might bring forth such responses as "around 6 PM," "when my husband gets home from work," or "during the evening television news broadcast." The question itself contains no words that are technical or difficult, but the question can be responded to in a variety of ways because the intent of the researcher is not apparent. The need for clarity is more critical in a questionnaire than in an interview schedule, because with a questionnaire respondents cannot ask for clarification.

Another issue relates to the respondents' ability to provide the requested information. Research participants are often reluctant to say "I don't know" or "I don't understand," perhaps out of embarrassment or perhaps to avoid appearing uncooperative. There are several techniques for wording a question in such a way that "don't know" responses may appear acceptable to respondents. Nevertheless, methodological research has shown that subjects are more willing to admit ignorance of some topic or the lack of any opinion when responding privately to a questionnaire rather than they are to admit it to an interviewer.

A related concern involves questions of a personal or sensitive nature. All questionnaires and interview schedules represent an intrusion on people's privacy. Instruments should always be designed to show courtesy, consideration, and appreciation to respondents. There are many techniques for the wording of questions that are designed to create an atmosphere of objectivity and nonjudgment. Nevertheless, questions of a highly sensitive nature (e.g., questions about drug use or extramarital sexual behavior) may be more comfortably answered on a questionnaire than in an interview situation.

Instrument Format

The appearance and layout of the schedule may seem a matter of minor administrative importance. However, a poorly designed format can have substantive consequences if respondents (or interviewers) become confused, miss questions, or answer questions that they should have omitted. The format is more important in the case of questionnaires since respondents are unfamiliar with the researcher's intent and will not usually have an opportunity to ask questions.

It is generally easier to follow the flow of an instrument if there is ample space and if response alternatives are aligned vertically. Respondents can be asked either to circle the appropriate answer or to place a check in the appropriate box, illustrated below as Methods A and B:

Are you a member of the American Nurses' Association?

Method A (Circling)	*Method B (Checking)*
1. Yes	1. [ ] Yes
2. No	2. [ ] No

Special care should be given to formatting *filter questions*, which are designed to route respondents through different sets of questions depending on their response to earlier questions. Probably the least confusing approach is to set off questions appropriate to only a subset of respondents from the main series of questions, as shown below.

4. Are you a member of the American Nurses' Association?

    [ ] Yes———┐

    [ ] No   ↓

                  5. If yes: For how many years have you been a member? _____years

6. Do you subscribe to any nursing journals?

    [ ] Yes

    [ ] No

There are alternative procedures, but they are more likely to give rise to difficulties. Instructions such as "skip to question 6" might be misunderstood by some respondents. It is also best to avoid forcing all readers to go through inapplicable questions. That is, question 5 in the example above could have been worded "If you are a member of ANA, for how long have you been a member?" The person who is not an ANA member might not be sure how to handle this question and might be annoyed at having to read through material that is not relevant. Again, it is much more important to have a well-formatted questionnaire than interview schedule. "Skip to" instructions are commonly used in interview schedules because interviewers are generally thoroughly trained in the use of the instrument.

Collection of Self-Report Data

Interview schedules and questionnaires require different skills and different considerations in their administration. Let us first consider the collection of data via questionnaires. Self-administered questionnaires can be distributed in a number of ways. The most convenient procedure is to administer the questionnaire to an intact group of respondents (e.g., a class of students) who complete the instrument simultaneously. This approach has the obvious advantage of maximizing the number of completions and allowing the researcher to clarify any possible misunderstandings about the instrument.

Personal delivery or pick-up of questionnaires to individual respondents is another alternative. The personal contact of the respondent with the research personnel seems to have a positive effect on the rate of questionnaires completed. The presence of a research worker also can be an advantage in terms of explaining and clarifying the study or particular questions. This method is, however, relatively time-consuming and expensive if delivery is made to respondents' homes.

Questionnaires are often mailed to respondents. The problem with this approach is that the response rates tend to be very low. Low response rates can cause major difficulties. When only a small subsample of respondents return their questionnaires, it may be unreasonable to assume that those who did respond were somehow "typical" of the sample as a whole. In other words, the researcher is faced with the possibility that those persons who did not complete a questionnaire would as a group have answered the questions differently from those who did return the schedule. In such a situation, it may be inappropriate to generalize the results of the study to the target population.

The use of *follow-up reminders* has been found to be effective in achieving higher response rates for mailed questionnaires. This procedure involves the mailing of additional letters urging nonrespondents to complete and return their schedules. Follow-up letters or notices are typically sent 2 to 3 weeks after the initial mailing. A number of techniques have been adopted for follow-ups, the simplest being a letter of encouragement to nonrespondents. It is preferable, however, to enclose a second copy of the questionnaire with the reminder letter since most people will have misplaced the original copy. Telephone follow-ups can be quite successful, but they are costly and involve a considerable amount of time.

The successful collection of interview data, in contrast to questionnaire data, is strongly dependent on interpersonal skills. A primary task of the interviewer is to put respondents at ease so that they will feel comfortable in expressing their honest opinions. The respondents' personal reaction to the interviewer can seriously affect their willingness to participate. The interviewer should strive to appear unbiased and to create a permissive atmosphere that encourages candor. The job of the interviewer is to serve as a neutral medium of communication.

The interviewer undoubtedly will find that obtaining complete and relevant responses is not always an easy matter. Respondents often reply to seemingly straightforward questions with irrelevant discussions or partial answers, or they may say "I don't know" to avoid giving their opinions on sensitive topics or to stall while they think over the question. In such cases the job of the interviewer is to *probe*. The purpose of a probe is to elicit more useful information from a respondent than was volunteered during the first reply. A probe can take many forms: sometimes it involves a repetition of the original questions and sometimes it is a long pause intended to communicate to respondents that they should continue. Frequently, it is necessary to encourage a more complete response by a nondirective supplementary question, such as "How is that?" or "Anything else?" or "Could you explain a bit further?" The interviewer must be careful to insert only neutral probes that do not influence the subject's response. The ability to probe well is perhaps the greatest test of an interviewer's skill.

The guidelines for handling telephone interviews are essentially the same as those for face-to-face interviews, although additional effort usually is required to build rapport over the telephone. In both cases, the interviewer should strive to make the interview a pleasant and satisfying experience in which respondents are made to feel as though the information they are providing is important.

Questionnaires vs. Interviews: An Assessment

Self-administered questionnaires offer a number of advantages over personal interviews, but they have some drawbacks as well. First, let us consider some of the strong points of questionnaires.

1. Questionnaires, relative to interviews, are generally much less costly and require less time and energy to administer. Group-administered questionnaires are clearly the least expensive and time-consuming of any

procedure. With a fixed amount of funds or time, a larger and more geographically diverse sample can usually be obtained with mailed questionnaires than with interviews.

2. Questionnaires, unlike interview schedules, offer the possibility of complete anonymity. Sometimes a guarantee of anonymity is crucial in obtaining candid responses, particularly if the questions are of a highly personal or sensitive nature. Anonymous questionnaires often result in a higher proportion of socially unacceptable responses (*i.e.*, responses in which the respondent admits to deviant behavior or an unpopular opinion) than do face-to-face interviews.

3. The absence of an interviewer assures that there will be no interviewer bias. Ideally, an interviewer is a neutral agent through whom questions and answers are passed. Studies have shown, however, that this ideal is difficult to achieve. Respondents and interviewers interact as human beings, and this interaction can affect the subject's responses. This problem clearly is not present for questionnaires.

Despite these advantages, the strengths of interviews far outweigh those of questionnaires. For most research purposes, interviews are superior to questionnaires, for the following reasons:

1. The response rate tends to be high in face-to-face interviews. Respondents are apparently more reluctant to refuse to talk to an interviewer who is directly in front of them than to discard or ignore a questionnaire.

2. There are many people who simply cannot fill out a questionnaire. Examples include young children, the blind, the very elderly, the illiterate, or the uneducated. Interviews, on the other hand, are normally feasible with most people.

3. Interviews offer a protection against ambiguous or confusing questions. The interviewer can determine whether questions have been misunderstood and clarify matters. In questionnaires, items that are misinterpreted may go undetected by the researchers, and thus the responses may lead to erroneous conclusions.

4. The information obtained from questionnaires tends to be somewhat more superficial than interview data. This situation is due partly to the fact that questionnaires ordinarily contain a preponderance of closed-ended items. Open-ended questions often engender resentment among questionnaire respondents, who dislike having to compose and write out a reply. Much of the richness and complexity of the human experience can be lost if closed-ended items are used exclusively. Furthermore, interviewers can enhance the quality of their data through judicious probing.

5. Interviews permit greater control over the sample in the sense that the interviewer knows whether or not the person being interviewed is the intended participant. It is common to have persons who receive questionnaires pass the schedule on to a friend, relative, secretary, and so forth. This kind of activity can change the characteristics of the sample.

6. Finally, face-to-face interviews have an advantage in their ability to produce additional data through observation. The interviewer is in a position to observe or judge the respondents' level of understanding, degree of cooperativeness, social class, life-style, and so forth. These kinds of information can be most useful in interpreting the responses.

It should also be pointed out that many of the advantages of face-to-face interviews also apply to telephone interviews. Complicated or detailed schedules clearly are not well suited for telephone interviewing but, for relatively brief instruments, the telephone interview combines the cheapness and the ease of administration of questionnaires with relatively high response rates.

Designing Self-Report Instruments

In an introductory textbook such as this, it is impossible to adequately describe the numerous techniques that have been developed to design high-quality self-report instruments. It is important for beginning researchers to recognize, however, that the construction of instruments that contain unambiguous, relevant, and diplomatically worded questions and that yield accurate and meaningful data is a task that requires considerable skill and artistry. Useful tips on how to design high-caliber instruments are provided in Bradburn and Sudman (1979), Polit and Hungler (1983), and Selltiz and associates (1976). In this section we present an overview of the instrument development process and then illustrate several types of closed-ended questions.

Steps in Instrument Development

A careful, well-developed schedule cannot be prepared in minutes or even in hours. A researcher interested in designing a useful and accurate instrument must devote considerable time to analyzing the research requirements and attending to minute details. If a researcher is sloppy or haphazard in designing an instrument, little confidence can be placed in the obtained data. Imagine how wary you might be in using a piece of technical equipment—say a sphygmomanometer—that had been designed in haste and inadequately tested. The following steps are normally required to develop a sound self-report instrument:

1. A decision must be made regarding instrument form. If the instrument is to be self-administered, the questions probably will be more structured and fewer open-ended questions will be necessary than if an interview were used.

2. Next, a decision is made regarding the type of information that needs to be collected. Direct questioning is particularly useful for obtain-

ing the following kinds of information: facts about the respondent or others known to the respondent (e.g., birth date, hospitalization history); beliefs (e.g., smokers' beliefs about the risks of lung cancer); attitudes and feelings (e.g., patients' fear of death); knowledge (e.g., nurses' knowledge about malpractice suits); and intentions (e.g., nursing students' intention to attend graduate school).

3. Questions for all relevant content areas are then drafted. Since there is a considerable variety of question types, there is ample room here for ingenuity and creativity. The wording of each question needs to be carefully monitored for clarity, sensitivity to the respondents' psychological state, freedom from bias, and (in questionnaires) reading levels. For closed-ended questions, careful attention must also be paid to the handling of response alternatives. The responses should adequately encompass all of the significant alternatives. Furthermore, the alternatives should be mutually exclusive. Ideally, alternatives should not be too lengthy since it is inefficient and cumbersome for subjects to read detailed replies. In general, the response alternatives should be approximately equal in length. If response A consists of 30 words and response B consists of 5 words, the respondents probably are subtly being told something about the researcher's point of view, which could influence their responses.

4. The questions are seldom written in their order of presentation, so the next step should be to decide how to sequence the questions. A questionnaire or interview schedule is not a random set of questions that the researcher pulls out of a hat. Some thought needs to be given to the sequencing of the questions so as to arrive at an order that is psychologically meaningful to respondents and encourages candor and cooperation. For example, the schedule should begin with questions that are interesting and motivating. The instrument also needs to be arranged in such a way that distortions and biases are minimized. The possibility that earlier questions will influence replies to the subsequent questions is an everpresent problem. Whenever both general and specific questions about a topic are to be included, the general question should be placed first to avoid putting ideas into people's heads. Once the questions have been ordered, the instrument can be formatted.

5. An introduction should then be written and, for questionnaires, instructions on how to complete the form should be prepared. Every schedule should be prefaced by some introductory comments about the nature and purpose of the study. In face-to-face or telephone interviews the introductory comments would normally be read to the respondents by the interviewer. In questionnaires the introduction usually takes the form of a cover letter accompanying the instrument. The introduction should be given considerable care and attention, since it represents the first point of contact between the researcher and potential respondents. The introduction would normally answer the following questions:

  . What is the purpose of the study? Why should the respondent spend time providing the information; that is, what contribution is the respondent making?

- How did the respondent come to be selected? Where did you get his or her name? (People are sometimes puzzled by or suspicious about being selected to participate in a study.)
- What will be done with the information? Will confidentiality or anonymity be maintained?
- What is the deadline for the return of the schedule (in the case of a questionnaire)? How should the respondent go about returning the questionnaire?
- Has the respondent been adequately thanked for participating in the study?

6. When a first draft of the instrument is in reasonably good order, it should be discussed critically with persons who are knowledgeable about the construction of questionnaires and with persons who are familiar with the substantive content of the schedule. The instrument should also be reviewed by someone who is capable of detecting technical difficulties, such as spelling mistakes, grammatical errors, and so forth. When these various persons have provided feedback, a revised version of the instrument can be pretested.

7. A *pretest* of an instrument is a trial run to determine, insofar as possible, its clarity, research adequacy, and freedom from bias. The pretest provides an opportunity for detecting at least gross inadequacies or unforeseen problems before going to the expense of a full-scale study. The pretest should be administered to persons who are similar to those who will ultimately participate in the study.

Examples of Closed-Ended Questions

It is often difficult to design good-quality closed-ended questions because the researcher must pay careful attention not only to the wording of the question but also to the content, wording, and formatting of the fixed alternatives. Nevertheless, the analytic advantages of closed-ended questions make it compelling to include at least some on most instruments. In this section we illustrate several different types of closed-ended questions.

The simplest type of closed-ended questions requires the respondent to make a choice between two alternatives. *Dichotomous items,* as such questions are called, are considered most appropriate for gathering factual information, as in the following example:

Have you ever taken a course in statistics?

( ) Yes

( ) No

Dichotomous items often are considered too restrictive by respondents, who may resent being forced to see an issue as either yes or no. Graded alternatives are preferable for opinion or attitude questions because they give the researcher more information and because they give the respondent the opportunity to be more accurate. A range of alternatives provides more information in that the researcher can measure intensity of feeling as well as direction. Multiple-choice questions most commonly offer three to five alternatives, as in the example below:

How important is it to you to work in a hospital that has ample opportunity for advancement?

( ) Extremely important
( ) Very important
( ) Somewhat important
( ) Not at all important

A special type of multiple choice is the "cafeteria" question, which asks respondents to select a response that most adequately states their view:

People have very different opinions about the use of estrogen replacement therapy for women in menopause. Which of the following statements best represents your point of view?

1. Estrogen replacement is dangerous and should be totally banned.
2. Estrogen replacement may have some undesirable side-effects that suggest the need for caution in its use.
3. I am undecided about my views on estrogen replacement therapy.
4. Estrogen replacement has many beneficial effects that merit its promotion.
5. Estrogen replacement is a wonder cure that should be administered routinely to menopausal women.

Rank-order questions ask respondents to rank their responses along a continuum from most favorable to least favorable (or most/least important, beneficial, familiar, etc.). They can be quite useful but need to be carefully handled because they are often misunderstood by respondents. Here is an example:

People value different things about life. Below is a list of principles or ideas that are often cited when people are asked to name the things that they value most. Please indicate the order of importance of these values to you by placing a "1" beside the most important, "2" beside the next most important, and so forth.

( ) Achievement and success
( ) Family relationships
( ) Friendships and social interaction
( ) Health
( ) Money
( ) Religion

Checklists are items that encompass several questions on a topic and require the same response format. Checklists are relatively efficient and easy for respondents to understand. Since checklists are difficult for an interviewer to read, they are used more frequently in self-administered questionnaires than in interviews.

A checklist is often a two-dimensional arrangement in which a series of questions is listed along one dimension (usually vertically) and response alternatives are listed along the other. It is this two-dimensional character that is being referred to when the term *matrix question* is used by some writers instead of the term "checklist." An example of a checklist follows:

Here are some characteristics of birth-control devices that are of varying importance to different people. How important a consideration has each of these been for *you* in choosing a birth-control method?

	Of Very Great Importance	Of Great Importance	Of Some Importance	Of No Importance
1. *Comfort*				
2. *Cost*				
3. *Ease of use*				
4. *Effectiveness*				
5. *Noninterference with spontaneity*				
6. *Safety to you*				
7. *Safety to partner*				

Scales

Self-report instruments frequently include one or more scales. A *scale* is a device designed to assign a numerical score in order to place subjects along a continuum with respect to the attribute being measured. The purpose of social–psychological scales is to quantitatively distinguish among people in terms of the degree to which they can be characterized by some trait. Scales have been constructed to discriminate among people with different attitudes, fears, motives, perceptions, personality traits, and needs.

Scales vary in their complexity, sophistication, and ability to make fine-grained distinctions. One of the simplest types of scales is referred to as a *graphic rating scale*. With graphic rating scales respondents are asked to give a judgment of something along an ordered dimension. The task is to place a check at the appropriate point along the line that extends from one extreme of the characteristic or dimension in question to the other extreme. Graphic rating scales are *bipolar* in nature because they specify

Table 11-1. An Example of a Likert Scale to Measure Attitudes Toward the Mentally Ill

DIRECTION OF SCORING*		SA	A	?	D	SD	(✓) Person 1	(X) Person 2
		RESPONSES†					SCORE	
+	1. People who have had a mental illness can become normal, productive citizens after treatment.		✓			X	4	1
−	2. People who have been patients in mental hospitals should not be allowed to have children.			X	✓		5	3
−	3. The best way to handle patients in mental hospitals is to restrict their activity as much as possible.		X		✓		4	2
+	4. Many patients in mental hospitals develop normal, healthy relationships with staff members and other patients.			✓	X		3	2
+	5. There should be an expanded effort to get the mentally ill out of institutional settings and back into their communities.	✓				X	5	1
−	6. Since the mentally ill cannot be trusted, they should be kept under constant guard.		X			✓	5	2
−	7. There is really very little that can be done to help a person once they have had a mental disorder.		X			✓	5	2
−	8. Too much money is being spent on research to help the mentally ill.	X				✓	5	1
+	9. Mental illness could happen to anyone.	✓			X		5	2

Table 11-1. (*Continued*)

DIRECTION OF SCORING*		RESPONSES†					SCORE	
							(✓) Person 1	(X) Person 2
		SA	A	?	D	SD		
+	10. The condition of most facilities for the mentally ill is critically in need of improvement.	✓		X			5	3
							46	19
	Total Score for Person 1 = 46 Total Score for Person 2 = 19							

*The researcher would not indicate the direction of scoring on a Likert scale administered to subjects. The scoring direction is indicated in this table for illustrative purposes only.
†SA—strongly agree; A—agree; ?—uncertain; D—disagree; SD—strongly disagree

the two opposite ends of a continuum. Here is an example of an item that might be used in a questionnaire to senior nursing students:
How would you rate the overall quality of your nursing preparation? (Place a check in the appropriate space on the scale.)

Excellent 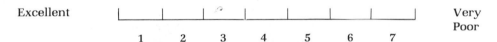 Very Poor

1   2   3   4   5   6   7

Graphic rating scales can be quite effective and are relatively easy to construct. Seven scale points are most commonly used, as in the example above, but five or nine might also be employed. Some researchers prefer to label one or more of the intermediary points to guide the respondent. In the illustration above, the position "4" could be labeled "fair."

More sophisticated scaling techniques have been developed in connection with the measurement of attitudes. The most common form of attitude measurement is the *Likert scale*, named after social psychologist Rensis Likert, who developed its use. A Likert scale consists of several declarative statements expressing a viewpoint on a topic. Respondents are asked to indicate the degree to which they agree or disagree with the opinion expressed in the statement. Table 11-1 presents a ten-item Likert scale for measuring attitudes toward the mentally ill.

Since Likert scales are used extensively, several features of these scales should be noted. First, 10 to 20 items are generally needed to form a good Likert scale. Second, neutral items or items with which most people would either agree or disagree should be omitted, since the point is to measure differences among people with different attitudes. Third, approximately equal numbers of positively and negatively worded statements should be used in order to avoid biasing the responses in one direction.

After the items are administered to respondents, the responses to the Likert scale must be scored. Typically, the responses are scored in such a way that endorsement of positively worded statements and nonendorsement of negatively worded statements are assigned a higher score. Table 11-1 illustrates what this procedure involves. The first statement is phrased such that agreement is indicative of a favorable attitude toward the mentally ill. The "+" in the first column of the table signifies that this is a positively worded item. We would, therefore, assign a higher score to a person agreeing with this statement than to someone disagreeing with it. Since the scale has a maximum of five points, we would give a "5" to someone strongly agreeing, "4" to someone agreeing, and so forth. The responses of two hypothetical respondents are shown by a check or an "X," and their score for each item is shown in the right-hand columns of the table. Person 1, who agreed with the first statement, is given a score of 4, while person 2, who strongly disagreed, is given a score of 1.

The second item is negatively worded: someone who agreed with the statement would tend to have a negative attitude toward the mentally ill. For this question, the scoring must be reversed, assigning a score of "1" to those who strongly agree, and so forth. This reversal is necessary so that a high score will consistently reflect positive attitudes toward the mentally ill. When each item has been handled in this manner, a person's total score can be determined by adding together individual item scores. The computation of total scores in this manner has led to the term *summated rating scale*, which is sometimes used to refer to Likert scales. The total scores of the two hypothetical respondents to the items in Table 11-1 are shown at the bottom of that table. These scores reflect a considerably more positive attitude toward the mentally ill on the part of person 1 than person 2.

Likert scales may appear to involve a lot of work and trouble, but they are actually quite powerful. The summation feature of these scales makes it possible to make very fine discriminations among persons with different points of view. A single Likert question allows people to be put into only five (or seven) categories. A ten-item scale, such as the one in Table 11-1, permits much finer gradations—from a minimum possible score of 10 (10 × 1) to a maximum possible score of 50 (10 × 5).

Another technique that one frequently encounters in research literature is known as the *semantic differential* (SD). The semantic differential is structurally very similar to a set of graphic rating scales. The respondent is asked to rate a given concept (*e.g.*, euthanasia, male nurses, integrated curriculum, 4-day work schedule) on a series of seven-point bipolar rating scales. The scales consist of bipolar adjectives, such as good–bad, important–unimportant, strong–weak, beautiful–ugly. An example of the format for a complete semantic differential is shown in Figure 11-1.

The semantic differential has the advantage of being highly flexible and easy to construct. The concept being rated can be virtually anything— a person, place, situation, abstract idea, controversial issue, and so forth. Furthermore, the concept can be a single word, a phrase, a sentence, or even a picture or sketch. Typically, several concepts are included on the same schedule so that comparisons can be made across concepts (if the same bipolar scales are used). For instance, a researcher may be interested in contrasting the reactions of respondents to the concepts of male nurse, female nurse, male physician, and female physician.

Extensive research with the SD technique has revealed that adjective pairs tend to cluster along three independent dimensions labeled Evaluation, Potency, and Activity. The most important group of adjectives are those that are Evaluative, such as valuable–worthless, good–bad, and fair– unfair. Potency adjectives include strong–weak and large–small, and examples of Activity adjectives are active–passive and fast–slow. The reason these three dimensions need to be considered separately is that a person's evaluative rating of a concept (such as a nurse practitioner) is independent of the activity or potency ratings of that concept. Two persons who associate high levels of activity with the concept of nurse practitioner might have divergent views with regard to how valuable they perceive the role to be. The researcher must decide whether to represent all three of these dimensions or whether only one or two are needed. Each dimension or aspect must be scored separately.

The scoring procedure for semantic differential responses is essen-

NURSE PRACTITIONERS

fair	7*	6	5	4	3	2	1		unfair
worthless	1	2	3	4	5	6	7		valuable
important									unimportant
pleasant									unpleasant
bad									good
cold									warm
responsible									irresponsible
successful									unsuccessful

*The score values would not be printed on the form administered to actual subjects. The numbers are presented here solely for the purpose of illustrating how semantic differentials are scored.

Figure 11-1. Example of a semantic differential

tially the same as for Likert scales. Scores from one to seven are assigned to each bipolar scale response. Usually, the positively worded adjective is associated with higher scores, so that a check to the extreme left for the fair–unfair combination in Figure 11-1 would be scored "7," and a check to the extreme right would be scored a "1." Note that in this figure the direction of the adjective pairs has been randomly reversed to prevent response biases. Thus, for the next set of adjectives, worthless–valuable, checks on the extreme right would be scored as "7." After proceeding in this fashion, subgroups of scale responses associated with the same dimension can be summed to yield a total score. Potentially, then, each concept could provide three scores (Evaluation, Potency, and Activity) if adjective pairs representing these three dimensions are included. In this example, only Evaluative adjectives are listed, so that all scale responses could be added together.

The development of accurate and meaningful scales is a more laborious and time-consuming process than the above discussion suggests. The person who designs Likert or other scales normally has the professional responsibility to assess the quality of data produced by these scales, and this assessment requires considerable technical sophistication. For this reason, novice researchers are generally encouraged to use or adapt existing scales. There are literally thousands of existing scales measuring a wide range of social–psychological traits already in existence, many of which have documentation of their validity, accuracy, response biases, and usages. In some cases it may be impossible to locate a scale for a particular trait of interest, but beginning researchers should be careful to exhaust all other possibilities before developing a new scale. Polit and Hungler (1983) provide some suggestions for locating existing scales and psychological tests.

Response Biases

Self-report instruments are susceptible to several common problems, the most troublesome of which are referred to as *response biases* or *response sets.*

One biasing influence on responses is a person's tendency to present a favorable image of himself or herself. The *social desirability response bias* refers to the tendency of some people to misrepresent their attitudes by giving answers that are consistent with prevailing social mores. This problem is a thorny one and often difficult to combat. Subtle, indirect, and delicately worded questioning sometimes can help to alleviate this response bias. The creation of a permissive atmosphere and provisions for respondent anonymity also encourage frankness.

Response biases are an especially difficult problem for social–psychological scales. One of the biases associated with Likert scales or semantic differentials is the *extreme-response set*. This biasing factor results from the fact that some people consistently express their attitudes in terms of extreme response alternatives (*e.g.*, "strongly agree"), while others characteristically endorse middle-range alternatives. This response style is a distorting influence in that extreme responses may not necessarily signify the most intense attitude toward the phenomenon under investigation. There appears to be little that a researcher can do to counteract this bias, although there are procedures for detecting its existence.

Some people have been found to agree with statements regardless of their content. In the research literature, these people are sometimes referred to as "yea-sayers"; the bias is known as the *acquiescence response set*. A less common problem is the opposite tendency for other people, called "nay-sayers," to disagree with statements independently of the question content. While there apparently are some people for whom such tendencies are stable and enduring personality characteristics, acquiescence and its opposite counterpart can often be avoided or minimized by the simple strategy of *counterbalancing* positively and negatively worded statements.

The effects of response biases should not be exaggerated, but it is important that researchers who are constructing a scale or using an existing one give these issues some thought. Consumers of research should also be alert to how response set biases could distort the results of studies based on self-report data.

Research Example

Schulte (1985) conducted a study on nurses' smoking behavior and attitudes toward nurses' smoking.* She developed a ten-page questionnaire that was distributed through the mail to a random sample of 1000 registered nurses residing in the state of New York. She enclosed self-addressed stamped envelopes so that respondents could easily respond. After 3 weeks a total of 415 questionnaires had been returned. The questionnaires had been numbered, enabling Schulte to identify the 585 nurses who had failed to reply; these nurses were sent a follow-up letter and a new questionnaire. Three weeks later the total number of returned questionnaires was up to 632, yielding a response rate of 63%.

Schulte's questionnaire covered several areas arranged in the following sequence: demographic and background information, attitudes toward nurses' smoking, history of smoking, age of initiation, attempts to reduce or discontinue smoking, perceived reasons for

---

*This example is fictitious.

smoking or nonsmoking, daily consumption, on-the-job smoking, knowledge of health risks associated with smoking, and perceived personal vulnerability to health risks. The questionnaire included mostly closed-ended questions, but open-ended questions were included concerning the nurses' reasons for smoking and nonsmoking.

One Likert scale was developed to measure attitudes toward nurses' smoking. The scale consisted of the following six items:

Nurses should set an example by not smoking.

Nurses can hurt their public image by smoking in public.

Nurses have just as much right as anyone else to smoke if they choose.

Nurses have a professional obligation not to smoke.

The public can hardly be expected to take smoking risks seriously if they see health-care workers such as nurses smoking.

Nurses who smoke are behaving irresponsibly.

Schulte's study has a number of strengths and weaknesses that deserve comment. Given the size and geographic dispersion of the sample throughout New York State, the use of questionnaires rather than face-to-face interviews was understandable. However, since the instrument was relatively brief and the issues were relatively nonintrusive and noncontroversial, a telephone interview would have been a preferable method. Perhaps Schulte did not have the resources to conduct a telephone interview, however.

Given Schulte's decision to use a mailed questionnaire, she took several commendable steps. First, she included a self-addressed stamped envelope, which is essential for an adequate response rate. Second, she boosted her response rate from 41.5% to 63.2% by sending follow-up letters to nonrespondents. Despite these efforts, however, nearly two out of five nurses in the sample failed to respond. Chances are that the 37% who did not respond were not a random subsample of the original 1000 nurses. One can imagine possible biases in opposing directions. Nonsmokers might have found the topic uninteresting and irrelevant, or perhaps found the instrument to be boring since so many questions were aimed at smokers only. Alternatively, some smokers may have been too embarrassed to respond or may have found the instrument too biased against smoking. In other words, the 37% who did not respond could overrepresent or underrepresent smokers, thereby giving a distorted picture of smoking behavior in nurses.

Several additional steps could have been taken to raise the response rate. A second follow-up letter would probably have resulted in a higher rate of return. Sometimes researchers offer incentives to study participants, such as monetary rewards or small "gifts." The best strategy would probably have been to call the 368 nonrespondents and conduct a telephone interview with them. Failing this, Schulte should at least have telephoned a random subsample of the nonrespondents (say 15%–20%) and administered the interview to them. This procedure would at least have provided information about the direction of the biases, if any. For example, if 30% of the 632 respondents were smokers, but 65% of the sampled nonrespondents were smokers, Schulte would have known that smokers were underrepresented among the nurses who returned the questionnaire.

With respect to the questionnaire itself, we can only make a few comments without seeing the actual instrument. First, the instrument appears to have been of a suitable length for a mailed questionnaire, and it covered a good mix of issues. Schulte wisely included mostly closed-ended items, and the use of open-ended questions to get at the nurses' reasons for their smoking behavior seems appropriate. The Likert scale, however, has some deficiencies. First, there are only six items, allowing for a maximum range of scores between 6 and 30. Ten or more items would have yielded more stable and discriminating results. Second, there is only one statement among the six that is not worded against smoking. To respondents, this kind of unbalanced scale suggests that the researcher believes it is wrong to smoke and may bias their responses against the admission of favorable smoking attitudes. This problem is worsened by the fact that the scale appeared early in the instrument, which possibly resulted in distortions of misrepresentations in subsequent sections. One further criticism is that Schulte developed her own Likert scale without, apparently, assessing its accuracy or validity. She possibly could have identified an existing scale and adapted it for use in her study. For example, there are several existing scales to measure attitudes toward smoking in general, which could have been modified to measure attitudes toward nurses' smoking. Finally, Schulte began the questionnaire by asking background questions (e.g., age, sex, employment status). These are rather dull questions and may have discouraged some people from responding. It is often best to put such demographic questions at the end of an instrument.

One final comment is that Schulte numbered the questionnaires, enabling her to send follow-up letters to nonrespondents only. This procedure was convenient administratively, but it precluded a guarantee of anonymity to respondents. Potentially this affected the response rate, but this is not likely in this particular case. The most ethically acceptable procedure is for the researcher to explain in the cover letter why the questionnaires are enumerated and to indicate that identifying information will be destroyed prior to data analysis.

Summary

Questionnaires and interviews are the methods used to obtain self-report information from subjects. The *interview schedule* is an instrument designed by the investigator to obtain verbal responses in either a face-to-face or telephone situation between an interviewer and the respondent. *Questionnaires* are self-administered in written form by the subjects. While there are many similarities between interview schedules and questionnaires, there are, nevertheless, some important differences.

Self-report data can be collected through instruments that range from the tightly structured (allowing little flexibility for the respondent) to the unstructured (allowing both respondent and questioner latitude in the framing of questions and answers). Questions themselves vary along this same dimension. *Open-ended questions* permit respondents to reply to questions in their own words. *Closed-ended* (or *fixed-alternative*) *questions* offer a number of alternative responses from which respondents are instructed to make a decision. Questionnaires are generally more structured than interviews so that respondents will not be burdened by composing and writing out lengthy responses.

One of the most problematic aspects of instrument construction is the wording of questions and response options. Questions must be clear and must take the respondents' intelligence and level of comprehension into account. This is particularly true for questionnaires, since no interviewer is available to clarify ambiguities.

Self-administered questionnaires can be distributed in various ways. Group administration to an intact group is the most convenient and economical procedure. The most common approach is to mail questionnaires to persons in their home or place of work. The main problem with mailed questionnaires is that many people fail to respond to them, leading to the risk of a biased sample. A number of techniques, such as the use of *follow-up reminders*, are designed to reduce the problem of nonresponse.

The collection of interview data depends quite heavily on the interpersonal skills of the interviewer. In order to secure participants' cooperation and trust, the interviewer must take pains to put people at ease. The interviewers should be thoroughly trained and familiar enough with the schedule so that they do not need to read questions from it. When respondents give incomplete or irrelevant replies to a question, the interviewer must use a technique known as *probing* to solicit additional information.

On the whole, interviews suffer from fewer weaknesses than questionnaires. Questionnaires are less costly and time-consuming than interviews, offer the possibility of anonymity, and run no risk of interviewer bias. However, interviews yield a higher response rate, are suitable for a wider variety of people, are less likely to lead to misinterpretations of questions, and provide richer data than do questionnaires.

Interview schedules and questionnaires are generally similar in terms of their development. First, some preliminary decisions must be made: the researcher needs to determine whether the data should be collected via interviews or questionnaires, how structured the schedule should be, and what type of information should be collected. Next, the questions should be drafted and put into a suitable sequence and format. An introduction should also be prepared. Finally, the draft of the instrument should be subjected to critical review and pretesting so that appropriate revisions can be made.

In designing self-report instruments, special attention needs to be paid to the construction of closed-ended items. Closed-ended questions can take a number of different forms. The simplest type of fixed alternative requires a choice between two options, such as "yes/no"; this type is referred to as *dichotomous items. Multiple-choice questions* provide respondents with a range of alternatives. *"Cafeteria" questions* are a special type of multiple-choice item in which respondents are asked to select a statement that best represents their view. Respondents are sometimes requested to *rank order* a list of alternatives along a continuum from (usually) most favorable to least favorable. A *checklist* groups together several questions that require the same response format and that can be answered by placing a check in the appropriate space. *Graphic rating scales* are devices for quantifying people's attitudes, views, and perceptions along a bipolar dimension (*e.g.*, important/unimportant).

Sophisticated scaling techniques have been developed to measure social–psychological characteristics, such as attitudes, motivations, personality traits, needs, and perceptions. *Scales* are tools for quantitatively measuring the degree to which people possess or are characterized by target traits or attributes. The most common form of attitude measure is the *Likert scale*, or *summated rating scale*. Likert scales present the respondent with a series of items (normally between 10 and 20) that are worded either favorably or unfavorably toward some phenomenon. Respondents are asked to indicate their degree of agreement or disagreement with each statement. The responses can then be combined to form a composite score, the aim of which is to signify the person's position, relative to that of others, on the attitudinal favorability/unfavorability continuum. A total score is derived by the summation of scores assigned to all items, which in turn are scored according to the direction of favorability expressed.

The *semantic differential* is a procedure for measuring the meaning of concepts to individuals and has been used widely in the area of attitude measurement. The technique consists of a series of graphic rating scales on which respondents are asked to indicate their reaction toward some phenomenon. Normally, 5 to 15 bipolar adjectival scales are included for each concept. The adjectives may be measuring an Evaluation (good–bad), Activity (active–passive), or Potency (strong–weak) dimension. Scoring of the semantic differential proceeds in a fashion similar to that of Likert scales.

The researcher interested in constructing self-report measures must contend with a number of difficulties, some of which are referred to as *response set biases.* This problem concerns the tendency of certain persons to respond to items in characteristic ways, independently of the item's content. The *social desirability response set* is a bias stemming from a person's desire to appear in a favorable light. The *extreme-response set* results when persons characteristically endorse extreme response alternatives. A third type of response bias is known as *acquiescence,* which designates a person's tendency to agree with statements regardless of their content. A converse problem arises less frequently when a person disagrees with most statements.

The researcher should give sufficient consideration to existing measures before embarking on a project to construct new scales. The development of good instruments is both arduous and time-consuming. Since literally thousands of existing measures are available, some effort should be made to identify potentially useful instruments that tap the variables of interest.

Study Suggestions

1. The underutilization of nursing skills because of voluntary nonemployment is sometimes the cause of some concern. Suppose that you were planning to conduct a statewide study of the plans and intentions of nonemployed registered nurses in your state. Would you adopt an interview or questionnaire approach? How structured would your schedule be? Why?

2. For the study suggested in No. 1 above, develop two open-ended and two closed-ended questions.

3. Suppose that the investigation of unemployed nurses were to be accomplished by means of a mailed questionnaire. Draft a cover letter to accompany the schedule.

4. Suppose that you were interested in studying the attitudes of men toward witnessing the birth of their children in a hospital delivery room. Develop five positively worded and five negatively worded statements that could be used in constructing a Likert scale for such a study.

5. List ten pairs of bipolar adjectives that would be appropriate for rating *all* of the following concepts for a semantic differential scale: cigarettes, alcohol, marijuana, heroin.

Chapter 12
Observational Methods

For certain types of research problems, an alternative to self-reports is direct observation by the researcher. Observational methods can be used fruitfully to gather a variety of information. To give the reader a flavor for the application of observational techniques, we list below several categories of information amenable to observations:

1. *Characteristics and Conditions of Individuals.* A broad variety of information about people's attributes and states can be gathered by direct observation. We refer here not only to relatively enduring traits of individuals, such as their physical appearance, but also to more temporary conditions, such as physiological symptoms that are amenable to observation. To illustrate this class of observable phenomena, the following could be used as dependent or independent variables in a nursing research investigation: the sleep or wake state of patients, the presence of edema in congestive heart failure, turgor of the skin in dehydration, the manifestation of decubitus ulcers, alopecia during cancer chemotherapy, or symptoms of infusion phlebitis in hospitalized patients.

2. *Verbal Communication Behaviors.* One of the most commonly observed types of human behavior is linguistic behavior. The content and structure of people's conversations are readily observable, easy to record, and, thus, are an obvious source of data. Among the kinds of verbal communications that a nurse researcher might be interested in observing are the relaying of information from nurses to patients, nurses' conversations with grieving relatives, dialogue among nursing faculty members discussing curriculum revisions, nurse–physician interactions, and exchange of information among nurses at change of shift report.

3. *Nonverbal Communication Behaviors.* People communicate their fears, wants, and emotions in many ways other than just with words. For nursing researchers, nonverbal communication represents an extremely promising area for research, since nurses are often called upon to be sensitive to nonverbal cues. The kinds of nonverbal behavior amenable to observational methods include facial expressions, touch, posture, gestures

and other body movements, and extralinguistic behavior (*i.e.*, the manner in which people speak, such as the intonation, loudness, and continuity of the speech).

4. *Activities.* There are many actions that constitute valuable data for nursing researchers. Activities that serve as an index of health status or physical and emotional functioning are particularly important. As illustrations, the following constitute the kinds of activities that lend themselves to an observational study: patients' eating habits and trends, bowel movements in postsurgical patients, self-grooming activities of nursing-home residents, length and number of visits by friends and relatives to hospitalized patients, and aggressive actions among children in the hospital playroom.

5. *Skill Attainment and Performance.* Nurses and nurse educators are constantly called upon to develop skills among clients and students. The attainment of these skills is often manifested behaviorally, such that an observational assessment is necessary. New types of nursing interventions designed to improve task performance lend themselves to an observational research project.

For example, a nursing researcher might want to observe the following kinds of behaviors: the ability of student nurses to properly insert a urinary catheter, the ability of stroke patients to scan a food tray if homonymous hemianopsia is present, the ability of diabetics to test their urine for sugar and acetone, or the ability of children to perform the Denver developmental screening tasks.

6. *Environmental Characteristics.* A person's surroundings may have a profound effect on her or his behavior and, therefore, a number of studies have explored the relationship between certain observable attributes of the environment on the one hand and human beliefs, actions, and needs on the other. A number of environmental attributes and conditions could play a role in observational nursing research studies, as in the following examples: the noise levels in different areas of a hospital, the existence of architectural barriers in the homes of disabled persons, or the cleanliness of the homes in a community.

As the above discussion suggests, observational methods are versatile with respect to the type of research problem for which these methods are appropriate. Two other aspects of observational methods deserve mention before going on to describe specific procedures. First, the researcher has flexibility in defining the observational unit, that is, the entity that will be observed. There are two basic approaches, which are perhaps best considered as the end-points of a continuum. The *molar approach* entails observing large units of behavior and treating them as a whole. For example, psychiatric nurse researchers might engage in a study of patient mood swings. A whole constellation of verbal and nonverbal behaviors might be construed as signaling aggressive behaviors, while another set might constitute passive behaviors. At the other extreme, the *molecular approach* uses small and highly specific behaviors as the unit of observation. Each movement, action, gesture, or phrase is treated as a separate entity, or perhaps broken down into even smaller units. The choice of approaches depends to a large degree on the nature of the problem and the preferences of the investigator. The molar approach is more susceptible to observer errors and distortions because of the greater ambiguity in the definition of the units. On the other hand, in reducing the observations to more concrete and specific activities, the investigator may lose sight of the activities that are at the heart of the inquiry.

Another area in which the researcher has some latitude concerns the relationship between the observer and the observed. There are two basic dimensions to be considered: intervention vs. nonintervention and concealment vs. nonconcealment. Intervention, as will be recalled from Chapter 6, concerns whether the researcher poses as a passive bystander or intervenes in some way to manipulate or control the research situation. Concealment refers to the researcher's openness in admitting to subjects that they are being observed as part of a scientific study.

The issue of concealment is one that has stirred much controversy in scientific circles. On the one hand, the ethical principle of informed consent is violated when people are not told they are subjects in a study. On the other hand, people under observation often fail to behave "normally," thereby jeopardizing the accuracy of the observations. The problem of behavioral distortions owing to the known presence of an observer has been called a reactive measurement effect or, more simply, *reactivity*. Concealment offers the researcher other advantages, even beyond the reduction of reactivity. Some people might deny a researcher the privilege of observing them altogether, so that the alternative to concealed observation might be no observation at all. Total concealment may, however, be difficult to attain except, perhaps, in highly structured or active settings.

Sometimes it is possible to establish a situation wherein subjects are aware of the researcher's presence but may not be aware of the investigator's underlying motives. This approach offers the researcher the opportunity of getting more in-depth information than is usually possible with totally concealed observation and may raise fewer ethical problems. On the other hand, a serious drawback of this second approach is the possibility that the interaction between the observer and the observed will alter the subjects' behavior. Even when the observed persons are unaware of being participants in a research study, there is always a risk that the researcher's presence will alter their normal activities, mannerisms, or conversations.

Concealed observations can be accomplished in the laboratory through the use of one-way mirrors. The subjects may or may not be told of the observation, or they may be given a false accounting of whom or what is being observed. Clearly, such procedures raise a number of ethical questions. Beyond ethical considerations, laboratory settings are particularly susceptible to external validity threats, since the subjects are likely to be highly self-conscious of their subject status.

In summary, observational techniques can be used to measure a broad range of phenomena. Both global behaviors and minute aspects of human activity can be used as the observational unit. The researcher can intervene or not, be concealed or not, and conduct the investigation in the laboratory or in a natural setting. Observation can also be done directly through the human senses or with the aid of technical apparatus, such as videotape, tape recorders, and equipment for enhancing physiological observations (e.g., x-rays and stethoscopes). Thus, observational methods are an extremely versatile approach to data collection.

Like self-report techniques, observational methods can vary in the degree of structure the researcher imposes. Structured and unstructured observational techniques are described below.

Unstructured Observational Methods

Unstructured observational methods generally involve the collection of large amounts of descriptive information that is analyzed qualitatively rather than quantitatively. The observer is guided by the research questions, but is not constrained to observe only certain classes of phenomena or to systematically count the appearance of certain types of behaviors. Anthropologists generally use unstructured observational techniques to gather their data.

Nurse researchers have sometimes used an unstructured approach known as *participant observation* to study nursing problems. Participant observation is a technique wherein a researcher participates in the functioning of the social group that is under investigation. In participant observation studies, the researcher maintains a high degree of contact and involvement with the subjects. The researcher gains entrance into a social group or social setting and typically shares in the experiences of the group. By occupying a participating role within a setting, the observer may have insights that would have eluded a more passive and concealed observer. Proponents of the participant observation approach claim that it represents both a source of data *and* a basis for understanding what the data mean. The participant observer strives to secure information within the contexts, experiences, structures, and symbols that are relevant to the subjects. The researcher endeavors not to interject his or her world views and meanings into the social situation under observation.

The participant observer typically places few restrictions on the types of data collected, in keeping with the goal of minimizing observer-imposed meanings and structure. Given this aim, the most common forms of record-keeping in participant observation studies are logs and field notes. A *log* is a record of events and conversations and usually is maintained on a daily basis by field workers. *Field notes* may include the daily log but tend to be much broader, more analytic, and more interpretive than a simple listing of occurrences. Field notes represent the participant observer's efforts to record information and to synthesize and understand the data.

The success of any participant observation study is highly dependent upon the quality of the logs and field notes. It is clearly essential to record observations while the researcher is still in the process of collecting information, since memory failures are bound to occur if there is too long a delay. On the other hand, the participant observer cannot perform the recording function by visibly carrying a clipboard, pens, and paper, since this procedure would ruin the observer's guise as an ordinary participating member of the group. The researcher, therefore, must develop the skill of making detailed mental notes that can later be committed to paper or recorded on tape.

Unstructured observational methods have been both criticized and lauded. Those researchers who support the use of unstructured methods point out that these techniques usually provide a deeper and richer understanding of human behaviors and social situations than is possible with more rigorous procedures. Participant observation is particularly valuable, according to this view, for its ability to "get inside" a particular situation and lead to a more complete understanding of its complexities. Advocates of qualitative observational research claim that structured, quantitatively oriented methods are too mechanistic and superficial to render a meaningful account of the intricate nature of human behavior.

Critics of the unstructured approach point out its serious methodological shortcomings. Observer bias and observer influence are prominent difficulties. Not only is there a concern that the observer may lose objectivity in recording actual observations, there is also the question that the observer will inappropriately sample events and situations to be observed. Memory distortions represent another possible source of inaccuracy.

In participant observation studies, one difficulty is that it may be impossible to gain entrance into a group and be accepted as a fellow member. Once the researcher begins to participate in a group's activities, the possibility of emotional involvement becomes a salient issue. The researcher in the new "member" role may fail to attend to many scientifically relevant aspects of the situation or may develop a myopic view on issues of importance to the group. Participant observation techniques, thus, may be an unsuitable approach to study problems when one suspects that the risks of identification are strong.

Structured Observational Methods

Structured observational methods differ from the unstructured techniques in the specificity of behaviors or events selected for observation, in the advanced preparation of record-keeping forms, and in the kinds of activities in which the observer engages. The creativity of structured observation lies not in the observation itself but, rather, in the formulation of a system for categorizing, recording, and encoding the observations and sampling the phenomena of interest.

Structured observations commonly involve the construction of a category system to which observed behaviors or characteristics can be assigned. A category system represents an attempt to designate in a systematic or quantitative fashion the qualitative behaviors and events transpiring within the observational setting. A well-designed category system provides observers with a common frame of reference and facilitates the process of accurately noting relevant phenomena. The basic type of category scheme is designed to be used as a checklist in which the observer records the absence or presence (or frequency of occurrence) of specified classes of events and behaviors.

One of the most important requirements of a category system is the careful and explicit definition of the behaviors to be observed. Each category must be explained in detail with an operational definition so that observers will have relatively clear-cut criteria for assessing the occurrence of the phenomenon in question. For example, Borgatta (1962) presented a category system for the observation of verbal communication and social interaction. The Interaction Process Score system involves a total of 18 categories of interactive behavior. Category 4, which designates the observed subject's "acknowledgement, understanding, or recognition" within a social interaction, is defined as follows:

This category includes all passive indicators of having understood or recognized the communication directed toward the recipient. The most common score for this category is a nod or saying "Uhuh," "Yes," "O.K.," "Mum," "Right," "Check," "I see," "That may be, but . . ." In general, items are scored into this category if they indicate the acceptance of an item of communication, but this does not require agreement with the communication, the presence of which would place the response in Category 5 (Borgatta, 1962, p. 273).

In developing the categorization scheme, the researcher must make a decision with regard to the exhaustiveness of the phenomena to be observed. Some category systems, such as Borgatta's interaction procedure, are constructed such that virtually all the observed behaviors can be classified into one, and only one, of several categories. Another example of an exhaustive system is the Downs and Fitzpatrick (1976) observation tool for analyzing body position and motor activity. Their instrument was developed with the objective that all postural and motor behavior could be classified into one or another of their categories. A contrasting technique is to develop a system in which only particular types of behavior are categorized. For example, if we were observing the aggressive behavior of autistic children, we might develop such categories as "strikes another child," "kicks or hits walls/floors," "calls other children names," "throws objects around the room," and so forth. In this more restricted category system, nonaggressive behaviors would not be classified. It might be pointed out that while nonexhaustive systems may be adequate for many research purposes, they run the risk of providing data that are difficult to interpret. When a large number of behaviors are unclassified, the investigator may have difficulty in placing the categorized behaviors into a proper perspective.

Virtually all category systems require that some inferences be made on the part of the observer, but there is considerable variability on this dimension. The Downs and Fitzpatrick observational instrument for body position and motor activity consists of a category system that requires only a modest amount of inference. For example, total body position is classified in one of six relatively straightforward categories: upright, lying down, leaning, sitting, leaning over, and kneeling. On the other hand, a system such as the one developed by Bales (1950) for observing verbal behavior in small groups contains such categories as "shows solidarity" and "shows tension release." Even when such categories are accompanied by detailed definitions and descriptions, there is clearly a heavy inferential burden placed upon the observer.

Checklists based on category systems represent a method for the observer to record the observed phenomena. The investigator uses the checklist to tally whether a behavior, event, or characteristic is present or not. There are two basic formats for observational checklists. The first approach, which is sometimes referred to as a *sign system*, begins with a listing of categories of behaviors that may or may not be manifested by the subjects. The observer's task is to watch for instances of the behaviors on the list. When a behavior occurs, the observer either places a checkmark beside the appropriate behavior to designate its occurrence or makes a cumulative tally of the number of times the behavior was witnessed. The product of this type of endeavor is a kind of demography of events transpiring within the observational period. A hypothetical example of a sign system for describing patients' ability to perform selected activities of daily living is presented in Table 12-1.

The second approach is to use the category system for separately analyzing ongoing and discrete elements of behavior. The task of the observer using this system is to place behaviors in only one category for each element. By element, we refer here to a unit of behavior, such as a sentence in a conversation. To illustrate, suppose that we were interested in studying the problem-solving behavior of a group of nurse educators develop-

Table 12-1. Examples of Categories for a Sign Analysis

HYGIENIC ACTIVITIES	EATING BEHAVIORS	DRESSING SKILLS
Washes hands	Eats with hand	Fastens buttons
Dries hands	Eats with spoon	Unfastens buttons
Washes extremities	Eats with fork	Fastens snaps
Brushes teeth	Cuts soft food	Unfastens snaps
Cleans fingernails	Cuts meat	Pulls up zipper
Brushes or combs hair	Drinks from a straw	Pulls down zipper
Shaves	Drinks from a cup	Ties shoelace
	Drinks from a cup	Unties shoelace
		Puts on eyeglasses
		Takes off eyeglasses
		Fastens buckle
		Unfastens buckle
		Puts in dentures
		Takes out dentures

ing curriculum plans. We might construct a category system such as the following: (1) information seeking; (2) information giving; (3) problem describing; (4) suggestion proposing; (5) suggestion opposing; (6) suggestion supporting; (7) summarizing; (8) miscellaneous. The observer would be required to classify every group member's contribution to the problem-solving process in terms of one of these eight categories and would normally record the speaker's name and to whom the communication was addressed. By employing such a system, it would be possible to analyze, for example, the relationship between a group member's role, status, or characteristics on the one hand and the types of problem-solving behaviors engaged in on the other. Checklists of this second type are more demanding of the observer than checklists based on the sign system, since the recording task is more continuous, and the categories are typically exhaustive.

Structured observational data can also be gathered through the use of rating scales. A *rating scale* is a tool that requires the observer to rate some phenomenon in terms of points along a descriptive continuum. The ratings usually are quantified during the subsequent analysis of the observational data.

Rating scales normally are used in one of two ways. The observer may be required to make ratings of behavior or events at frequent intervals throughout the observational period in much the same way that a checklist would be used. Alternatively, the observer may use the rating scales to summarize an entire event or transaction after the observation is completed.

Let us consider an example. Suppose that we were interested in comparing the behaviors of nurses working in intensive care units with those of nurses in other units. After 15-minute observation sessions, the observer might be asked to rate the perceived anxiety level of the nursing staff in each unit as a whole or that of individual members. The rating-scale item might take the following form:

According to your perceptions, how tense were the nurses in the observed unit?

1. Extremely relaxed
2. Rather relaxed
3. Somewhat relaxed
4. Neither relaxed nor tense
5. Somewhat tense
6. Rather tense
7. Extremely tense

The same information could be solicited using a graphic rating scale format:

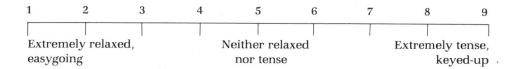

Rating scales can also be used as an extension of category systems wherein the observer records not only the occurrence of some behavior but also some qualitative aspect of it, such as its magnitude or intensity. The Downs and Fitzpatrick (1976) instrument for motor activity once again provides a good example. Their category scheme is comprised of eight body-movement categories: head active, right arm active, left arm active, both arms active, right leg active, left leg active, both legs active, and both arms and legs active. Observers must both classify the subjects' activity in terms of these categories *and* rate the intensity of the movement on a three-point scale: minimally active, moderately active, and very active. When rating scales are coupled with a category scheme in this fashion, considerably more information about the phenomena under investigation can be obtained. The disadvantage of this approach is that it places an immense burden on the observer, particularly if there is an extensive amount of activity.

Observational Sampling

Observational methods rarely involve the recording of all behaviors or activities that take place in a given situation. The investigator must generally make some decisions about how and when the system will be applied. Observational sampling methods represent a mechanism for obtaining representative examples of the behavior being observed without having to observe an entire event.

The most frequently used system is the *time-sampling method*. This procedure involves the selection of time periods during which the observations will take place. The time frames may be systematically selected (e.g., every 30 seconds at 2-minute intervals) or may be selected at random. As a hypothetical example, suppose we were studying the interaction patterns of mothers and their handicapped children. Some of the mothers have received specific preparation from a community health nurse for dealing with their conflict over the child's dependence–independence needs, while a control group of mothers has not received this preparation. In order to examine the effects of this intervention, the behavior of the mothers and children are observed in a playground setting. During a 1-hour observation period, we decide to sample behaviors rather than to observe the entire session. For the sake of simplicity, let us say that 3-minute observations will be made. If we use a systematic sampling approach, we would observe for 3 minutes, then cease observing for a prespecified period, say 3 minutes. Using this scheme, a total of ten 3-minute observations would be made. A second approach is to randomly sample 3-minute periods from the total of 20 such periods in an hour. The decision with regard to the length and number of periods comprising a suitable sample must be influenced by the aims of the research. In establishing time units, one of the most important considerations is determining what a psychologically meaningful time frame would be. A good deal of pretesting and experimentation with different sampling plans is essential in developing or adapting observational strategies.

Event sampling is a second system for obtaining a set of observations. This approach selects integral behaviors or events of a prespecified type for observation. Event sampling requires that the investigator either have some knowledge of the occurrence of events or be in a position to wait for their occurrence. Examples of "integral events," which may be suitable for event sampling, include shift changes of nurses in a hospital, cast removals of pediatric patients, epileptic seizures, and cardiac arrests in the emergency room. This sampling approach is preferable to time sampling when the events of principal interest are infrequent throughout the day and are at risk of being missed if specific time-sampling frames are established. However, when behaviors and events are relatively frequent, time sampling does have the virtue of enhancing the representativeness of the observed behaviors.

Evaluation of Observational Methods

The field of nursing is particularly well suited for observational research. Nurses are often in a position to watch people's behaviors and may by training be especially sensitive observers. There are many nursing problems that are better suited to an observational approach than to self-report techniques. Whenever people cannot be expected to describe adequately their own behaviors, observational methods may be needed. This may be the case when people are unaware of their own behavior (*e.g.*, manifesting preoperative symptoms of anxiety), when people are embarrassed to report their activities (*e.g.*, displays of aggression or hostility), when behaviors are emotionally laden (*e.g.*, grieving behavior among the bereaved), or when people are not capable of articulating their actions (*e.g.*, young children or the mentally ill).

Observational methods have an intrinsic appeal with respect to their ability to directly capture a record of behaviors and events. Furthermore, there is virtually no other data-collection method that can provide the depth and variety of information as observation. With this approach, human beings—the observers—are used as "measuring instruments" and provide a uniquely sensitive and intelligent (if fallible) tool.

Several of the shortcomings of the observational approach have already been mentioned. These include possible ethical difficulties, reactivity of the observed when the observer is conspicuous, and lack of consent to being observed. Unquestionably, however, one of the most pervasive problems is the vulnerability of observational data to distortions and biases. A number of factors interfere with objective observations: (1) emotions, prejudices, attitudes, and values of the observer may result in faulty inference; (2) personal interest and commitment may color what is seen in the direction of what the observer wants to see; (3) anticipation of what is to be observed may affect what is observed; and (4) hasty decisions before adequate information is collected may result in erroneous classifications or conclusions.

Several specific types of observational bias can be mentioned. One bias is referred to as the *enhancement of contrast effect*. The observer may tend to distort the observation in the direction of dividing the content into clear-cut entities. The converse effect—a bias toward *central tendency*—occurs when extreme events are distorted toward a middle ground. Other biases are in a category described as *assimilatory*. The observer may tend to distort observations in the direction of identity with previous inputs. This problem would have the effect of biasing records in the direction of regularity and orderliness.

Rating scales are susceptible to several distinct types of error. The *halo effect* refers to the tendency of the rater to be influenced by one characteristic in rating other nonrelated characteristics. For example, if we formed a very positive general impression of a person, we would probably be likely to rate that person as "intelligent," "loyal," and "dependable" simply because these traits are positively valued. Rating scales may reflect the personality traits of the observer. The *error of leniency* is the tendency for the observer to rate everything positively, and the *error of severity* is the contrasting tendency to rate too harshly.

Such biases probably cannot be eliminated completely, but they can be minimized through the careful training of observers. Normally, detailed instructions and examples should be prepared for the observers. Training sessions are useful for clarifying any ambiguities, for explaining how to deal with marginal cases, and for alerting the observers to the need to perceive familiar behaviors within the constraints imposed by the observation schedule. During the training session, observers should perform a trial run so that difficulties can be detected. During a practice session, the comparability of the observers' recordings should be assessed. That is, two or more observers should watch a trial event or situation, and the notations on the checklist or rating scales should be compared. This procedure is referred to as an evaluation of *interrater reliability* and will be described more fully in the next chapter.

Research Example

Owens (1984) studied hospitalized patients' requests for nursing assistance in relation to their age, sex, and number of daily outside visitors.* Subjects for the study were 100 patients on a medical–surgical unit of a 650-bed hospital in New Jersey. All 100 subjects were patients admitted for relatively routine procedures, such as appendectomies; none was terminally ill. Observations were made by the nursing staff, who were instructed to record verbatim all requests that the subjects made during a 24-hour period and all instances of patients' use of the call button. At the end of each shift, each nurse rated the patient on several dimensions, such as talkative/not talkative; hostile/friendly; and in no pain/in great pain.

Each request was then categorized according to a sign system that Owens had developed. The categories included the following: request for pain medication; request for beverage; request for food; request for environmental change (*e.g.*, temperature or light adjustment); request for reading material, TV, or radio; request for assistance in getting in/out of bed; and request for dialogue or emotional support. Owens performed all of the categorization herself based on the nurses' verbatim accounts.

Owens found that the number of patients' requests was unrelated to their sex and age, although there were age and sex differences in the type of requests made. Patients with no visitors made significantly more requests than patients with one or more visitors on the day of the observation and were also somewhat more likely to be rated as unfriendly.

Owens' choice of an observational approach seems reasonable. Given Owens' aim of learning about patients' actual behavior (*i.e.*, requests for

---

*The example is fictitious.

assistance from the nursing staff), it would not have been appropriate to ask patients about the frequency and type of requests they had made. Self-reports would have been subject to distortions of memory lapses and misreporting. Patients might also have a different notion than the researcher about what constitutes a "request."

Owens elected to use a highly structured observational scheme. Again, this choice appears to be sound: the investigator was interested in fairly specific phenomena that lent themselves easily to enumeration. The use of both a category system and rating scales also seems to have been a good choice for capturing information about the quantity and quality of patients' requests.

Despite these strengths, Owens' study could have been improved. First, consider the possibility of reactivity. It is likely that patients were not informed about their participation while the data were being collected. While this procedure may raise some ethical questions, it nevertheless seems justifiable: the privacy of the patients was not, after all, being seriously threatened, and patients would undoubtedly have altered their interactions with the nursing staff if they had known that their dialogue was being scrutinized. Thus, Owens' procedure of having nurses record patients' requests after they were made (i.e., after leaving the patients' rooms) eliminated the problem of reactivity stemming from the patient. But what about the reactivity of the nurses? The nurses knew exactly what the researcher was studying and could have communicated "cues" to the patients in subtle or not so subtle ways. The nurses' nonverbal behavior could have either encouraged or discouraged patients' requests for assistance.

Two other problems relate to the use of the nurses as the observational recorders. First, without adequate training the nurses could misinterpret the researcher's definition of "requests." Second, the nurses were required to report verbatim the patients' requests, an activity that is by no means easy to do. The nurses probably did not accurately remember the wording of the patients' questions.

From a methodological point of view, the best procedure would have been to unobtrusively tape record all nurse–patient dialogue. In addition to providing accuracy and eliminating the risk of nurse reactivity, the use of a recording device would have permitted more fine-grained analyses of the content and tone of the requests. However, this would be ethically problematic. Perhaps the researcher could have told both the nursing staff and subjects about the presence of recording equipment and described only in broad terms the nature of the study (e.g., to better understand patient–nurse communication patterns).

Owens sampled an entire 24-hour period for all 100 subjects. It would probably have been wiser to sample 1-hour segments over a 48- to 72-hour interval. A single day may not have adequately represented the range of patient requests during a hospital stay and could also have been atypical in terms of visitation.

Owens elected to look only at patient communication that took the form of requests for assistance. The sign system presumably covered all types of requests, but no other patient conversation. While the decision to use such a nonexhaustive category scheme is understandable, it does have the disadvantage of failing to provide a context for understanding patient behavior. If a patient made 15 requests in 1 day, it might be useful to know whether these requests represented *all* patient-initiated communication or only a small fraction of it.

Categorization of the requests according to the sign system was handled centrally by Owens rather than by individual nurse observers. This approach has the advantage of not having different biases produced by multiple observers. However, it does mean that any biases went undetected. Owens would have been well advised to have a second person categorize the requests (or at least a portion of them) to determine interobserver agreement.

With respect to this latter issue, the use of nurses from all three shifts who rated patients' communication on several dimensions was a strong point of the study. The use of tape recorders to record actual dialogue would have provided yet another opportunity to independently verify nurses' observations. In summary, then, Owens' research was fairly well-conceived but could also have been improved with relatively little additional effort.

Summary

Observational methods are techniques for acquiring information for research purposes through the direct observation and interpretation of phenomena in the environment. Observation plays an important role in most scientific disciplines, and nursing research and practice are no exceptions. In conducting an observational study, the researcher must select an appropriate *unit of analysis*. The *molar approach* entails the observation of large segments of behaviors and events as integral units. The *molecular approach*, on the other hand, treats small, specific actions as separate entities.

The investigator must also make decisions about the nature of the relationship between the observer and the subjects. The decisions relate primarily to the two dimensions of *concealment* and *intervention*. Concealment refers to the degree to which the observed persons are aware that they are being observed or that they are the subjects of a research study. The problem of behavioral distortions stemming from the presence of an observer (known as *reactivity*) is a major reason for making concealed or inconspicuous observations. Intervention refers to the degree to which the investigator structures the observational setting in line with research demands as opposed to being a passive observer.

Observational techniques vary along a continuum from tightly structured procedures to loose and unstructured ones. One type of *unstructured observation* is referred to as *participant observation*, a method that has been used widely by anthropologists and sociologists. The researcher in a participant observation study gains entry into the social group of interest and participates to varying degrees in its functioning. The participant observer endeavors to obtain information about the dynamics of the social group within the subject's own frame of reference, without imposing a preconceived structure based on the researcher's world view. This approach places relatively few restrictions on the types or amount of data collected. *Logs* of daily events and *field notes* of the observer's experiences and interpretations constitute the major data-collection instruments. Unstructured methods can yield extremely rich and useful information, particularly when used by insightful observers, but are subject to a number of methodological difficulties.

Structured observational methods impose a number of constraints upon the observer for the purpose of maximizing observer accuracy and objectivity and for obtaining an adequate representation of the phenomenon of interest. Two types of record-keeping forms are used most commonly by observers in structured situations. *Checklists* are tools for recording the appearance or frequency of prespecified behaviors, events, or characteristics. Checklists are based on the development of *category systems* for encoding the observed phenomena.

Checklists are used to tally whether the phenomenon described by a category is present or not. One type of checklist is based on the *sign system* and is used as a demographic record of the types of behavior that occurred during the observational session. A second format is used to analyze ongoing events and activities. This second type of checklist either classifies an element of behavior according to the predetermined category system or assigns activities occurring within a designated time frame to the appropriate category.

Rating scales are the second most common record-keeping tool for structured observations. The observer using a rating scale is required to rate some phenomenon according to points along a dimension that is typically bipolar (*e.g.*, passive/aggressive or excellent health/poor health). Ratings are made either during the observational setting at specific intervals (*e.g.*, every 5 minutes) or after the observation is completed.

Most structured observations make use of some form of *sampling plan* for selecting the behaviors, events, and conditions to be observed. The most frequently used approach is *time sampling*, which involves the specification of the duration and frequency of both the observational periods and the intersession intervals. *Event sampling* selects integral behaviors or events of a special type for observation.

Observational techniques are versatile and offer an important alternative to self-report techniques. Nevertheless, human perceptual and judgmental errors can pose a serious threat to the validity and accuracy of observational information. Thorough training of observers is critical to the successful conduct of observational research.

Study Suggestions

1. Suppose you were interested in observing the behavior of fathers in the delivery room during the birth of their first child. Identify the observer/observed relationship among the concealment/intervention dimensions that you would recommend adopting for such a study and defend your recommendation. What are the possible drawbacks of your approach and how might you deal with them?

2. Would a psychiatric nurse researcher be well suited to conduct a participant observation study of the behavior of psychiatric nurses and their interactions with clients? Why or why not?

3. A nurse researcher is planning to study temper tantrums displayed by hospitalized children. Would you recommend using a time-sampling approach? Why or why not?

4. Suppose you were interested in studying pain-related behaviors using observational methods. Develop some categories of behavior that could be used for classifying the observations.

Chapter 13
Reliability and Validity

As we have seen in the preceding chapters, there are many different methods of measuring research variables and collecting scientific data. Each method has a number of strengths as well as weaknesses. Scientists have devised methods to formally assess the adequacy of data-collection instruments. Both producers and consumers of research need to make judgments about the quality of instruments in order to draw conclusions about research findings. This chapter reviews the criteria and procedures for assessing measurement tools. We turn first to some basic concepts from the theory of measurement error.

Errors of Measurement

No measuring tool is infallible. Values and scores obtained from even the best of instruments contain a certain margin of error. One can think of every obtained score or piece of data as consisting of two parts—an error component and a true component. This can be written symbolically as follows:

$$\text{Observed score} = \text{True score} \pm \text{Error}$$
$$or$$
$$X_0 = X_T \pm X_E$$

The "observed score" could be, for example, a patient's heart rate or a nursing student's score on a self-concept test. The "X_T" stands for the true value that would be obtained if it were possible to arrive at an infallible measure. The *true score* is a hypothetical entity; it can never be known because measures are *not* infallible, though its value can be estimated. The final term in the equation is the *error of measurement*. The difference between true and obtained scores is the result of factors that affect the measurement and, therefore, result in distortions.

Decomposing obtained scores in this fashion brings to light an important point. When a researcher measures an attribute of interest, he or she is also measuring attributes that are not of interest. The true score component is what one hopes to isolate; the error component is a composite of other factors that are also being measured, contrary to the desires of the researcher. This concept can be illustrated with an exaggerated example. Suppose a researcher were measuring the weight of ten people on a spring scale. As each subject stepped on the scale, our fictitious researcher places a hand on the subject's shoulder and applies some pressure. The resulting measures (the X_0s), will all be biased in an upward direction, because the scores reflect the influence of both the subject's actual weight (X_T) and the researcher's pressure (X_E).

Many factors contribute to errors of measurement. Among the most common are the following:

1. *Situational Contaminants.* Scores can be affected by the conditions under which they are produced. The subject's awareness of an observer's presence (the reactivity problem) is one source of bias. The anonymity of the response situation, the friendliness of the researchers, or the location of the data gathering can all affect a subject's responses. Other environmental factors, such as temperature, humidity, lighting, time of day, and so forth, can represent sources of measurement error.

2. *Response-Set Biases.* A number of relatively enduring characteristics of the respondents can interfere with accurate measures of the target attribute. Response sets, such as social desirability, extreme responses, and acquiescence, are potential problems in self-report measures, particularly psychological scales (see Chap. 11).

3. *Transitory Personal Factors.* A person's scores may be influenced by a variety of nonenduring personal states, such as fatigue, hunger, anxiety, mood, and so forth. Temporary personal factors can alter people's scores by influencing their motivation to cooperate, act "naturally," or do their best.

4. *Administration Variations.* Alterations in the methods of collecting data from one subject to the next could result in variations in obtained scores that have little to do with variations in the target attribute. For example, if some physiological measures are taken before a feeding and others are taken postprandially, then measurement errors can potentially occur.

5. *Instrument Clarity.* If the directions for obtaining measures are vague or poorly understood, then scores may reflect this ambiguity and misunderstanding. For example, questions in a self-report instrument may sometimes be interpreted differently by different respondents, leading to a distorted measure of the critical variable.

6. *Response Sampling.* Sometimes errors are introduced as a result of the sampling of items used to measure an attribute. For example, a nursing student's score on a 100-item test of general nursing knowledge will

be influenced to a certain extent by *which* 100 questions are included on the examination.

This list is not exhaustive but does illustrate that data are susceptible to measurement error from a variety of sources.

Reliability

The *reliability* of a measuring instrument is a major criterion for assessing its quality and adequacy. Essentially, the reliability of an instrument is the degree of consistency with which it measures the attribute it is supposed to be measuring. If a scale gave a reading of 120 pounds for a person's weight 1 minute and a reading of 150 pounds the next minute, we would naturally be wary of using that scale because the information would be unreliable. The less variation an instrument produces in repeated measurements of an attribute, the higher its reliability. Thus, reliability can be equated with the stability, consistency, or dependability of a measuring tool.

Another way of defining reliability is in terms of accuracy. An instrument can be said to be reliable if its measures accurately reflect the "true" measures of the attribute under investigation. This definition links reliability to the issues raised in our discussion of measurement error. We can make this relationship clearer by stating that an instrument is reliable to the extent that errors of measurement are absent from obtained scores. In other words, a reliable measure is one that maximizes the true-score component and minimizes the error component.

These two ways of approaching the concept of reliability (consistency and accuracy) are not so different as they might at first appear. The example of the scale that produced variable weight readings illustrates this point. Let us suppose that the true weight of a subject is 125 pounds, but that two independent measurements yielded 120 and 150 pounds. In terms of the equation presented in the previous section, we could express the measurements as follows:

$$120 = 125 - 5$$
$$150 = 125 + 25$$

The errors of measurement for the two trials are -5 and 25, respectively. These errors produced scores that are both inconsistent and inaccurate. We must conclude that our fictitious spring scale is highly unreliable.

Scientists can place little confidence in their findings if the instruments they use are of questionable reliability. Therefore, it has become a customary procedure for developers of new instruments to estimate the reliability of their tools before making them available for general use. Instruments that are psychological or behavioral in nature are in particular need of pretesting and trial runs. It should be pointed out, however, that an instrument's reliability is not a fixed entity. *The reliability of an instrument is not a property of the instrument, but rather of the instrument when administered to a certain sample under certain conditions.* A scale developed to measure dependence in hospitalized adults in the United States may be unreliable for use with hospitalized adolescents, with the elderly in nursing homes, and so forth.

What are the implications of this fact for researchers? First, in selecting a measuring tool one should always learn about the characteristics of the group with whom or for whom the instrument was developed. If the original group was similar to the researcher's target group, then the reliability estimate provided by the developer is probably a reasonably good index of the instrument's accuracy and consistency for the new study. Other things being equal, one should always choose a measure with demonstrated high reliability. However, the prudent scientist is not satisfied with an instrument that will "probably" be reliable in his or her study. A recommended procedure is to compute estimates of reliability whenever data are collected for a scientific investigation, except perhaps for physiological measures that are relatively impervious to random fluctuations stemming from personal or situational factors.

The reliability of a measuring tool can be assessed in several different ways. The method chosen depends to a certain extent on the nature of the instrument but also on the aspect of the reliability concept that is of greatest interest. Three aspects that have received major quantitative attention are stability, internal consistency, and equivalence.

Stability

The *stability* of a measure refers to the extent to which the same results are obtained on repeated administrations of the instrument. The estimation of reliability here focuses on the instrument's susceptibility to extraneous factors from one application to the next.

Assessments of the stability of a measuring tool are derived through procedures referred to as *test–retest reliability.* The researcher administers the same test to a sample of people on two occasions and then compares the scores obtained. The comparison procedure is performed objectively by computing a *reliability coefficient,* which is a numerical index of how reliable the test is.

In order to explain what a reliability coefficient is and how to interpret it, we must pause to briefly explain the concepts underlying the statistic known as the *correlation coefficient.** We have pointed out repeat-

---

*Computational procedures and additional information about correlation coefficients (Pearson r) are presented in Chapter 16.

edly in this text that the scientist's job is to detect and explain the relationships among phenomena: Is there a relationship between anxiety and illness? Is a nurse's age related to his or her attitudes toward the nurse practitioner role? The correlation coefficient is an important tool for quantitatively describing the magnitude and direction of a relationship. The computation of this index does not concern us here. It is more important to understand how to "read" a correlation coefficient.

Two variables that are obviously related to one another are height and weight. On the average, tall people tend to weigh more than short people. We would say that the relationship between height and weight was perfect if the tallest person in the world was the heaviest, the second tallest person was the second heaviest, and so forth. The correlation coefficient summarizes how "perfect" a relationship is. The possible values for a correlation coefficient range from a −1.00 through 0.0 to +1.00. If height and weight were *perfectly* correlated, the correlation coefficient expressing this relationship would be 1.00. Since the relationship exists but is not perfect, the correlation coefficient is probably in the vicinity of .50 or .60.

When two variables are totally unrelated, the correlation coefficient is equal to zero. One might anticipate that a woman's dress size is unrelated to her intelligence. Large women are as likely to perform well on tests of ability as small women. The correlation coefficient summarizing such a relationship would presumably be in the vicinity of 0.0.

Correlation coefficients running between 0.0 and −1.00 express what is known as *inverse* or *negative relationships.* When two variables are inversely related, increments in one variable are associated with decrements in the second variable. Let us suppose that there is an inverse relationship between a nurse's age and attitude toward abortion. This means that, on the average, the *older* the nurse, the *less* favorable the attitude. If the relationship were perfect (*i.e.*, if the oldest nurse had the least favorable attitude and so on), then the correlation coefficient would be equal to −1.00. In actuality, the relationship between age and abortion attitudes is probably quite modest—in the vicinity of −.20 or −.30. A correlation coefficient of this magnitude describes a weak relationship wherein older nurses tend to be unfavorable and younger persons tend to be favorable toward abortion, but a "crossing of lines" is not unusual. That is, many younger nurses oppose abortion while many older nurses defend it.

Now we are prepared to discuss the use of correlation coefficients to compute reliability estimates. In the case of test–retest reliability, a sample of subjects is exposed to the administration of the instrument on two occasions. Let us say we are interested in the stability of a scale to measure leadership potential in nurses. Since leadership potential might be presumed to be a fairly stable attribute, we would expect a measure of it to yield consistent scores on two separate testings. As a check on the instrument's stability, the scale is administered to a sample of ten people 3

Table 13-1. Fictitious Data for Test–Retest of a Leadership Potential Scale

SUBJECT NUMBER	TIME 1	TIME 2	
1	55	57	
2	49	46	
3	78	74	
4	37	35	
5	44	46	
6	50	56	
7	58	55	
8	62	66	
9	48	50	
10	67	63	r = .95

weeks apart. Some fictitious data for this example are presented in Table 13-1. It can be seen that, by and large, the differences in the scores on the two testings are not large. The reliability coefficient for test–retest estimates is the correlation coefficient between the two sets of scores. In this example, the computed reliability coefficient is .95, which is quite high. The higher the coefficient, the more stable the measure. For most purposes, reliability coefficients above .70 are considered satisfactory.

The test–retest approach to estimating reliability has certain disadvantages. One problem is that many traits of interest *do* change over time, independently of the stability of the measure. Attitudes, behaviors, moods, knowledge, physical condition, and so forth can be modified by intervening experiences between the two testings.

Stability estimates also suffer from other problems. One possibility is that the subjects' responses on the second administration will be influenced by the memory of their responses on the first administration, regardless of their actual inclinations on the second day. This memory interference will result in a spuriously high reliability coefficient. Another difficulty is that subjects may actually change as a result of the first administration. Finally, people may object to being measured with the same instrument twice. If they find the procedure boring on the second occasion, their responses could be haphazard, resulting in a spuriously low estimate of stability.

In summary, the test–retest approach is a procedure for estimating the stability of a measure over time. On the whole, reliability coefficients tend to be higher for short-term retests than for long-term retests (i.e., those greater than 1 or 2 months) because of actual changes in the attribute being measured. Stability indexes are most appropriate for relatively enduring characteristics, such as personality, abilities, and so forth. Owing to other problems with test–retest estimates, however, instrument developers should not rely exclusively on this approach to assess the instrument's reliability.

Internal Consistency

Ideally, scales designed to measure an attribute are composed of a set of items, all of which are measuring the critical attribute and nothing else. On a scale to measure the decision-making abilities of nurses, it would be inappropriate to include an item that is a better measure of empathy than skill in decision making. An instrument may be said to be *internally consistent* or *homogeneous* to the extent that all of its subparts are measuring the same characteristic.

The internal-consistency approach to estimating an instrument's reliability is probably the most widely used method among researchers today. The reason for the popularity of the procedures described below is not only that they are economical (they require only one test administration), but also that they are the best means of assessing one of the most important sources of measurement error, which is the sampling of items.

One of the oldest methods for assessing internal consistency is the *split-half technique*. In this approach, the items comprising a test or scale are split into two groups, scored independently, and the scores on the two half-tests are used to compute a correlation coefficient. To illustrate this procedure, the fictitious scores from the first administration of the leadership potential scale are reproduced in the first column of Table 13-2. For the sake of simplicity, we will say that the total instrument consists of 20 questions. In order to compute a split-half reliability coefficient, the items must be divided into two groups of ten. While a large number of possible "splits" are possible, the most widely accepted procedure is to use odd items versus even items. One half-test, therefore, consists of items 1, 3, 5, 7, 9, 11, 13, 15, 17, and 19, while the remaining items comprise the second half-test. The scores on the two halves for our example are shown in the second and third columns of Table 13-2. The correlation coefficient describing the relationship between the two half-tests is an estimate of the

Table 13-2. Fictitious Data for Split-half Reliability of a Leadership Potential Scale

SUBJECT NUMBER	TOTAL SCORE	ODD-NUMBERS SCORE	EVEN-NUMBERS SCORE	
1	55	28	27	
2	49	26	23	
3	78	36	42	
4	37	18	19	
5	44	23	21	
6	50	30	20	
7	58	30	28	
8	62	33	29	
9	48	23	25	
10	67	28	39	r = .67

internal consistency of the leadership potential scale. If the odd items are measuring the same attribute as the even items, then the reliability coefficient should be high. The correlation coefficient computed on the fictitious data is .67.

The correlation coefficient computed on split-halves of a measure tends to systematically underestimate the reliability of the entire scale. Other things being equal, longer scales are more reliable than shorter ones. The correlation coefficient computed on the data in Table 13-2 is an estimate of reliability for a 10-item instrument, not a 20-item instrument. To overcome this difficulty, a formula has been developed for adjusting the correlation coefficient to give an estimate of reliability for the entire test. The correction equation, which is known as the *Spearman–Brown prophecy formula*, is as follows:

$$r^1 = \frac{2r}{1 + r}$$

where r = the correlation coefficient computed on the split-halves
r^1 = the estimated reliability of the entire test

Using the formula, the reliability for our hypothetical 20-item measure of leadership potential would be as follows:

$$r^1 = \frac{(2)(.67)}{1 + .67} = .80$$

The split-half technique is easy to use and eliminates most of the problems associated with the test–retest approach. More sophisticated and accurate methods of computing internal consistency estimates have been developed (*e.g.*, the *Kuder–Richardson formula 20* and *Cronbach's alpha*) and are described in texts on psychometrics, such as that of Nunnally (1978).

In summary, indices of homogeneity or internal consistency estimate the extent to which different subparts of an instrument are equivalent in terms of measuring the critical attribute. The split-half technique frequently has been used to estimate homogeneity, but other methods are increasingly preferred. None of these approaches take into consideration fluctuations over time as a source of unreliability.

Equivalence

A researcher may be interested in estimating the reliability of a measure via the equivalence approach under one of two circumstances: (1) when different observers or researchers are using an instrument to measure the same phenomena; or (2) when two presumably parallel instruments are administered at about the same time. In both situations, the aim is to determine the consistency or equivalence of the instrument(s) in yielding measurements of the same traits in the same subjects.

In the chapter on observational methods it was pointed out that a potential weakness of this data-collection approach is the fallibility of the observer. Even when great care is taken to design an observational system that minimizes the possibility of error, the researcher should assess the reliability of the instrument. In this case, the instrument includes both the category system developed by the researcher and the observer making the measurements.

Interrater (or *interobserver*) *reliability* is estimated by having two or more trained observers watching some event simultaneously and independently recording the relevant variables according to a predetermined plan or coding system. The resulting records can then be used to compute an index of equivalence or agreement. Several procedures for arriving at such an index are possible. For certain types of observational data, correlation techniques may be suitable. That is, a correlation coefficient may be computed to demonstrate the strength of the relationship between one observer's ratings and another's.

Another procedure is to compute reliability as a function of agreements, using the following equation:

$$\frac{\text{Number of agreements}}{\text{Number of agreements} + \text{Disagreements}}$$

The second situation in which the equivalence of measures is evaluated is when two alternative, parallel forms of a single instrument are available. In such a case, the two forms should be administered to a sample of persons in immediate succession, randomly alternating the order of presentation of the forms. The correlation coefficient between the two sets of scores would be an index of reliability of equivalence. This procedure is adopted to determine whether the two instruments are, in fact, measuring the same attribute. The researcher uses this technique to assess the errors of measurement resulting from errors in item sampling.

Validity

The second important criterion by which an instrument's quality is evaluated is its validity. *Validity* refers to the degree to which an instrument measures what it is supposed to be measuring. When an instrument to measure the attitudes of nurses toward the mentally retarded has been developed, how can its designer really know that the resulting scores validly reflect these attitudes?

The reliability and validity of an instrument are not totally independent qualities of an instrument. *A measuring device that is not reliable cannot possibly be valid.* An instrument cannot validly be measuring the attribute of interest if it is erratic, inconsistent, and inaccurate. An unreliable tool would be "measuring" too many other factors associated with random error to be considered a valid indicator of the target variable. However, an instrument can be reliable without being valid. Suppose we had the idea to measure anxiety in patients by measuring the circumference of their wrists. We could obtain highly accurate, consistent, and precise measurements of their wrist circumference, but such measures would not be valid indicators of anxiety. Thus, the high reliability of an instrument provides no evidence of its validity for an intended purpose; the low reliability of a measure *is* evidence of low validity.

Like reliability, validity has a number of different aspects and assessment approaches. Unlike reliability, however, the validity of an instrument is extremely difficult to establish. Solid evidence supporting the validity of most psychologically oriented measures is almost never available. Below we discuss several routes to evaluating an instrument's validity.

Content Validity

Content validity is concerned with how adequately covered the content area of an instrument is. Content validity is of most relevance to people designing a test to measure knowledge in a specific content area. In such a context the validity question being asked is "How representative are the questions on this test of the universe of all questions that might be asked on this topic?" Suppose we were interested in testing the knowledge of a group of lay people about the danger signals of cancer identified by the American Cancer Society. To be representative, or content valid, the questions on the test should include items from each of the seven danger signals or "CAUTION":

Change in bowel or bladder habits

A sore that does not heal

Unusual bleeding or discharge

Thickening or lump in breast or elsewhere

Indigestion or difficulty in swallowing

Obvious change in wart or mole

Nagging cough or hoarseness

The issue of content validity sometimes arises in conjunction with measures of attributes other than knowledge, such as in attitudinal measures, but the developers of attitude scales are usually more concerned with other aspects of validity.

The content validity of an instrument is necessarily based on judgment. There are no objective methods of assuring the adequate content coverage of an instrument. Experts in the content area may be called upon to analyze the items to see if they adequately represent the hypothetical content universe in the correct proportions. The test-maker, in writing or selecting items for inclusion in an instrument, should aim to build in content validity by careful planning and the careful execution of a plan.

Criterion-Related Validity

The *criterion-related approach* to validity assessment is a pragmatic one. The researcher attempting to establish the criterion-related validity of an instrument is not seeking to ascertain how well the tool is measuring a theoretical trait. The emphasis is on establishing the relationship between the instrument and some other criterion. The instrument, whatever abstract attribute it is measuring, is said to be valid if its scores correlate highly with some criterion.

The essential component of the criterion-related approach to validation is the availability of a reasonably reliable and valid criterion with which the measures on the target instrument can be compared. This is, unfortunately, seldom easy. If we were developing an instrument to predict the nursing effectiveness of nursing students, we might use subsequent supervisory ratings as our criterion. How can we be sure that these ratings are themselves valid and reliable? In fact, there is probably a good chance that the ratings are not dependable and consistent. The supervisory ratings would themselves be in need of validation. Usually the researcher must be content with less-than-perfect criteria.

Once the criterion is established, the validity can be assessed easily and straightforwardly. The scores on the instrument are correlated with scores on the criterion variable. The magnitude of the correlation coefficient is a direct indicator of how valid the instrument is. To illustrate, suppose a team of nurse researchers developed a scale to measure professionalism among nurses. They administer the instrument to a sample of nurses and at the same time ask the nurses to indicate how many articles they have published in professional journals. The latter variable was chosen as one of many potential objective criteria of professionalism. Fictitious data are presented in Table 13-3. The correlation coefficient of .83 indicates that the "professionalism scale" is a reasonably good predictor of the number of published articles a nurse has authored. Whether the scale is really measuring professionalism is a somewhat different issue—an issue that is the concern of construct validation.

Sometimes a distinction is made between two types of criterion-

Table 13-3. Fictitious Data for Criterion-Related Validity Example

SUBJECT	SCORE ON PROFESSIONALISM SCALE	NUMBER OF PUBLICATIONS	
1	25	2	
2	30	4	
3	17	0	
4	20	1	
5	22	0	
6	27	2	
7	29	5	
8	19	1	
9	28	3	
10	15	1	$r = .83$

related validity. The distinction is not a very important one, but the terms are used frequently enough to warrant their mention. *Predictive validity* refers to the adequacy of an instrument in differentiating between the performance or behaviors of subjects on some future criterion. When a school of nursing correlates the incoming SAT scores of students with subsequent grade-point averages, the predictive validity of the SATs for nursing school performance is being evaluated. *Concurrent validity* refers to the ability of an instrument to distinguish persons who differ in their present status on some criterion. For example, a psychological test to differentiate between those patients in a mental institution who can and cannot be released could be correlated with current behavioral ratings of health-care personnel. The difference between predictive and concurrent validity, then, is the difference in the timing of obtaining measurements on a criterion.

Validation by means of the criterion-related approach is most often used in applied or practically oriented research. Criterion-related validity is helpful in assisting decision-makers by giving them some assurance that their decisions will be effective, fair, and, in short, valid.

Construct Validity

Validating an instrument in terms of *construct validity* is one of the most difficult and challenging tasks that a researcher faces. Construct validity is concerned with the following questions: What is this measuring device actually measuring? Is the construct under investigation being adequately measured with this instrument? Unfortunately, the more abstract the concept, the more difficult it is to establish the construct validity of the measure; at the same time, the more abstract the concept, the less suitable it is to validate a measure by the criterion-related approach. What objective criterion is there for such concepts as empathy, grief, role conflict, separation anxiety, and so forth?

Construct validation can be approached in several ways, but there is always an emphasis on logical analysis and the testing of relationships predicted on the basis of theoretical considerations. Constructs are usually explicated in terms of other concepts; therefore, the researcher should be in a position to make predictions about the manner in which the construct will function in relation to other constructs. One common approach to construct validation is the *known-groups technique*. In this procedure, groups that are expected to differ on the critical attribute because of some known characteristic are administered the instrument. For instance, in validating a measure of fear of the labor experience, one might contrast the scores of primiparas and multiparas. Since one would expect that women who had never given birth would experience more fears and anxiety than pregnant women who had already had children, one might question the validity of the instrument if such differences did not emerge. There is not necessarily an expectation that the differences will be very great. It would be expected that some primiparas would feel no anxiety at all, while some multiparas would express some fears. On the whole, however, it would be anticipated that some group differences would be reflected in the scores.

A significant advance in the area of construct validation is the procedure developed by Campbell and Fiske (1959) known as the *multitrait–multimethod matrix method*. This procedure makes use of the concepts of convergence and discriminability. *Convergence* refers to evidence that different measures of a single construct yield similar results. Different approaches to measurement should converge on the construct if the various measures are valid. *Discriminability* refers to the ability to differentiate the construct being measured from other similar constructs. Campbell and Fiske have argued that evidence of both convergence and discriminability should be brought to bear in the construct-validity question. A more detailed description of this technique is presented in Polit and Hungler (1983).

In addition to the known-groups technique and the multitrait–multimethod procedure, there are other approaches to construct validation. A method that does not have a special name to identify it consists of an examination of relationships based on theoretical predictions. A researcher might reason as follows: According to theory, construct X is positively related to construct Y; instrument A is a measure of construct X, and instrument B is a measure of construct Y; scores on A and B are correlated positively, as predicted by the theory; therefore, it is inferred that A and B are valid measures of X and Y. This logical analysis is fallible and does not constitute proof of construct validity but is important as a type of evidence, nevertheless.

In summary, construct validation employs both logical and empirical procedures. Like content validity, construct validity requires a judgment pertaining to what the instrument is measuring. Unlike content validity, however, the logical operations required by construct validation are typically linked to a theory or conceptual framework. Construct validity and criterion-related validity share an empirical component, but in the latter case there is usually a pragmatic, objective criterion with which to compare a measure, rather than a second measure of an abstract theoretical construct.

Other Criteria for Assessing Measures

Reliability and validity are the two most important aspects to consider in evaluating a measuring instrument. If a measure can be shown to be reasonably reliable and valid for a specific purpose, then the researcher's confidence in the results of a study will be enhanced. High reliability and validity are a necessary, though not sufficient, condition for good scientific research.

Sometimes a researcher needs to consider other qualities of an instrument in addition to its validity and reliability. These additional criteria are by no means a substitute for reliability and validity but may in some cases be equally important. In many research situations, however, the criteria discussed below may be irrelevant or unimportant.

1. *Efficiency*. Instruments of comparable reliability and validity may still differ in their efficiency. An instrument that requires 10 minutes of a subject's time to measure his or her self-concept is efficient in comparison with an instrument to measure the same attribute that requires 30 minutes to complete. One aspect of efficiency is the number of items incorporated in an instrument. It was mentioned earlier that long instruments tend to be more reliable than shorter ones. There is, however, a point of diminishing returns. Other things being equal, it is desirable to select as efficient an instrument as possible.

2. *Sensitivity*. The sensitivity of an instrument determines how discriminating its measurements will be between persons with differing amounts of an attribute. Using a yardstick marked off in feet only, it would not be possible to discriminate between a person who is 5 feet 8 inches tall and one who is 6 feet 3 inches tall: both would be measured as 6 feet, measuring to the nearest foot. There are statistical procedures that permit a researcher to enhance the sensitivity of paper-and-pencil measures by assessing the degree to which each item is contributing to the instrument's power to make discriminations. These *item-analysis techniques* are described in detail in texts on measurement and psychometric theory.

3. *Objectivity*. Objectivity refers to the degree to which two independent users of an instrument obtain identical or similar scores for the

same subject. Physiological instruments tend to be high on objectivity. Observational measures are more susceptible to subjectivity. Instruments generally should be designed to be as objective as possible.

4. *Speededness.* For most types of instruments, the researcher should be sure that adequate time is allowed to obtain complete measurements without rushing the measuring process.

5. *Reactivity.* The instrument should, insofar as possible, avoid affecting the attribute that is being measured.

6. *Simplicity.* Other things being equal, a simple instrument is more desirable than a complex instrument inasmuch as complicated measures run a greater risk of errors.

In conclusion, it is probably fair to say that the development of adequate measuring tools is the single most pressing problem in the field of nursing research—as it is in such fields as education, psychology, sociology, and other disciplines concerned with human behavior. One of the greatest challenges facing this generation of nurse researchers is the construction and utilization of reliable, valid, and sensitive criterion measures of nursing outcomes.

Research Example

Hare (1984) developed a scale that measured feelings of loneliness and social isolation among the elderly.* She developed 12 Likert statements, 6 of which were worded positively and the other 6 of which were worded negatively. Examples from each category are (1) "I have lots of friends with whom I am close." and (2) "Sometimes days go by without my having a real conversation with someone." Hare administered a pretest of her instrument to 50 men and women aged 60 to 70 living independently in the community. She estimated the reliability of the scale using Cronbach's alpha, which yielded a reliability coefficient of .61.

Hare took two steps to validate her scale. First, she asked two geriatric nurses to examine the 12 items to assess the scale's content validity. These experts suggested some wording changes on three items and recommended replacing one of the items. Next, after the instrument was pretested she compared the scores of widows and widowers with people who were either married or had never been married. Her rationale was that the widowed would probably feel lonelier as a group than the nonwidowed. Her expectation was confirmed. Hare concluded that her scale was reasonably valid and reliable.

*This example is fictitious.

Hare took some reasonable steps in constructing her scale and assessing its quality. One must wonder, however, whether her new scale was really needed. Several scales for measuring social integration, loneliness, and "disengagement" in old age already exist, and their quality has been assessed and documented. Perhaps Hare rejected these other scales for one reason or another, although it is questionable whether her instrument represented any improvement.

Hare's scale was counterbalanced for negative and positive statements, thereby reducing the risk of measurement error attributable to such response sets as the acquiescence response bias. On the face of it, it would appear that she included a sufficient number of items to yield discriminating scores. She used a sophisticated procedure to estimate internal consistency, Cronbach's alpha, which is the best method available for Likert scales.

However, the reliability of Hare's scale could and should be improved. The reliability coefficient of .61 suggests that there is considerable measurement error. There are several steps that Hare can take to try to raise the reliability. First, she should make sure that each item on her scale is doing the job it was intended to do. Remember that scales are designed to discriminate among people who possess different amounts of some trait, in this case social isolation. If Hare identifies one or more items for which there is little variability (*i.e.*, most respondents either agree or disagree), then the item should be discarded. It is probably not measuring social isolation if everyone responds the same way.

Next, Hare should make sure that her scoring procedure is correct. Her assignment of scores is based on a *judgment* of what is a positively and negatively worded item. Respondents with high scores should agree with the positively worded items and disagree with the negatively worded ones. If substantial numbers of persons did the opposite, either the item should be eliminated or perhaps the scoring should be reversed. If people with high scores are divided in their agreement with an item, this may be caused by ambiguity in the wording of that question, so perhaps the statement could be revised.

Another step involves making sure that each item is measuring social isolation and not some other concept (such as morale or anxiety). This can be done judgmentally, although there are some sophisticated analytic procedures that are more objective.

Finally, Hare should consider lengthening the scale. Other things being equal, longer scales are more reliable than shorter ones. Hare must be careful, though, to add only items that measure social isolation.

Hare's efforts to validate her scale also deserve comment. Her first step was to consider the content validity of the scale. Having two knowledgeable persons examine the scale was undoubtedly a good thing to do. Nevertheless, it cannot be said that this activity made the scale valid. Content validity is not really as relevant for social–psychological scales as it is for, say, achievement tests. For variables such as social isolation, there is simply no well-defined domain from which items can be sampled. If Hare had used only the content-validity approach, she would have done little to establish her scale's validity.

As a second step, Hare used the known-groups technique. The data she obtained provided some useful evidence regarding the scale's validity. However, after making some of the revisions suggested above to improve the scale's reliability, Hare would do well to gather some additional data to support the scale's validity. For example, one might suspect that people would feel less socially isolated if they reported having kin living within a 20-mile radius; had visited with a friend within a 72-hour period preceding the completion of the scale; and were active members of a club, church group, or other social organization. If Hare took these additional steps to establish the reliability and validity of her scale, she could be justifiably confident that her scale was of a reasonably high quality.

Summary

Few, if any, measuring instruments used by researchers are pure or infallible. Rather, the "scores" obtained by the measuring tools may be decomposed into two parts—a true score and an error component. The *true score* is a hypothetical entity that represents the value that would be obtained if it were possible to arrive at a "perfect" measure. The *error component*, or *error of measurement*, represents the inaccuracies present in the measurement process. Sources of measurement error include situational contaminants, response-set biases, and transitory personal factors.

One important characteristic of a measuring tool is its *reliability*, which refers to the degree of consistency or accuracy with which an instrument measures an attribute. The higher the reliability of an instrument, the lower the amount of error present in the obtained scores. There are several empirical methods for assessing various aspects of an instrument's reliability. The *stability* aspect, which concerns the extent to which the instrument yields the same results on repeated administrations, is evaluated by *test–retest* procedures. The *internal consistency* or *homogeneity* aspect of reliability refers to the extent to which all of the instrument's subparts or items are measuring the same attribute. Internal consistency may be evaluated using either the *split-half reliability technique* or *Cronbach's alpha method*. When the focus of a reliability assessment is on establishing equivalence between observers in rating behaviors, estimates of *interrater reliability* may be obtained. The reliability of an instrument is partly a function of its length, the adequacy of the sampling of items, and the procedure used for obtaining the reliability coefficient.

Validity refers to the degree to which an instrument measures what it is supposed to be measuring. *Content validity* is concerned with the sampling adequacy of the content being measured. *Criterion-related validity* focuses on the relationship or correlation between the instrument and some outside criterion. *Construct validity* refers to the adequacy of an instrument in measuring the abstract construct of interest. One approach to assessing the construct validity of a measuring tool is the *known-groups technique,* which contrasts the scores of groups that are presumed to differ on the attribute. Another construct validity approach is the *multitrait–multimethod matrix technique,* which is based on the concepts of *convergence* and *discriminability.*

While high reliability and validity are essential criteria for assessing the quality of an instrument, other characteristics of the tool may also be important. Other criteria for evaluating a measuring tool include its efficiency, sensitivity, objectivity, speededness, reactivity, and simplicity.

Study Suggestions

1. Explain in your own words the meaning of the following correlation coefficients:

a. The relationship between intelligence and grade-point average was found to be .72.

b. The correlation coefficient between age and gregariousness was −.20.

c. It was revealed that patients' compliance with nursing instructions was related to their length of stay in the hospital (r = −.50).

2. Suppose the split-half reliability of an instrument to measure attitudes toward contraception was .70. Calculate the reliability of the full scale by using the Spearman–Brown formula.

3. Suppose a nurse researcher constructed an instrument to measure anxiety in ICU nurses. The instrument was then administered to 100 nurses immediately after the completion of their shifts. Identify some of the possible sources of measurement error.

4. A nurse researcher developed a new Likert scale to measure physicians' attitudes toward nurse practitioners. She used the test–retest approach to estimate the instrument's reliability and found it to be .87. Comment on the scale's reliability.

5. Suppose a nurse researcher who developed a scale to measure limitations in functional ability calculated an internal consistency coefficient of .51. Comment on the scale's reliability and validity.

6. What types of groups do you feel might be useful to employ for a known-groups approach to validating a measure of (a) emotional maturity; (b) attitudes toward alcoholics; (c) territorial aggressiveness; (d) job motivation; and (e) subjective pain?

Chapter 14
Quantitative Measurement

The previous section of this book reviewed a variety of methods of collecting research data. The terms "measurement" and "measuring instrument" were used repeatedly without a detailed discussion of the technical or analytic properties of data-collection measures. In this chapter we begin to discuss the quantitative aspects of instruments in preparation for the material on data analysis.

Measurement Principles

Measurement may be defined as follows: "Measurement consists of rules for assigning numbers to objects to represent quantities of attributes" (Nunnally, 1978, p. 2). In our private lives, we develop our own rules for measuring things, but as researchers we must either adopt well-specified rules (as in the case of measuring body temperature in terms of Fahrenheit degrees) or explicitly formulate new ones. Let us consider various aspects of the definition of measurement and the measurement process.

Quantification and Measurement

The above definition of measurement states that numbers are assigned to objects to quantify their attributes. Quantification is intimately associated with measurement and with the whole research process. While a few studies employ qualitative procedures for analyzing research information, the vast majority of scientific research uses quantitative data.

There is an often-quoted statement by an early American psychologist, L. L. Thurstone, that advances a position assumed by most researchers: "Whatever exists, exists in some amount and can be measured." The notion underlying this statement is that attributes of objects are not constant: they vary from day to day, from situation to situation, or from one

255

person to another. This variability is capable of a numerical expression that signifies *how much* of an attribute is present in the subject. Quantification is used to communicate that amount.

The purpose of assigning numbers, then, is to differentiate between persons or objects that possess varying degrees of the critical attribute. If nurse X is a more effective nurse than nurse Y, then the first nurse should have a higher "score" for effectiveness than the second. The crucial problem is determining *how much* higher the score should be in order to accurately reflect the differences that exist.

Rules and Measurement

Numbers must be assigned to objects according to specified rules rather than haphazardly. Quantification in the absence of rules would be meaningless. The rules for measuring temperature, weight, pressure, and other physical attributes are widely known and accepted. Rules for measuring many variables for nursing research studies, however, have to be invented. Whether the data are collected through observation, a self-report questionnaire, a projective test, or some other method, the researcher must specify under what conditions and according to what criteria the numerical values are to be assigned to the characteristic of interest.

Let us take a simple example to clarify this point. Suppose we were studying attitudes toward sex roles and asked nurses to express their extent of agreement with the following statement:

Basically, women are too emotional and dependent to be placed in
positions of authority.
( ) Strongly agree
( ) Agree
( ) Slightly agree
( ) Undecided
( ) Slightly disagree
( ) Disagree
( ) Strongly disagree

This question measures some aspect of a person's attitude toward traditional roles for women in our society. The responses can be quantified by developing a system for assigning numbers to them. It should be stressed that *any* rule would satisfy the definition of measurement. We could assign the value of 30 to "strongly agree," 27 to "agree," and 20 to "slightly agree," but there appears to be little justification for doing so. Therefore, in measuring attributes we must strive not only to develop rules, but also to develop good, meaningful rules. A simplified scheme of assigning a 1 to "strongly agree" and a 7 to "strongly disagree" is probably the most defensible procedure for the question at hand. This "rule" would quantitatively differentiate, in increments of one point, between people who have seven different reactions to the statement.

In developing a new set of rules for measuring attributes, the researcher seldom knows in advance if his or her rules really are the best ones possible. In essence, a new set of measurement rules constitutes a researcher's hypothesis about how an attribute functions and varies. The adequacy of the hypothesis—that is, the worth of the measuring tool— needs to be assessed, as described in the preceding chapter.

Measurement and Reality

The concepts we employ and the rules we develop to quantify those concepts must be linked to the real world. To state this requirement somewhat more technically, the measurement procedures must be isomorphic to reality. The term *isomorphic* signifies equivalence of or similarity between two phenomena. A measurement tool cannot be of scientific utility unless the measures resulting from it have some rational correspondence with reality.

Perhaps the isomorphism criterion strikes the reader as self-evident. Yet researchers continuously face the risk that their instruments are not accurately and validly reflecting real-world phenomena. Failures to meet the requirement for isomorphism generally stem from (1) inadequate conceptualization or definition of attributes, (2) inappropriate rules for assigning numbers to objects, or (3) both of these deficiencies.

To illustrate this point, suppose the Scholastic Aptitude Test (SAT) is administered to ten people, who obtain the following scores: 345, 395, 430, 435, 490, 505, 550, 570, 620, 640. These values are shown at the top of Figure 14-1. Let us further suppose that "in reality," the true scores of these same ten persons in terms of a hypothetical perfect test of scholastic aptitude would be as follows: 360, 375, 430, 465, 470, 500, 550, 610, 590, 670. These values are shown at the bottom of Figure 14-1. This figure shows that, while not perfect, the actual examination came fairly close to representing the "true" scores of the ten subjects. Two obtained scores matched exactly the hypothetical true scores, and no score was off by more than 40 points. Only two subjects (H and I) were improperly ordered as a result of the actual test. This example illustrates a measure whose isomorphism with reality can be considered high but improvable.

The researcher almost always works with fallible measures. Measuring instruments that measure psychological concepts are less likely to correspond to "reality" than physical measures, but few instruments are immune from error. A person's "true score" on an attribute can never be known, of course, but reliability procedures can be used for estimating the instrument's success in satisfying the isomorphism criterion.

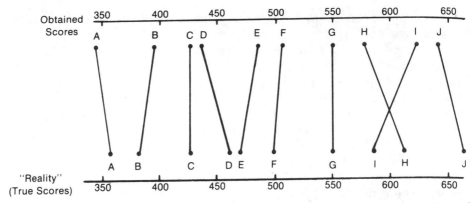

Figure 14-1. Relationship between obtained and true scores for a hypothetical set of test scores

Advantages of Measurement

What exactly does measurement accomplish that nonmeasurement does not? The previous section dealt with some fundamental principles of measurement without explaining in much detail why measurement is such an important scientific tool. In this section we examine some answers to the question of what the function of measurement is in science.

Before noting the major advantages of measurement, consider what researchers would work with in its absence. What would happen, for example, if there were no measures of height, temperature, blood pressure, or stress? All that would be left is intuition, guesses, personal judgment, and subjective evaluations. With this thought in mind, many of the advantages described below should be apparent.

Objectivity

One of the principal strengths of measurement is that it removes much of the guesswork in gathering scientific data. An objective measure is one that can be independently verified by other researchers. Two persons measuring the weight of a subject using the same scale would be likely to get identical or highly similar results. Two persons scoring a standardized personality test would be likely to arrive at identical scores for the attribute of introversion. Not all scientific measures are completely objective, but most are likely to incorporate rules for minimizing subjectivity.

In addition to the objectivity that is often built into the measure itself, quantification enhances objectivity in another respect. The numerical results of measurement are amenable to analytic procedures in which subjectivity is all but nonexistent. With purely qualitative information, the organization and analysis are likely to be judgmental.

Precision

Quantitative measures make it possible to obtain reasonably precise information. Instead of describing John as "rather tall," we can depict him as a man who is 6 feet 1½ inches tall. If we chose, or if the research requirements demanded it, we could obtain even more precise height measurements. Because of the possibility for precision, the researcher's task of differentiating among objects that possess different degrees of an attribute becomes considerably easier.

Communication

Measurement constitutes a language of communication. Science is not a private enterprise, engaged in solely to amuse or satisfy the curiosity of isolated researchers. Communication among scientists is essential if a knowledge base is to be developed. Inasmuch as numbers are less vague than words, quantitative measurement does a reasonably good job of communicating information to a broad audience of people. If a researcher reported that the average oral temperature of a sample of postoperative patients was "somewhat high," different readers might develop different conceptions about the physiological state of the sample. However, if the researcher reported an average temperature of 99.5° F, there is no possibility of ambiguity and subjective interpretations.

Levels of Measurement

Scientists have developed a classification system for categorizing different types of measures. This classification system is important because the analytic operations that can be performed on data depend on the measurement level employed. Four major classes, or levels, of measurement have been identified.

Nominal Measurement

The lowest level of measurement is referred to as *nominal measurement*. This level involves the assignment of numbers to simply classify characteristics into categories. For many attributes, we can do no more than to perform this sorting function. Examples of variables amenable to nominal measurement include gender, ethnicity, religion, eye color, blood type, nationality, and nursing specialty.

The numbers assigned in nominal measurement are not intended to convey any quantitative implications. If we establish a rule to classify male subjects as 1 and female subjects as 2, the numbers in and of themselves have no meaning. The number 2 here clearly does not mean "more than" or "better than" 1. It would be perfectly acceptable to reverse the code and use 1 for female subjects and 2 for male subjects. The numbers are merely symbols that represent two different values of the gender attribute. Indeed, instead of numerical symbols we could as easily have chosen alphabetical symbols, such as M and F. We recommend, however, thinking in terms of numerical categories, because the subsequent analysis of data will be simplified if such a procedure is adopted when a computer is employed.

Nominal measurement provides no information about an attribute except that of equivalence and nonequivalence. If we were to "measure" the gender of Tom, Mary, Susan, and Jim, we would—according to the rule stated above—assign them the codes 1, 2, 2, and 1, respectively. Tom and Jim are considered equivalent, at least with respect to the target attribute, but they are not equivalent to the other two subjects.

The basic requirements for measuring attributes on the nominal scale are that the classifications must be mutually exclusive and collectively exhaustive. For example, if we were measuring ethnicity, we might establish the following scheme: 1 = whites, 2 = blacks, 3 = Hispanics. Each subject must be classifiable into one and only one of these categories. The requirement for collective exhaustiveness would not be met if, for example, there were several respondents of Chinese descent in the sample.

The numbers used in nominal measurement cannot be treated mathematically. While it might make perfectly good sense to determine the average weight of a sample of subjects, it is meaningless to calculate the average gender of a sample. However, the elements assigned to each category can be enumerated, and statements can be made about the frequency of occurrence in each class. In a sample of 50 patients, we might find 30 men and 20 women. We could also say that 60% of the sample were male and 40% were female. However, no further mathematical operations would be permissible with data from nominal measures.

It might strike some readers as odd to think of the categorization procedure we have been describing as measurement. If our definition of measurement is recalled, however, it can be seen that nominal measurement does, in fact, involve the assignment of numbers to attributes according to rules. The rules are not sophisticated, to be sure, but they are rules nonetheless.

Ordinal Measurement

The next level in the measurement hierarchy is *ordinal measurement*. Ordinal measurement permits the sorting of objects on the basis of their standing relative to each other on a specified attribute. This level of measurement goes beyond a mere categorization: the attributes are ordered according to some criterion. If a researcher were to order subjects from the heaviest to the lightest, or the tallest to the shortest, or the most efficient to the least efficient, then we would say that an ordinal level of measurement had been used.

The fundamental difference between nominal and ordinal measurement is that in the latter case information about not only equivalence but also relative standing or ordering among objects is implied. When we assign numbers to a person's religious affiliation, the numbers have no inherent meaning or significance. We could develop a scheme whereby Catholics were assigned to category 1, Jews to 2, Protestants to 3, and all others to 4. This nominal measuring scheme is absolutely arbitrary. Now, consider this scheme for measuring a client's ability to perform activities of daily living: 1—completely dependent, 2—needs another person's assistance, 3—needs mechanical assistance, 4—completely independent. In this case the measurement is ordinal. The numbers are not arbitrary: they signify incremental ability to perform the activities of daily living. The persons assigned a value of four are equivalent to each other with regard to their ability to function and, relative to those in all the other categories, have more of that attribute. In fact, the following relationship can be stated: $4 > 3 > 2 > 1$.

Ordinal measurement does not, however, tell us anything about how much greater one level of an attribute is than another level. We do not know if being completely independent is "twice as good" as needing mechanical assistance; neither do we know if the difference between needing another person's assistance and needing mechanical assistance is the same as that between needing mechanical assistance and being completely independent. Ordinal measurement only tells us the relative ranking of the levels of an attribute.

As in the case of nominal scales, the types of mathematical operations permissible with ordinal-level data are rather restricted. Averages are generally meaningless with rank-order measures. Frequency counts, percentages, and several other statistical procedures to be discussed in Chapter 15 are appropriate for analyzing ordinal-level data.

Interval Measurement

Interval measurement occurs when the researcher can specify both the rank ordering of objects on an attribute and the distance between those objects. Most psychological and educational tests are based on interval scales. The Scholastic Aptitude Test (SAT) is an example of this level of measurement. A score of 550 on the SAT is higher than a score of 500, which in turn is higher than 450. In addition to providing this rank-order information, a difference between 550 and 500 on the test is presumably equivalent to the difference between 500 and 450.

Interval measures, then, are more informative than ordinal measures. One piece of information that interval measures fail to provide is the absolute magnitude of the attribute for any particular object. The Fahrenheit scale for measuring temperature illustrates this point. A temperature of 60° F is 10 degrees warmer than 50° F. A 10-degree difference similarly separates 40° F and 30° F, and the two differences in temperature are equivalent. However, it cannot be said that 60° F is twice as hot as 30° F, or three times as hot as 20° F. The Fahrenheit scale, then, is not a measure of temperature in absolute units. The assignment of numbers to temperature on the Fahrenheit scale involves an arbitrary zero point. Zero on the thermometer does not signify a total absence of heat. In interval scales, there is no real or rational zero point.

The use of interval scales greatly expands the researcher's analytic possibilities. The intervals between numbers can be meaningfully added and subtracted: the interval between 10° F and 5° F is 5 degrees, or $10 - 5 = 5$. This same operation could not be performed with ordinal measures. Because of this capability, interval-level data can be averaged. It is perfectly reasonable, for example, to compute an average daily temperature for hospitalized patients from whom temperature readings are taken four times a day. Most sophisticated statistical procedures require that measurements be made on an interval scale.

Ratio Measurement

The highest level of measurement is the *ratio scale*. Ratio scales are distinguished from interval scales by virtue of having a rational, meaningful zero. Measures on a ratio scale provide information about (1) the rank ordering of objects on the critical attribute, (2) the intervals between objects, and (3) the absolute magnitude of the attribute for the object. Many physical measures provide ratio-level data. A person's height and weight, for example, are measured on a ratio scale. It is perfectly acceptable to say that someone who weighs 200 pounds is twice as heavy as someone who weighs 100 pounds.

Since ratio scales have an absolute zero, all arithmetic operations are permissible. One can meaningfully add, subtract, multiply, and divide numbers on a ratio scale. Consequently, all of the statistical procedures suitable for interval-level data are also appropriate for ratio-level data. Ratio measurement constitutes the measurement ideal for scientists but is probably an unattainable ideal for the vast majority of attributes of a psychological or behavioral nature.

Comparison of the Levels

The four levels of measurement presented in this section constitute a hierarchy, with ratio scales at the pinnacle and nominal measurement at the base. The major characteristics of each level have been discussed, but several additional points are in order.

Researchers generally should strive to construct measuring instruments on as high a level of measurement as possible. This guideline is based on two considerations: higher levels of measurement yield more information and they are amenable to more powerful and sensitive analytic procedures than lower levels. When one moves from a higher to a lower level of measurement, there is always an information loss. Let us look at an example relating to data on the weight of a sample of people. Table 14-1 presents fictitious data for ten subjects. The first column shows the ratio-level data, that is, the actual weight in pounds. The ratio measure gives us complete information about the absolute weight of each subject and the differences in weights between all pairs of subjects.

In the second column the original data have been converted to interval measures by assigning a score of zero to the lightest person, the score of 5 to the person 5 pounds heavier than the lightest person (Darlene), and so forth. Note that the differences in pounds are equally far apart, even though they are at different parts of the scale. The data no longer tell us, however, anything about the absolute weights of the persons in this sample. Terry, the lightest person, might be a 10-pound infant or a 200-pound Weight Watcher.

In the third column of Table 14-1, ordinal measurements were devel-

Table 14-1. Fictitious Data for Four Levels of Measurement

	RATIO LEVEL	INTERVAL LEVEL	ORDINAL	NOMINAL
Bill	180	70	10	2
Terry	110	0	1	1
Doug	165	55	8	2
Ingrid	130	20	5	1
Lee	175	65	9	2
Darlene	115	5	2	1
Helen	125	15	4	1
Tom	150	40	7	1
Mark	145	35	6	1
Nancy	120	10	3	1

oped by rank-ordering the sample from the lightest, who was assigned the score of 1, to the heaviest, who was assigned the score of 10. Now even more information is missing. The data provide no indication of how much heavier Bill is than Terry. The difference separating them might be as little as 5 pounds or as much as 150 pounds.

Finally, the last column presents nominal measurements in which all subjects were classified as either "heavy" or "light." The criterion applied in categorizing people was arbitrarily set as a weight either greater than 150 pounds (2), or less than/equal to 150 pounds (1). The available information is very limited. Within any one category, there are no clues as to who is heavier than whom. With this level of measurement, Bill, Doug, and Lee are considered equivalent. They are equivalent with regard to the attribute "heavy/light" as defined by the classification criterion.

This example illustrates that at every successive level in the measurement hierarchy there is a loss of valuable information. It also illustrates another point: when one has information at one level, one can always manipulate the data to arrive at a lower level, but the converse is not true. If we were only given the nominal measurements, it would be impossible to reconstruct the actual weights. Researchers seldom collapse information to arrive at lower-level data, but it is important to recognize the greater flexibility possible with ratio and interval measures than with ordinal and nominal measures.

One final point should be mentioned. It is not always a straightforward task to identify the level of measurement for a particular instrument. Usually, nominal measures and ratio scales are discernible with little difficulty, but the distinction between ordinal and interval measures is more problematic. Some methodologists argue that most psychological measures that are treated as interval measures are really only ordinal measures. The majority of writers seem to believe that, while such instruments as IQ tests and personality measures produce data that are, strictly speaking, ordinal level, the distortion introduced by treating them as interval measures is too small to warrant an abandonment of powerful statistical analyses.

Research Example

Stevens (1985) explored factors that might be related to leadership ability in head nurses and nursing administrators.* He distributed a questionnaire that included a 20-item "Leadership Potential" scale to a sample of 500 nurses who had a supervisory role in 25 hospitals in the Midwest. The scale had been shown to have high levels of validity and reliability when administered to other samples of

---

*This example is fictitious.

nurses. The independent variables measured in the questionnaire were as follows: age (under 30/30–40/over 40); sex; membership in ANA (yes/no); number of years of presupervisory experience; number of continuing-education units in previous 12 months; number of nursing journals subscribed to (none/1–2/3 or more); type of basic nursing preparation (diploma, associate's degree, baccalaureate degree); and advanced degrees held (yes/no). Stevens found that scores on the leadership potential scale were highest among nurses in the 30-to-40 age range, among those with the most years of presupervisory experience, and among those with a graduate-level degree.

Stevens' study involved the collection of data at every level of measurement. Variables measured on the nominal scale included sex, membership in ANA, type of training, and attainment of a graduate degree. Age and nursing-journal subscriptions were measured on an ordinal scale: in each case the investigator created three categories that ranked the responses in an ascending hierarchy. (Some people might argue that type of educational preparation is also an ordinal scale, but to justify this one would have to assume that the major underlying difference between the three programs was number of years of preparation). The dependent variable, leadership potential, was measured with a 20-item scale that we can presume to yield interval-level data. Finally, variables measured on a ratio scale included years of presupervisory experience and number of continuing-education units.

For the most part, Stevens measured his variables on the highest scale possible. There were, however, two exceptions—age and number of journal subscriptions. Both could have been measured on a ratio scale but were measured in such a way that only ordinal-level data were gathered. It is interesting that in this case the analysis revealed a pattern that suggests some collapsing of information was desirable. Nurses in the 30-to-40 age range scored higher than both younger *and* older nurses on the leadership potential scale. Perhaps this relationship (sometimes referred to as a *curvilinear relationship*) between age and leadership potential would have gone undetected had the investigator analyzed the dependent variables in relation to actual age by computing a correlation coefficient. Still, this does not justify Stevens' decision to ask for the data in a precategorized form. After all, with the actual ages he could always have categorized after the fact. It may be, in fact, that Stevens came to some misleading conclusions. Perhaps the nurses with maximum leadership potential are aged 35 to 40, but it would be impossible to discover this using Stevens' precoded scheme. Furthermore, Stevens would not even be able to adequately describe the age of his sample. He would not be able to report that the average age of the nurses was, say, 38.2. With ordinal-level data he could only tell us that, say, 56% of his sample were between the ages of 30 and 40. In short, analytic possibilities were curtailed by not using the highest level of measurement possible.

Summary

Measurement consists of a set of rules according to which numerical values are assigned to objects to represent varying degrees of some attribute. Strictly speaking, we do not measure "things," but rather some abstract characteristic of things, such as height, weight, pain, and so on. The quantification aspect of measurement usually focuses on developing a numerical system to indicate how much of the critical attribute the object possesses. This quantification process is not performed haphazardly, but rather according to well-formulated rules. The researcher must strive to locate or develop measures that are *isomorphic* with reality; that is, there must be some correspondence between or equivalence of the actual attributes and the measurements of them.

Measurement offers the research scientist a number of benefits. Objectivity is enhanced through measurement, inasmuch as it permits observations to be independently verified by other researchers. Greater precision can be attained through measurement than through casual observation, making it easier for the researcher to differentiate among the varying degrees of an attribute possessed by objects. Measurement also constitutes an important channel of communication among scientists.

Measures can be categorized into one of four levels: nominal, ordinal, interval, and ratio. *Nominal measurement* classifies characteristics of attributes into mutually exclusive and collectively exhaustive categories. Nominal measurements, which represent the lowest level of measurement, cannot be manipulated mathematically. *Ordinal measurement* involves the sorting of objects on the basis of their relative standing to each other on a specified attribute. Ordinal-level data yield rank-orderings among objects. *Interval measurements* indicate not only the rank-ordering of objects on an attribute, but also the amount of distance between each object. Distances between numerical values on the interval scale represent equivalent distances in the attribute being measured. *Ratio measurements*, which constitute the highest form of measurement, are distinguished from interval measurements by virtue of having a rational zero point. Since ratio scales have an absolute zero, all arithmetic operations are permissible. In general, researchers should strive to measure key variables on as high a measurement scale as possible.

Study Suggestions

1. Read a research report in a recent issue of *Nursing Research*. Was the level of measurement used by the author the highest possible? If not,

explain how the researcher could have attained a higher level of measurement than was used.

2. For each of the following variables, specify the highest level of measurement that you feel would ordinarily be attainable: number of siblings, rank in class, color of urine specimen, time to first voiding for postoperative patients, faculty status (*i.e.*, professor, instructor), attitude toward abortion, exposure to genetic counseling, length of stay in hospital, diastolic blood pressure, hospital nursing positions, sleeping state, anxiety level.

3. Below are fictitious data for the length in centimeters of ten newborns. Convert this information to interval, ordinal, and nominal measurements. *ordinal*   *Nominal*   *interval*

a. 45 cm 1   1   0
b. 52 cm 3   2   7
c. 61 cm 9   3   16
d. 49 cm 2   1   4
e. 60 cm 8   3   15
f. 58 cm 7   2   13
g. 63 cm 10   3   18
h. 58 cm 6   2   13
i. 53 cm 1   2   8
j. 57 cm 5   8   12

Part V
Analysis of Research Data

Chapter 15
Introduction to Data Analysis

The data collected in the course of a research project do not in and of themselves answer the research questions or test the research hypotheses. The data are generally too numerous to be meaningfully understood by a quick perusal of the information. The research data need to be processed and analyzed in some systematic fashion so that trends and patterns of relationships can be detected.

There are two broad approaches to the analysis of research data: qualitative and quantitative. The type of approach used is linked to the nature of the data collected. *Quantitative data*, as the term suggests, consist of numerical (quantified) information, such as body temperatures, grade-point averages, blood pressure readings, scores on a Likert scale measuring attitudes toward estrogen replacement therapy, and so on. *Qualitative data*, on the other hand, consist of detailed descriptions of people, events, situations, or observed behavior. Examples of qualitative materials include the field notes from a participant observer, descriptions written on medical records, and historical letters and diaries.

The distinction between qualitative and quantitative data is not, however, as clear-cut as it may at first appear. Qualitative materials *can* be quantified and therefore subjected to quantitative analysis. For example, suppose we asked patients to describe in their own words the quality of the nursing care they were receiving. We could quantify the materials in a number of ways: we could *count* the number of specific complaints mentioned, we could *code* for the presence or absence of a complaint about the time required for the nurses to respond to a call, or we could *rate* the description in terms of overall favorableness toward the care received.

Whether or not qualitative data *should* be quantified and analyzed using statistical procedures is a different issue. Some investigators argue that everything can be measured (quantified), and that statistical analysis is the only scientifically acceptable method of determining, in an objective manner, the relationships among variables. Other researchers argue that

271

qualitative materials are richer than numbers and offer more potential for understanding relationships; they also assert that, since data collection and coding procedures are not immune to subjectivity, the use of numbers merely disguises potential bias and gives the illusion of objectivity.

We are inclined to disagree with both of the extremes in this controversy. We believe that an understanding of human behaviors, problems, and characteristics is best advanced by the judicious and combined use of both qualitative and quantitative data. In any event, researchers should have sufficient understanding of the limitations and advantages of both analytic approaches so that they can make an informed choice of method and so that they can render a meaningful critique of the work of other investigators.

The vast majority of scientific research continues to use quantitative analysis in processing data. Therefore, in the next two chapters we focus on quantitative methods. The next section, however, discusses qualitative procedures.

Qualitative Analysis

Qualitative analysis uses as data detailed and free-flowing descriptions derived from a variety of sources. The most common forms of data collection for qualitative analysis, however, are through participant observation, unstructured interviews, and written records. Qualitative methods are more appropriately applied to certain types of research problems than to others. There is general agreement that qualitative data are not appropriate for establishing causality, rigorously testing hypotheses, or determining the opinions of a large population. The unsuitability of qualitative methods for these purposes is based in part on the difficulties of analysis. Another problem, however, is that qualitative methods tend to yield vast amounts of data from small samples that are generally not selected at random. Therefore, the generalizability of the conclusions is often questionable.

We must stress that these shortcomings of qualitative research are offset by some important advantages. There are four major purposes for qualitative techniques:

1. *Description.*   When little is known about a group of people, an institution, or some social phenomenon, in-depth interviewing or participant observation are good ways to learn about them. For example, suppose we wanted to learn about the experiences of deinstitutionalized mental patients. How do these people live? What factors facilitate or impede improved mental health? How do they cope with the transition to a new environment? For this type of study, a survey approach might not be feasible or profitable.

2. *Hypothesis Generation.*   A researcher using qualitative techniques often has no explicit *a priori* hypotheses. The collection of in-depth information about some phenomenon might, however, lead to the formulation of hypotheses that could be tested more formally in subsequent research. For example, through in-depth interviews a researcher could investigate the reasons for discontinued use of oral contraceptives among teenage girls. Open-ended discussion with a sample of girls might lead the researcher to hypothesize that girls whose boyfriends have complained about the pill's side-effects on the girls (*e.g.*, weight gain, moodiness, headaches) are more likely to stop using the pill than girls whose boyfriends have not made such complaints.

3. *Understanding Relationships and Causal Processes.*   Quantitative methods often demonstrate that variables are systematically related to one another, but they often fail to provide insights about *why* the variables are related. For example, suppose we found that special care unit nurses had higher self-esteem than other nurses. Qualitative methods might yield some understanding about the mechanisms underlying this relationship.

4. *Illustrating Descriptions or Relationships.*   Qualitative materials can be useful as illustrations in a quantitatively focused study. Suppose a researcher were studying stress and coping behavior among recently divorced women. The researcher, in analyzing the quantitative materials, might conclude that 80% of the sample had experienced considerable distress in the postseparation period, and 30% had sought professional assistance for that stress. These facts are interesting, but the following (real) excerpt, illustrating a report of stress, would add a perspective that the numbers alone could not provide:

> I've had a lot of emotional problems since my husband left. I can't foresee the future and I don't want to because I don't think I could keep my sanity if I knew what was ahead. Sometimes when I wake up in the morning I just lie there staring at the ceiling, thinking about everything I've been through, and I'll think, "What am I here for? What's the use of going on? Will anything in my life ever go right for me?"

Excerpts such as this are clearly richer than the statistic indicating that 80% of divorced women experience distress. However, how does one analyze such information so that it can be presented in an objective and systematic way? There are, in fact, no rules for analyzing and presenting qualitative data. It is largely because of this fact that qualitative methods have sometimes been described as "soft." The absence of systematic analytic procedures makes it difficult for the researcher engaged in a qualitative analysis to present conclusions in such a way as to convince other scientists of their validity. Although there are no explicit rules for analyzing qualitative materials, we present below some guidelines that are designed to provide some internal checks on the conclusions that are derived. We include in these guidelines a procedure described by Becker (1970) as quasi-statistical analysis, as well as procedures normally associated with content analysis. *Content analysis* is a method that has been devised for yielding objective and systematic descriptions of communications and written materials.

The analysis of qualitative materials generally begins with a search for themes. For example, if we were studying women's decisions to switch from breast-feeding to a bottle formula, we might find that one theme had to do with feelings of failure vis-a-vis the baby's nutritional needs. Another theme might relate to the impracticality of breast-feeding. The thematic analysis is usually carried a step further by looking for themes that emerge in relation to other variables. For example, do certain themes for discontinuing breast-feeding emerge among primiparous women, while others emerge in multiparous women? The search for themes is essentially a search for commonalities among people and for differences across subgroups.

The next step involves a validation of the understandings that the thematic exploration provides. In this step, the concern is whether the themes inferred are an accurate representation of the subjects' perspectives. Several procedures can be used in this validation step. If there is more than one researcher working on a study, debriefing sessions in which the themes are reviewed and specific cases discussed can be highly productive. Multiple perspectives cannot ensure the validity of the themes but can minimize any idiosyncratic biases. Using an iterative approach can also be helpful; that is, the researcher derives themes from descriptive materials, goes back with the themes to see if the materials fit, and then refines the themes as necessary. In some cases it might also be appropriate to review the thematic analysis with a few of the subjects who generated the data originally. That is, respondents can be presented with the preliminary thematic analysis and encouraged to contradict or support this analysis.

In the next step a more formal categorization system is developed and the descriptive materials are coded according to this system. It is at this point that "quasi-statistics" come into play. *Quasi-statistics* are essentially an accounting system: the researcher tabulates the frequency with which certain themes, relations, or insights are supported by the data. A more robust use of quasi-statistics involves the additional step of counting the frequency with which the themes, relations, and understanding fail to be supported by the data.

Next, usually on a theme-by-theme basis, the researcher summarizes the understandings gleaned from the qualitative analysis. Here, illustrative quotes or excerpts from field notes are essentially used as evidence in support of the researcher's propositions. When a draft summary is completed, the validity of the descriptions is assessed by comparing the description with the frequency information. Negative cases should then be reviewed to determine what bearing they have, if any, on the researcher's propositions. Finally, the descriptions are revised as necessary by integrating the insights derived from the validity check.

It should be clear that qualitative analysis is an exceedingly laborious and time-consuming enterprise, and for that reason the samples tend to be small. Rarely are unstructured interviews conducted with more than 100 to 200 people. Surveys, on the other hand, may involve thousands of respondents.

The fact is that, in our current state of knowledge about human characteristics and behavior, we need both in-depth information and information from a broad representation of people. We need exploratory, detailed research and rigorous hypothesis-testing studies. Both quantitative and qualitative methods are essential to advancing our understanding. In fact, we are inclined to regard a study that triangulates multiple data-collection methods and multiple analytic strategies as potentially the most fruitful type of research endeavor.

Quantitative Analysis: Elementary Descriptive Statistics

Statistical methods are techniques for rendering quantitative information meaningful and intelligible. Without the aid of statistics, the quantitative data collected in a research project would be little more than a chaotic mass of numbers. Statistical procedures enable the researcher to reduce, summarize, organize, evaluate, interpret, and communicate numerical information.

A knowledge of basic statistical methods is indispensable for those who want to keep abreast of research developments in their field. Many people are intimidated by statistics because they feel that they are "no good at math." It is not necessary to have a strong mathematical talent to profit from the advantages of statistical analysis. In order to apply and interpret statistics, one need only to have basic arithmetic skills and logical thinking ability. In the remainder of this chapter and in the one that follows, the emphasis will be on how to use statistics appropriately in different research situations and how to understand what they mean once they have been applied.

Statistics usually are classified as either descriptive or inferential. *Descriptive statistics* are used to describe and synthesize data obtained from empirical observations and measurements. Averages and percentages are examples of descriptive statistics. Actually, when such indices are calculated on data from a population, they are referred to as *parameters*. A descriptive index from a sample is called a *statistic*. Most scientific questions are about parameters, but researchers usually must be content to calculate statistics to estimate these parameters. Various types of descriptive statistics are discussed below.

Frequency Distributions

Raw data that are neither analyzed nor organized are overwhelming. It is not even possible to discern general trends until some order or structure is imposed on the data. Consider the 60 numbers presented in Table 15-1. Let us assume that these numbers represent the scores of 60 industrial nurses on a 30-item test to measure knowledge about industrial alcoholism and drug abuse. Visual inspection of the numbers in this table is not too helpful in understanding how the nurses performed. The data are too numerous to make much sense of them in this form.

Frequency distributions represent a method of imposing some order on a mass of numerical data. A *frequency distribution* is a systematic arrangement of numerical values from the lowest to the highest, together with a count of the number of times each value was obtained. The fictitious test scores of the industrial nurses are presented as a frequency distribution in Table 15-2. It should be apparent that this organized arrangement makes it convenient to see at a glance what the highest and lowest scores are, where the bulk of scores tend to cluster, and what the most common score is. None of this was easily discernible before the data were organized.

The construction of a frequency distribution is simple. It consists basically of two parts—the classes of observations or measurements (the Xs) and the frequency or count of the observations falling in each class (the fs). The observations are listed in numerical order in one column and the corresponding frequencies are listed in another. The only requirement for a frequency distribution is that the classes of observation must be mutually exclusive and exhaustive. The sum of the numbers appearing in the frequency column must be equal to the size of the sample. In less verbal terms, $\Sigma f = n$, which translates as the sum of (signified by the Greek letter sigma, Σ) the frequencies equals the sample size, n. It is often useful to display not only the frequency counts for different values, but also the percentages of the total, as shown in the fourth column of Table 15-2.

Rather than listing frequencies in tabular form, some researchers prefer to display their data graphically. Graphs have the advantage of being able to communicate a lot of information almost instantaneously. A widely used type of graph is known as a *frequency polygon*. Frequency

Table 15-1. Test Scores for Industrial Nurses

22	27	25	19	24	25	23	29	24	20
26	16	20	26	17	22	24	18	26	28
15	24	23	22	21	24	20	25	18	27
24	23	16	25	30	29	27	21	23	24
26	18	30	21	17	25	22	24	29	28
20	25	26	24	23	19	27	28	25	26

Table 15-2. Frequency Distribution of Test Scores

SCORE (X)	TALLIES	FREQUENCY (f)	PERCENT
15	|	1	1.7
16	||	2	3.3
17	||	2	3.3
18	|||	3	5.0
19	||	2	3.3
20	||||	4	6.7
21	|||	3	5.0
22	||||	4	6.7
23	⊞⊞	5	8.3
24	⊞⊞||||	9	15.0
25	⊞⊞||	7	11.7
26	⊞⊞|	6	10.0
27	||||	4	6.7
28	|||	3	5.0
29	|||	3	5.0
30	||	2	3.3
		$N = 60 = \Sigma f$	$100\% = \Sigma \%$

polygons are easy to construct and interpret. First, scores are placed on a horizontal dimension, with the lowest value on the left, ascending to the highest value on the right. Next, the vertical dimension is used to designate the frequency count or, alternatively, percentages. The numbering of the vertical axis usually begins with zero. Then, a dot corresponding to the frequency is placed above each score, as shown in Figure 15-1. It is conventional to connect the figure to the base (zero line) at the score below the minimum value obtained and above the maximum value obtained. In this particular example, however, the graph is terminated at 30 and brought down to the base at that point with a dotted line, because 30 was the highest possible score on the nurses' test of knowledge.

Shapes of Distributions

A set of data can be completely summarized in terms of three characteristics—the shape of the distribution, central tendency, and variability. The latter two characteristics will be dealt with in subsequent sections.

A distribution is said to be *symmetrical* in shape if, when folded over, the two halves of a frequency polygon would be superimposed. In other words, symmetrical distributions consist of two halves that are mirror images of one another. Both distributions shown in Figure 15-2 are symmetrical. With real data sets, the distributions are rarely as perfectly sym-

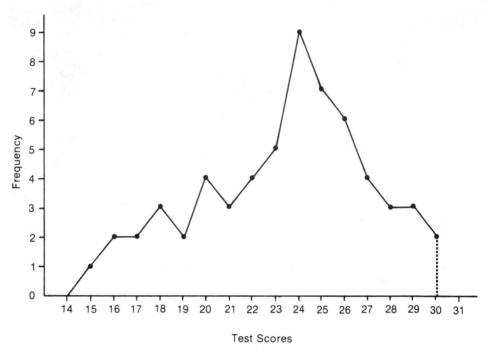

Figure 15-1. Frequency polygon of test scores

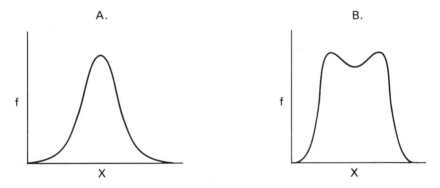

Figure 15-2. Examples of symmetrical distributions

metrical as shown in this figure. However, minor discrepancies are often ignored in trying to briefly characterize the shape of a distribution.

Nonsymmetrical distributions are described as being *skewed*. In skewed distributions, the peak is "off center" and one tail is longer than the other. Distributions that are skewed are usually described in terms of the direction of the skew. When the longer tail is pointed toward the right, the distribution is said to be *positively skewed*. The first part of Figure 15-3 depicts a positively skewed distribution. If, on the other hand, the tail points to the left, the skew is described as negative. A *negatively skewed* distribution is illustrated in the second graph in Figure 15-3. An example of an actual attribute that is positively skewed is personal income. Most people have low to moderate incomes, with only a few people in very high income brackets at the tail of the distribution. An example of a negatively skewed attribute is age at death. Here, the bulk of people are at the upper end of the distribution, with relatively few people dying at an early age.

A second aspect of a distribution's shape is its modality. A *unimodal* distribution is one that has only one peak or high point, whereas a *multimodal* distribution has two or more peaks. The most common type of multimodal distribution is one with two peaks, which is called *bimodal.* Graph A in Figure 15-2 is unimodal, as are both graphs in Figure 15-3. A bimodal distribution is illustrated in graph B of Figure 15-2. It should be noted that symmetry and modality are completely independent aspects of a distribution. Knowledge of skewness does not tell you anything about how many peaks the distribution has.

Some distributions are encountered so frequently that special labels are used to designate them. Of particular interest in statistical analysis is the distribution known as the *normal curve* (sometimes called a *bell-shaped curve).* In terms of the descriptions introduced above, a normal curve is one that is symmetrical, unimodal, and not too peaked, as illustrated by the distribution in graph A of Figure 15-2. Many physical and psychological attributes of human beings been found to approximate a normal distribution. Examples include height, intelligence, birthweight, and grip strength. As we will see in the next chapter, the normal curve plays a central role in inferential statistics.

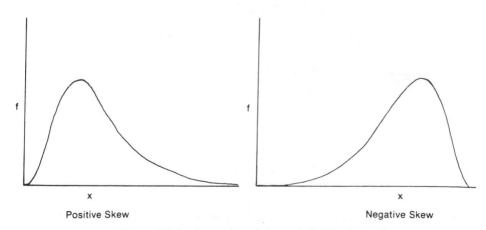

Positive Skew   Negative Skew

Figure 15-3. Examples of skewed distributions

Central Tendency

Frequency distributions are an important means of imposing order on a set of raw data and of clarifying group patterns. For many purposes, however, a group pattern is of less interest to a researcher than an overall summary of a group's characteristics. The researcher usually asks such questions as "How does the typical nurse feel about euthanasia?" or "How much information does the average high school student have about nutrition?" Such questions seek a single number that best represents a whole distribution of measures. Such indices of "typicalness" are referred to as measures of *central tendency*. To lay persons, the term *average* is normally used to designate central tendency. Researchers seldom use this term because it is too ambiguous, inasmuch as there are three commonly used kinds of averages, or indices of central tendency—the mode, the median, and the mean. Each can be used as an index to represent a whole set of measurements.

The Mode. The *mode* is that numerical value in a distribution that occurs most frequently. The mode is not computed, but rather arrived at through inspection of a frequency distribution. In the following distribution of numbers, one can readily determine that the mode is 53:

50   51   51   52   53   53   53   53   54   55   56

The score of 53 was obtained four times, a higher frequency than for any other number. In the example used earlier in this chapter, the mode of the test scores of industrial nurses is 24 (see Table 15-2). The mode, in other words, identifies the most "popular" score. The mode is seldom used in research reports as the only index of central tendency, because it is unsuitable for further computation and is also rather unstable. By unstable we mean that modes tend to fluctuate widely from one sample drawn from a population to another sample drawn from the same population. The uses of the mode, therefore, are quite limited.

The Median. The *median* is that point in a distribution above which and below which 50% of the cases fall. As an example, consider the following set of values:

2   2   3   3   4   5   6   7   8   9

The value that divides the cases exactly in half is 4.5, which is the median for this set of numbers. The point that has 50% of the cases above and below it is halfway between 4 and 5. An important characteristic of the median is that it does not take into account the quantitative values of individual scores. The median is an index of average *position* in a distribution of numbers. The median is insensitive to extreme values. Let us take the previous example to illustrate this point, making only one small change:

$$2 \quad 2 \quad 3 \quad 3 \quad 4 \quad 5 \quad 6 \quad 7 \quad 8 \quad 99$$

Despite the fact that the last value has been increased from 9 to 99, the median remains unchanged at 4.5. Because of this property, the median is often the preferred index of central tendency when the distribution is skewed and when one is interested in finding a "typical" value.

The Mean. The *mean* is the point on the score scale that is equal to the sum of the scores divided by the number of scores. The mean is the index of central tendency that is usually referred to as an average. The computational formula for a mean—which everyone knows, but whose symbols need to be learned—is as follows:

$$\overline{X} = \frac{\Sigma X}{n} \qquad \text{where } \overline{X} = \text{the mean}$$

$$\Sigma = \text{the sum of}$$
$$X = \text{each individual raw score}$$
$$n = \text{the number of cases}$$

Let us apply the above formula to calculate the mean weight of eight subjects whose individual weights are as follows:

$$85 \quad 109 \quad 120 \quad 135 \quad 158 \quad 177 \quad 181 \quad 195$$

$$\overline{X} = \frac{85 + 109 + 120 + 135 + 158 + 177 + 181 + 195}{8} = 145$$

Unlike the median, the mean is affected by the value of every score. If we were to exchange the 195-pound subject for one weighing 275 pounds, the mean would increase from 145 to 155. A substitution of this kind would leave the median unchanged.

Comparison of the Mode, Median, and Mean. The mean is unquestionably the most widely used measure of central tendency. Most of the important tests of statistical significance, which will be dealt with in the next chapter, are based on the mean. When researchers work with interval-level or ratio-level measurements, the mean rather than the median or mode is almost always the statistic reported.

Of the three indices of central tendency, the mean is the most stable. This means that if repeated samples were drawn from a given population, the means would vary or fluctuate less than the modes or medians.

Because of its stability, the mean is the most reliable estimate of the central tendency of the population.

The mean is the most appropriate index in situations in which the concern is for totals or combined performance of a group. If a school of nursing were comparing two incoming classes in terms of scores on the Scholastic Aptitude Test, then the calculation of two means would be in order. Sometimes, however, the primary concern is learning what a "typical" value is, in which case a median might be preferred. In efforts to understand the economic well-being of United States citizens, for example, we would get a distorted impression of the financial status of the typical person by considering the mean. The mean in this case would be inflated by the wealth of a small minority. The median, on the other hand, would reflect more realistically how the average person fared financially.

Variability

Although measures of central tendency are of immense importance in descriptions of data, averages do not give a total picture of a distribution. Two sets of data with identical means could be different from one another in several respects. For one thing, two distributions with the same mean could be very different in shape; they could be skewed in opposite directions, for example. The characteristic of concern in this section is how spread out or dispersed the data are. The variability of two distributions could be quite different, while the mean values could be identical.

The concept of variability is concerned with the degree to which the subjects in a sample vary from one another with respect to the critical attribute. Consider the two distributions in Figure 15-4, which represent the hypothetical scores of students from two high schools on the Scholastic Aptitude Test. Both distributions have an average of 500, but the outcomes are clearly different. In school A, there is a wide range of obtained scores—from scores below 300 to some above 700. This school has many students who performed among the best, but it also has many students who did relatively poorly. In school B, on the other hand, there are few low scores but also few outstanding students. School A is said to be more *heterogeneous* than school B, while school B may be described as more *homogeneous* than school A.

In order to describe a distribution adequately, there is a need for a measure of variability that expresses the extent to which scores deviate from one another. Several such indices have been developed. Two of these, the range and standard deviation, are described below.

The Range. The *range* is simply the highest score minus the lowest score in a given distribution. In the examples shown in Figure 15-4, the

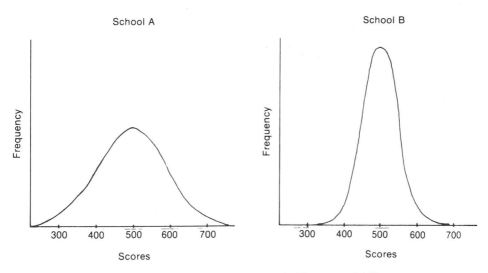

Figure 15-4. Two distributions of different variability

range for school A is approximately 500 (750–250), while the range for school B is approximately 300 (650–350). The range indicates the distance on the score scale between the lowest and highest values.

The chief virtue of the range is the ease with which it can be computed. As an index of variability, the shortcomings of the range outweigh this modest advantage. The range, being based on only two scores, is a highly unstable index. From sample to sample drawn from the same population, the range tends to fluctuate considerably. Another difficulty with the range is that it completely ignores variations in scores between the two extremes. In school B of Figure 15-4, suppose that one "deviant" student obtained a score of 250 and another obtained a score of 750. The range of both schools would then be 500, despite obvious differences in the heterogeneity of scores. For these reasons, the range is used largely as a gross descriptive index and is typically reported in conjunction with, not instead of, other measures of variability.

Standard Deviation. The most widely used measure of variability is the *standard deviation* (SD). Like the mean, the standard deviation takes into consideration every score in a distribution.

What is needed in a variability index is some way of capturing the degree to which scores deviate from one another. The standard deviation is such an index. The first step in calculating a standard deviation is to compute *deviation scores* for each subject. A deviation score (usually symbolized with a small x) is the difference between an individual score and the mean. If a person weighed 150 pounds and the sample mean was 140,

Table 15-3. Computation of a Standard Deviation

RAW SCORE (X)	DEVIATION SCORE (x)	DEVIATION SCORE SQUARED (x^2)
4	-3	9
5	-2	4
6	-1	1
7	0	0
7	0	0
7	0	0
8	1	1
9	2	4
10	3	9
$\Sigma X = 63$	$\Sigma x = 0$	$\Sigma x^2 = 28$

Mean $= 63/9 = 7$

$$SD = \sqrt{\frac{28}{8}} = \sqrt{3.50} = 1.87$$

the person's deviation score would be $+10$. Symbolically, the formula for a deviation score is $x = X - \overline{X}$.

Since what one is essentially looking for in an index of variability is a kind of "average" deviation, one might think that a good variability index could be arrived at by totaling the deviation scores and then dividing by the number of cases. This gets us close to a good solution, but the difficulty is that the sum of a set of deviation scores is always zero. Table 15-3 presents an example of deviation scores computed for nine numbers. As shown in the second column, the sum of the xs is equal to zero. The deviations above the mean always balance exactly those deviations below the mean.

The standard deviation overcomes this problem by squaring each deviation score before summing. After dividing by the number of cases, one takes the square root to bring the index back to the original units. The formula for the standard deviation is as follows:

$$SD = \sqrt{\frac{\Sigma x^2}{n - 1}}$$

The standard deviation has been completely worked out in the example in Table 15-3. First, a deviation score is calculated for the nine raw scores by subtracting the mean ($\overline{X} = 7$) from each of them. The third column shows that each deviation score is squared, thereby converting all values to positive numbers. The squared deviation scores are summed ($\Sigma x^2 = 28$)

and divided by the number of cases less 1 ($n - 1 = 8$), and a square root is taken to yield a standard deviation of 1.87.*

A standard deviation is typically more difficult for students to interpret than other statistics, such as the mean or range. In the example above we calculated a standard deviation of 1.87. One might well ask, 1.87 *what?* What does the number mean? We will try to answer these questions from several vantage points. First, as we already know, the standard deviation is an index of how variable the scores in a data set are. If two distributions had a mean of 25, but one had a standard deviation of 7 while the other had a standard deviation of 3, we would immediately know that the second sample was more homogeneous (*i.e.*, scores were less variable).

A convenient way to conceptualize the standard deviation is to think of it as an average of the deviations from the mean. The mean tells us the single best point for summarizing an entire distribution, while a standard deviation tells us how much, on the average, the scores deviate from that mean. A standard deviation might thus be interpreted as an indication of our degree of error when we use a mean to describe an entire data set.

When the distribution of scores is normal, it is possible to say even more about the standard deviation. A normal curve, it will be recalled, is a symmetric, unimodal curve. There are approximately three standard deviations above and below the mean with normally distributed data. To illustrate some further characteristics, suppose that we had a normal distribution of scores in which the mean was 50 and the standard deviation was 10. Such a distribution is shown in Figure 15-5. In a normal distribution such as this, a fixed percentage of cases fall within certain distances from the mean. Sixty-eight percent of all cases fall within one standard deviation of the mean. In this example, nearly seven out of every ten scores fall between 40 and 60. Ninety-five percent of the scores in a normal distribution fall within two standard deviations from the mean. Only a handful of cases—about 2% at each extreme—lie more than two standard deviations from the mean. Using this figure, we can see that a person who obtained a score of 70 got a higher score than about 98% of the sample.

In sum, the standard deviation is a useful index of variability that can be used to describe an important characteristic of a distribution and to interpret the score or performance of a person vis-a-vis others in the sam-

---

*Occasionally, one will find a reference to an index of variability known as the *variance*. The variance is simply the value of the standard deviation before a square root has been taken. In other words:

$$\text{Variance} = \frac{\Sigma x^2}{n - 1} = \text{SD}^2$$

In the above example, the variance is 1.87^2, or 3.50.

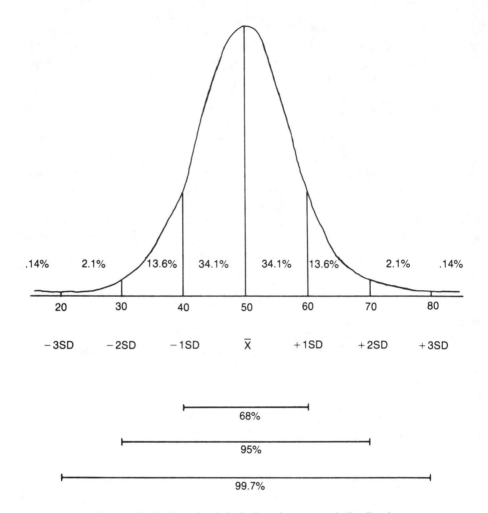

Figure 15-5. *Standard deviations in a normal distribution*

ple. Like the mean, the standard deviation is a stable estimate of a population parameter and is used extensively in more advanced statistical procedures. The standard deviation is the preferred measure of a
distribution's variability. The standard deviation should only be computed, however, with interval-level or ratio-level data.

Bivariate Descriptive Statistics: Contingency Tables and Correlation

The discussion has so far focused on a description of single variables.
The mean, mode, standard deviation, and so forth are all used in describing data for one variable at a time. We have been examining what is
referred to as *univariate* (one-variable) *statistics.* As stressed repeatedly

throughout this text, research usually is concerned with relationships between variables. What is needed then, is some method of objectively describing relationships. In this section we will look at *bivariate* (two-variable) *descriptive statistics.*

Contingency Tables. A *contingency table* is a two-dimensional frequency distribution in which the frequencies of two variables are cross-tabulated. Suppose we had data on subjects' sex and responses to a question on whether they were nonsmokers, light smokers, or heavy smokers. We might be interested in learning if there is a tendency for members of one sex to smoke more heavily than members of the opposite sex. Some fictitious data on these two variables are presented in Table 15-4. The best way to organize the data in a manner that highlights the research question is to construct a contingency table.

A contingency table for the data in Table 15-4 is presented in Table 15-5. Six "cells" are created by placing one variable (sex) along the vertical dimension and the other variable (smoking status) along the horizontal dimension. The system of bars and cross hatches can then be used to tabulate the number of subjects belonging in each cell. The first subject, who has a code of 1 for sex and 1 for smoking status, would be marked in the upper lefthand cell, and so on. After all subjects have been "assigned" to the appropriate cells, the frequencies can be tabulated and percentages computed. This simple procedure allows us to see at a glance that, in this

Table 15-4. Fictitious Data on Sex/Smoking Relationship

*SUBJECT SEX**	*SMOKING STATUS†*	*SUBJECT SEX*	*SMOKING STATUS*	*SUBJECT SEX*	*SMOKING STATUS*
1	1	2	2	2	1
2	3	2	3	1	1
2	1	1	1	2	2
1	2	2	2	1	2
1	1	1	2	1	1
2	2	1	1	2	2
2	1	1	3	2	3
2	3	1	2	2	3
1	1	2	2	2	2
2	3	2	1	1	2
1	2	1	3	1	1
1	3	2	3	2	1
1	1	1	1	1	2
2	3	1	3	2	2
2	1	1	2		

*1 = female; 2 = male
†1 = nonsmoker; 2 = light smoker; 3 = heavy smoker

Table 15-5. Contingency Table for Sex/Smoker Relationship

	NONSMOKER (1)		LIGHT SMOKER (2)		HEAVY SMOKER (3)		
Female (1)	⊬⊬⊬ ⊬⊬⊬ 10	22.7%	⊬⊬⊬ ||| 8	18.2%	|||| 4	9.1%	22
Male (2)	⊬⊬⊬ | 6	13.6%	⊬⊬⊬ ||| 8	18.2%	⊬⊬⊬ ||| 8	18.2%	22
	16		16		12		44

particular sample, women were more likely to be nonsmokers and less likely to be heavy smokers than men. The use of contingency tables usually is restricted to nominal data or to ordinal data that have few levels or ranks. In the present example, sex is a nominal measure and smoking status is an ordinal measure. We will encounter contingency tables again in the chapter on inferential statistics.

Correlation. The most common method of describing the relationship between two measures is through *correlation* procedures. The computation of a correlation coefficient is normally performed with either ordinal, interval, or ratio data. Correlation coefficients were briefly described in Chapter 13, and this section extends that discussion.

The correlation question is "To what extent are two variables related to each other?" For example, to what extent are height and weight related? To what degree are nursing effectiveness and grades in nursing school related? These questions can be answered by the calculation of an index that describes the relationship.

A quantitative index known as the correlation coefficient expresses both the magnitude and direction of a bivariate relationship. It may be recalled from Chapter 13 that correlations can be either positive or negative in direction. A positive correlation is obtained when high values on one variable are associated with high values on the second variable. A negative relationship is one in which high values on one variable are related to low values on the other. The correlation coefficient is an index whose values range from -1.00 for a perfect negative correlation, through zero for no relationship, to $+1.00$ for a perfect positive correlation. Relationships are described as "perfect" when it is possible to know precisely a person's score on one variable by knowing his or her score on the other. All correlations that fall between 0.0 and -1.00 are negative, while all correlations that fall between 0.0 and $+1.00$ are positive. The higher the absolute value of the coefficient (*i.e.*, the value disregarding the sign), the stronger the relationship. A correlation of $-.80$, for instance, is stronger than a correlation of $+.20$.

The most commonly used correlation index is the *product moment correlation coefficient,* also referred to as the *Pearson r.* This coefficient is computed when the variables being correlated have been measured on either an interval or ratio scale. The calculation of the r statistic is rather laborious and seldom performed by hand.*

Perfect correlations (+1.00 and −1.00) are extremely rare in research with humans. It is difficult to offer guidelines on what should be interpreted as strong or weak relationships. This determination depends, to a great extent, on the nature of the variables. If we were to measure patients' body temperatures both orally and rectally, a correlation of .70 between the two measurements would probably be considered low. For most variables of a social or psychological nature, however, an *r* of .70 is quite high.

Research Example

Aufderheide (1985) conducted a descriptive study of the effects of bedmaking activities on the vital signs of bed-ridden hospitalized patients.+ Heart rate, temperature, and blood pressure measurements were taken for 50 patients immediately before and after the beds were made. Patients were also asked to rate their discomfort during the bedmaking on a three-point scale—very comfortable (3), somewhat uncomfortable (2), and not uncomfortable (1). Information about the patients' backgrounds was obtained from hospital records.

Aufderheide computed a variety of descriptive statistics from her data. She reported that her sample tended to be middle-aged (mean age of 49), predominantly male (68%), and predominantly white (86%). The before–after vital signs data were presented as follows (see table, next page):

---

*For those who may wish to understand how a correlation coefficient is computed, we offer the following formula:

$$r_{xy} = \frac{\Sigma(X - \overline{X})(Y - \overline{Y})}{\sqrt{[\Sigma(X - \overline{X})^2][\Sigma(Y - \overline{Y})^2]}}$$

where r_{xy} = the correlation coefficient for variables X and Y

X = an individual score for variable X
$\overline{X}$ = the mean score for variable X
Y = an individual score for variable Y
$\overline{Y}$ = the mean score for variable Y
Σ = the sum of

+This example is fictitious.

	BEFORE BEDMAKING		AFTER BEDMAKING	
	Mean	SD	Mean	SD
Systolic Blood Pressure	140.9	16.4	168.2	28.3
Diastolic Blood Pressure	80.3	10.1	92.0	15.7
Heart Rate	65.2	7.8	76.6	9.9
Temperature	99.1	0.8	99.2	0.8

The changes in blood pressure readings led Aufderheide to conclude that the bedmaking activities were mildly stressful to these bed-ridden patients. This interpretation was supported by her finding that the mean discomfort rating was 2.5. Aufderheide further learned that changes in blood pressure and heart rate were moderately correlated with the patients' age (e.g., for heart rate changes, $r = .39$), suggesting that older people were somewhat more stressed by the bedmaking activities than younger ones.

Aufderheide did a reasonably good job of summarizing the data collected in her study through the use of descriptive statistics. She was able to communicate, succinctly and clearly, the demographic characteristics of her sample, the physiological state of patients before and after bedmaking, their subjective reaction of discomfort, and the relationship between age and elevations in blood pressure and heart rate.

For the most part, Aufderheide chose the statistic that was best suited to a particular variable, given its level of measurement. She appropriately reported means and standard deviations for her ratio-level physiological measures. For nominal-level data (e.g., sex and ethnicity/race), she reported percentages for the modal (most frequently observed) response. She reported a Pearson's r between two ratio-level measures, age and heart rate changes. The one variable for which an inappropriate statistic was chosen was the patients' ratings of discomfort. It is not reasonable to assume that this three-point rating scale produced interval-level data. With such an ordinal scale, it would have been better to report either the median or the modal response, or the percentage of cases for each value.

Given the descriptive purposes of her study, Aufderheide should probably have presented either a frequency distribution or, even better, a frequency polygon of the physiological data. We can see by looking at the above table that both the means and the standard deviations increased after bedmaking. In other words, the average blood pressure and heart rate measures (but not temperatures) went up and variability became greater (the measures became more dispersed). We know nothing, unfortunately, about whether the distributions were skewed or unimodal. It would have been interesting to have before–after data superimposed on a single frequency polygon to see if the shape of the distribution, as well as its central tendency and variability, had changed after bedmaking.

Summary

Qualitative analysis involves the organization and summarization of detailed descriptive materials. *Quantitative analysis* involves the processing of numerical information through statistical procedures. Both approaches can be useful in nursing research, although qualitative analysis has more limited applications. Qualitative analysis essentially involves a search for major themes and relations, and a validation of thematic insights. *Quasi-statistics*, which is a system of counting both positive and negative cases relating to an insight, is one method of assessing the validity of qualitative descriptions.

Descriptive statistics enable the researcher to reduce, summarize, and describe data obtained from quantified observations and measurements. Raw data that have not been organized or analyzed are difficult, if not impossible, to interpret and communicate to others. A *frequency distribution* is one of the easiest methods of imposing some order on a mass of numbers. In a frequency distribution, numerical values are ordered from the lowest to the highest, with a count of the number of times each value was obtained. *Frequency polygons* are a common method of displaying frequency information graphically.

A set of data may be completely described in terms of the shape of the distribution, central tendency, and variability. The most important attributes of the distribution's shape are its symmetry and modality. A distribution is *symmetrical* if its two halves are mirror images of each other. A *skewed distribution*, by contrast, is nonsymmetrical, with one "tail" longer than the other. The modality of a distribution refers to the number of peaks present: a *unimodal* distribution has one peak, while a *multimodal* distribution has more than one high point.

Measures of *central tendency* are indices, expressed as a single number, that represent the "average" or typical value of a set of scores. The *mode* is the numerical value that occurs most frequently in the distribution. The *median* is that point on a numerical scale above which and below which 50% of the cases fall. The *mean* is the arithmetic average of all the scores in the distribution. In general, the mean is the preferred measure of central tendency because of its stability and its usefulness in further statistical manipulations.

Variability refers to the spread or dispersion of the data. Measures of variability include the range and the standard deviation. The *range* is the distance between the highest and lowest score values. The most commonly used measure of variability is the *standard deviation* (SD). This index is calculated by first computing *deviation scores*, which represent the degree to which the scores of each person deviate from the mean. The standard deviation is designed to indicate how much, on the average, the scores deviate from the mean. A related index, the *variance*, is equal to the standard deviation squared.

Bivariate descriptive statistics describe the degree and magnitude of relationships between two variables. A *contingency table* is a two-dimensional frequency distribution in which the frequencies of two variables are cross-tabulated. When the scores have been measured on an ordinal, interval, or ratio scale, it is more common to describe the relationship between two variables with correlational procedures. A *correlation coefficient* can be calculated to express in numerical terms the direction and magnitude of a relationship. The values of the correlation coefficient range from −1.00 for a perfect negative correlation, through 0.0 for no relationship, to +1.00 for a perfect positive correlation. The most frequently used correlation coefficient is the *product-moment correlation coefficient*, also referred to as the *Pearson r*.

Study Suggestions

1. Construct a frequency distribution for the following set of scores, obtained from a scale to measure attitudes toward primary nursing:

32	20	33	22	16	19	25	26	25	18
22	30	24	26	27	23	28	26	21	24
31	29	25	28	22	27	26	30	17	24

2. What are the mean, median, and mode for the following set of data? Compute the range and standard deviation.

13   12   9   15   7   10   16   8   6   11

3. Two hospitals are interested in comparing the tenure rates of their nursing staff. Hospital A finds that its present staff has been employed for a mean of 4.3 years, with a standard deviation of 1.5. Hospital B, on the other hand, finds that its nurses have worked there for a mean of 5.4 years, with a standard deviation of 4.2 years. Discuss what these results signify.

4. Suppose a researcher has conducted a study of lactose intolerance in children. The data revealed that 22 boys and 16 girls have lactose intolerance, out of a sample of 60 children of each sex. Construct a contingency table and calculate the percentages for each cell in the table. Discuss the meaning of these statistics.

Chapter 16
Bivariate Inferential Statistics

Descriptive statistics such as means, standard deviations, and correlation coefficients are useful for summarizing univariate and bivariate sets of data. Usually, however, the researcher needs to do more than simply describe data obtained from a sample. Normally, subjects selected to participate in a research project are only a sample of people drawn from a population with certain characteristics. *Inferential statistics* provide a means for drawing conclusions about a population, given the data obtained from the sample. Inferential statistical reasoning would help us with such questions as "What can I conclude about the differential need for health education among women over age 25 (the population) after having found in a sample of 500 women that 50% of college-educated women, but only 20% of high-school-educated women, practiced breast self-examination?" With the assistance of inferential statistics, researchers make judgments about or generalize to a large class of persons based on information from a limited number of subjects.

Sampling Distributions

If a sample is to be used as a basis for making estimates of population characteristics, then it is clearly advisable to obtain as representative a sample as possible. As we saw in Chapter 9, random samples (*i.e.*, probability samples) are the most effective means of securing representative samples. Inferential statistical procedures are based on the assumption of random sampling from populations.

Even when random sampling is used, however, it cannot be expected that the sample characteristics will be identical with those of the population. Suppose we had a population of 30,000 nursing-school applicants who just completed the Scholastic Aptitude Test. By using descriptive statistics on the scores, we find that the mean for the entire population is 500 and the standard deviation (SD) is 100. Now, let us suppose that we do not know these parameters, but that we must estimate them by using the scores from a random sample of 25 students. Should we expect to find a mean of exactly 500 and an SD of 100 for this sample? It would be extremely unlikely to obtain identical values. Let us say that instead we calculated a mean of 505. If a completely new sample were drawn and another mean computed, we might obtain a value such as 497. The tendency for the statistics to fluctuate from one sample to another is known as *sampling error*.

A researcher actually works with only *one* sample on which statistics are computed and inferences made. But to understand inferential statistics we must perform a small mental exercise. With the population of 30,000 nursing-school applicants, consider drawing a sample of 25 students, calculating a mean and standard deviation, replacing the 25 students, and drawing a new sample. Each mean computed in this fashion will be considered a separate piece of data. If we draw 5000 such samples, we will have 5000 means or data points, which could then be used to construct a frequency polygon, as shown in Figure 16-1. This kind of distribution has a special name: it is called a *sampling distribution of the mean*. A sampling distribution is a theoretical rather than actual distribution, because in practice one does not draw consecutive samples and plot their means.

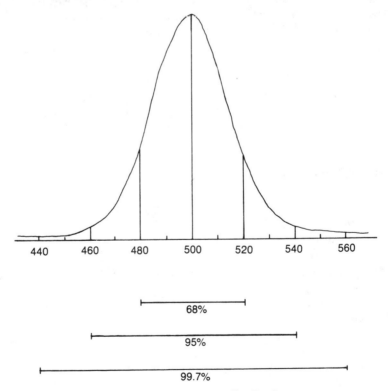

Figure 16-1. Sampling distribution

The concept of a theoretical distribution of sample means is basic to much of inferential statistics.

Characteristics of Sampling Distributions

Statisticians have been able to demonstrate that sampling distributions of means follow a normal curve. Furthermore, the mean of a sampling distribution comprised of an infinite number of sample means is equal to the population mean. In the present example, the mean of the sampling distribution is 500, the same value as the mean of the population.

In the preceding chapter we discussed the standard deviation in terms of percentages of cases falling within a certain distance from the mean. When scores are normally distributed, 68% of the cases fall between +1 SD and −1 SD from the mean. Since a sampling distribution of means is normally distributed, we can make the same type of statement. The probability is 68 out of 100 that any randomly drawn sample mean lies within the range of values between + 1 SD and −1 SD of the mean on the sampling distribution. The problem, then, is to determine the value of the standard deviation of the sampling distribution.

Standard Error of the Mean

The standard deviation of a theoretical distribution of sample means has a special name. It is called the *standard error of the mean*. The word "error" signifies that the various means comprising the distribution contain some error in their estimates of the population mean. The term "standard" indicates the magnitude of a standard, or average, error. The smaller the standard error—that is, the less variable the sample means— the more accurate are those means as estimates of the population value.

Since one does not ever actually construct a sampling distribution, how can its standard deviation be computed? Fortunately, there is a formula for estimating the standard error of the mean from the data from a single sample. It has been shown that the value of the standard error (symbolized as $s_{\bar{x}}$) has a systematic relationship to the standard deviation of the population and to the size of the samples drawn from it. The population standard deviation is estimated by the sample standard deviation to yield the following equation:

$$s_{\bar{x}} = \frac{SD}{\sqrt{n}}$$

where SD = the standard deviation of the sample
n = sample size
$s_{\bar{x}}$ = standard error of the mean

If we use this formula to calculate the standard error of the mean in our present example, we obtain the following:

$$s_{\bar{x}} = \frac{100}{\sqrt{25}} = 20$$

The standard deviation of the sampling distribution is 20, as shown in Figure 16-1. This statistic is an estimate of how much sampling fluctuation or sampling error there would be from one sample mean to another.

We can now use these calculations to estimate the probability of drawing a sample with a certain mean. With a sample size of 25, the chances are about 95 out of 100 that the mean would fall between the values of 460 and 540. Only 5 times out of 100 would the mean of a randomly selected sample exceed 540 or be less than 460. In other words, only 5 times out of 100 would we be likely to draw a sample in which the mean is wrong (*i.e.*, deviates from the population mean) by more than 40 points.

From the formula for the standard error of the mean, it can be shown that, in order to increase the accuracy of our estimate of the population mean, we need only increase the sample size. Suppose that instead of using a sample of 25 nursing-school applicants to estimate the average SAT score, we used a sample of 100 students. With this many students, the standard error of the mean would be as follows:

$$s_{\bar{x}} = \frac{100}{\sqrt{100}} = 10$$

In such a situation, the probability of obtaining a sample mean greater than 520 or less than 480 would be about 5 in 100. The chances of drawing a sample with a mean very different from that of the population are reduced as the sample size increases, because large numbers promote the likelihood that extreme cases will cancel each other out.

Hypothesis Testing

Statistical inference consists of two major types of techniques—estimation of parameters and hypothesis testing. *Estimation procedures* are used to estimate a single population characteristic, such as the mean value of some attribute (*e.g.*, the mean creatinine level of patients 24 hours after a kidney transplant operation). Estimation procedures, however, are not particularly common, because researchers are more typically interested in relationships between two or more variables than in estimating the accuracy of a single sample value. For this reason, we focus on hypothesis testing and refer those interested in estimation procedures to a text on statistics.

Statistical *hypothesis testing* provides researchers with objective criteria for deciding whether their hypotheses should be accepted as true or rejected as wrong. Suppose a nurse researcher hypothesized that maternity patients exposed to a teaching film on breast-feeding would continue breast-feeding longer than mothers who did not see the film. The researcher subsequently learns that the mean number of days of breast-feeding is 131.5 for 25 experimental-group subjects and 112.1 for 25 comparison-group subjects. Should the researcher conclude that the hypothesis has been supported? True, the group differences are in the predicted direction, but the results might simply be due to sampling fluctuations. In other words, the two groups might differ in their commitment to breast-feeding, independent of having seen the film; other groups of 25 subjects might not be so different. Statistical hypothesis testing helps researchers to make objective decisions about the results of their studies. Scientists need such a mechanism for helping them decide which outcomes are likely to reflect only chance differences between groups and which are likely to reflect true hypothesized effects.

The Null Hypothesis

The procedures used in testing hypotheses are based on rules of negative inference. This logic often seems somewhat awkward and peculiar to beginning researchers, so we will try to convey the concepts with a concrete illustration. In the above example, a nurse researcher showed the teaching film to only half the mothers and found that, on average, those who had seen the film breast-fed longer than those who had not. There are two explanations for this outcome: (1) the experimental treatment was successful in encouraging breast-feeding or (2) the differences were due to chance factors (such as differences in the pretreatment characteristics of the two groups).

The first explanation is the researcher's scientific hypothesis, but the second explanation is known as the *null hypothesis.* The null hypothesis is a statement that there is no actual relationship between variables and that any such observed relationship is only a function of chance, or sampling fluctuations. The need for a null hypothesis lies in the fact that statistical hypothesis testing is basically a process of disproof or rejection. It is not possible to prove directly that the first explanation—the scientific hypothesis—is correct. But it is possible to show that the null hypothesis has a high probability of being incorrect, and such evidence lends support to the scientific hypothesis. The rejection of the null hypothesis, then, is what the researcher seeks to accomplish through statistical tests. Although null hypotheses are accepted or rejected on the basis of sample data, the hypothesis is made about population values. The real interest in testing hypotheses, as in all statistical inference, is to use samples to draw conclusions about relationships within the population.

Type-I and Type-II Errors

The researcher's decision about whether to accept or reject the null hypothesis is based on a consideration of how probable it is that observed differences are due to chance alone. Since information about the entire population is not available, it is not possible to flatly assert that the null hypothesis is or is not true. The researcher must be content with the knowledge that the hypothesis is either probably true or probably false. We make statistical inferences based on incomplete information, so that there is always a risk of making an error.

There are two types of errors that a researcher can make: (1) the rejection of a true null hypothesis and (2) the acceptance of a false null hypothesis. The possible outcomes of a researcher's decision are summarized in Figure 16-2. An investigator makes a *Type-I error* by concluding that the null hypothesis is false when it is in fact true. For instance, if we concluded that the experimental treatment was effective in promoting breast-feeding when in actuality observed sample differences were due only to sampling fluctuations, then we would have made a Type-I error. In the reverse situation, we might conclude that observed differences in number of days of breast-feeding were due to chance, when in fact the experimental treatment did have an effect. This situation, in which a false null hypothesis is accepted, is an example of a *Type-II* error.

Level of Significance

The researcher does not know when an error in statistical decision making has been committed. The truth or falseness of a null hypothesis could only be definitively ascertained by collecting information from the entire population, in which case there would be no need for statistical inference.

The degree of risk in making a Type-I error is controlled by the researcher. The selection of a *level of significance* determines the chance

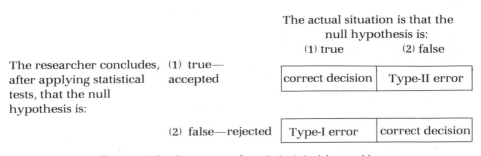

Figure 16-2. Outcomes of statistical decision making

of making this type of error. Level of significance is the phrase used to signify the probability of making a Type-I error.

The two most frequently used levels of significance are .05 and .01. If we say we are using a .05 significance level, this means that we are accepting the risk that out of 100 samples, a true null hypothesis would be rejected five times. With a .01 significance level, the risk of making a Type-I error is *lower:* in only one sample out of 100 would we erroneously reject the null hypothesis. The minimum acceptable level for significance level in scientific research is .05.

Naturally, researchers would like to reduce the risk of committing both types of error. Unfortunately, lowering the risk of making a Type-I error increases the risk of making a Type-II error.* The stricter the criterion we use for rejecting a null hypothesis, the greater the probability that we will accept a false null hypothesis. There is a kind of trade-off that the researcher must consider in establishing criteria for statistical decision making.

Tests of Statistical Significance

Within a hypothesis testing framework, the data collected in a study are used to compute a test statistic. For every test statistic there is a related theoretical distribution. Hypothesis testing uses theoretical distributions to establish "probable" and "improbable" values for the test statistics, which are in turn used as a basis for accepting or rejecting the null hypothesis.

A simple example will illustrate the process. Suppose a researcher wanted to test the hypothesis that the average SAT score for students applying to nursing schools was higher than that for all students taking the SAT in the state, whose mean score was 500. The null hypothesis is that there is no difference in the mean population scores of students who did or did not apply to nursing school. Let us say that the mean score for a sample of 100 nursing-school applicants was 525, with an SD of 100. Using statistical procedures, we can assess the likelihood that a mean score of this size represents a chance fluctuation from the population mean of 500.

In hypothesis testing, one assumes that the null hypothesis is true and then gathers evidence to disprove it. Assuming a mean of 500 for the nursing-applicant population, a sampling distribution can be constructed with a mean of 500 and an SD equal to approximately 10 ($s_{\bar{x}} = 100/\sqrt{100}$), as shown in Figure 16-3. Based on our knowledge of normal distribution characteristics, we can determine "probable" and "improbable" values of

---

*The probability of making a Type-II error can be calculated but is a complex topic beyond the scope of this book.

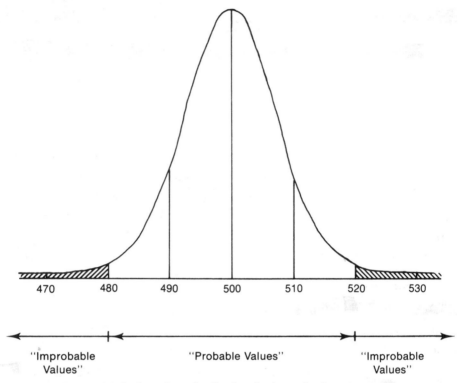

470   480   490   500   510   520   530

"Improbable   "Probable Values"   "Improbable
 Values"   Values"

Figure 16-3. Sampling distribution for hypothesis test example

sample means drawn from the nursing-school-applicant population. If, as is assumed, the population mean is actually 500, then 95% of all sample means would fall between 480 and 520. The obtained sample mean of 525 is "improbable" if the null hypothesis is correct and if we use as our criterion of "improbability" a significance level of .05. We would reject, therefore, the null hypothesis that the mean of the nursing-school-applicant population equals 500. We would not be justified in saying that we have "proven" the research hypothesis, because the possibility of having made a Type-I error remains.

Researchers reporting the results of hypothesis tests often say that their findings were *statistically significant*. This terminology has a very precise meaning. The word "significant" should not be given the familiar interpretation of "important" or "meaningful." In statistics, significant means that the obtained results are not likely to have been due to chance, at some specified level of probability. A nonsignificant outcome means that any observed differences or relationships could have been the result of a chance fluctuation.

The example used in this section was highly contrived, for researchers rarely know the value for the mean of the entire population. The use of theoretical distributions to determine "probable" and "improbable" values of a test statistic, however, is common to all tests of statistical significance.

Parametric and Nonparametric Tests

A distinction can be made between two classes of statistical tests. The bulk of the tests that we will consider in this chapter—and also the majority of tests used by researchers—are called *parametric tests*. Parametric tests are characterized by three attributes: (1) they focus on population parameters; (2) they require measurements on at least an interval scale; and (3) they involve several other assumptions about the variables under consideration, such as the assumption that the variables are normally distributed in the population.

Nonparametric tests may be contrasted with parametric tests in terms of several of these characteristics. This second class of statistical tests is not based on the estimation of parameters. Nonparametric methods also involve less restrictive assumptions about the shape of the distribution of the critical variables. Finally, nonparametric tests are usually applied when the data have been measured on a nominal or an ordinal scale.

Statisticians disagree about the utility and virtues of most nonparametric tests. Purists insist that if the strict requirements of parametric tests are not met, then parametric procedures are inappropriate. Many statistical research studies have shown, however, that the violation of the assumptions for parametric tests usually fails to affect statistical decision making or the number of errors made. The more moderate position in this debate, and the one that we feel is reasonable, is that nonparametric tests are most useful when (1) the data under consideration cannot in any manner be construed as interval-level measures or (2) the sample is very small. Parametric tests are more powerful and offer more flexibility than nonparametric tests and are, for these reasons, generally preferred.

Overview of Hypothesis Testing Procedures

In the pages that follow, various types of statistical procedures for testing research hypotheses are examined. The emphasis throughout is on explaining applications of statistical tests rather than on describing actual computations. One computational example is worked out to illustrate that numbers are not just "pulled out of a hat." However, calculators and computers have virtually eliminated the need for manual calculations. The advanced researcher is urged to pursue other references for a fuller appreciation of statistical techniques. In this basic text on research methods, our primary concern is to alert researchers to the potential use (or misuse) of statistical tests for different purposes.

While each of the statistical tests described in the remaining sections of this chapter has a particular application and can be used only with particular kinds of data, the overall process of testing hypotheses is basically the same. The steps are essentially as follows:

1. *Determine the test statistic to be used.* Is a parametric test justified? How large is the sample? What level of measurement was used for the measures? The summarization in Table 16-6 (see "Overview of Various Statistical Tests") may help in the selection of an appropriate test.

2. *Select the level of significance.* The .05 level will usually be acceptable. If a more stringent test is required, the significance level may be set at .01 or .001.

3. *Compute a test statistic.* Using the values from the collected data, calculate a test statistic using the appropriate computational formulas. Or, alternatively, have the computer calculate the statistic.

4. *Calculate the degrees of freedom.* The term *degrees of freedom* is a concept used throughout hypothesis testing to refer to the number of observations free to vary about a parameter. The concept is too complex for full elaboration here, but fortunately the computation is extremely easy.

5. *Compare the test statistic to a tabled value.* Theoretical distributions have been developed for all test statistics. These theoretical distributions enable the researcher to discover whether obtained values are beyond the range of what is "probable" if the null hypothesis were true. That is, at some probability level specified by the researcher, the obtained value of the test statistic reflects a true relationship between variables, and not just a relationship that occurred in the sample by chance. The researcher examines a table appropriate for the test used, obtains the tabled value by entering the table at a point corresponding to the relevant degrees of freedom and level of significance, and compares the tabled value to the computed value of the statistic. If the tabled value is smaller than the absolute value of the computed test statistic, then the results are statistically significant. If the tabled value is larger, then the results are nonsignificant.

When a computer is used to perform the calculations, the researcher generally only needs to follow the first step and then make the necessary commands to the computer. The computer will calculate the test statistic, the degrees of freedom, and the *actual* probability that the relationship being tested is due to chance. For example, the computer may print that the probability (p) of an experimental group doing better on a measure of postoperative recovery than the control group on the basis of chance alone is .025. This means that fewer than 3 times out of 100 (or only 25 times out of 1000) would a difference between the two groups as large as the one obtained reflect haphazard sampling differences rather than differences resulting from an experimental intervention. This computed probability level can then be compared with the investigator's desired level of significance. In the present example, if the significance level desired were .05, the results would be said to be significant, because .025 is more stringent than .05. If .01 were the significance level, the results would be nonsignificant (sometimes abbreviated NS). Any computed probability level greater than .05 (e.g., .20) indicates a nonsignificant relationship—that is, one that could have occurred on the basis of chance alone in more than 5 out of 100 samples. In the sections that follow, a number of specific statistical tests and their applications are described.

Testing Differences Between Two Group Means

A very common research situation is the comparison of two groups of subjects on the dependent variable of interest. For instance, we might wish to compare the scores of an experimental and control group of patients on a measure of physical function. Or perhaps we would be interested in contrasting the average length of hospitalization for a sample of maternity patients in urban versus rural hospitals. This section will describe methods for testing the statistical significance of differences between two group means.

The basic parametric procedure for testing differences in group means is the *t-test*. A distinction must be drawn between the case in which the two groups are independent (such as an experimental and control group, or male versus female subjects) or dependent (as when a single group yields pretreatment and posttreatment scores). Procedures for handling independent samples are described below to illustrate the computation of a test statistic.

Suppose that a researcher wanted to test the effect of a special workshop on nursing students' attitudes toward the elderly. A sample of 20 students is randomly drawn from a sophomore class of nursing students. Of these 20 students, 10 are randomly assigned to an experimental group, which will be exposed to the special workshop. The remaining 10 students comprise the control group, which will not attend the workshop. At the end of the experiment, both groups are administered a scale measuring attitudes toward the elderly. The null hypothesis being tested is that the two groups have the same attitudes; the research hypothesis is that the experimental group has more positive attitudes. In order to test this research hypothesis, a statistic known as the *t*-statistic must be computed. With independent samples, such as in the present example, the formula is as follows:

$$t = \frac{\overline{X}_A - \overline{X}_B}{\sqrt{\dfrac{\Sigma x_A^2 + \Sigma x_B^2}{n_A + n_B - 2}\left(\dfrac{1}{n_A} + \dfrac{1}{n_B}\right)}}$$

Table 16-1. Computation of the t-Statistic for Independent Samples

| | EXPERIMENTAL GROUP A | | | CONTROL GROUP B | | |
	(1)	(2)	(3)	(4)	(5)	(6)
	Scores (X_A)	Deviation Scores (x_A)	Deviation Scores Squared (x_A^2)	Scores (X_B)	Deviation Scores (x_B)	Deviation Scores Squared (x_B^2)
	30	5	25	23	4	16
	27	2	4	17	−2	4
	25	0	0	22	3	9
	20	−5	25	18	−1	1
	24	−1	1	20	1	1
	32	7	49	26	7	49
	17	−8	64	16	−3	9
	18	−7	49	13	−6	36
	28	3	9	21	2	4
	29	4	16	14	−5	25
	$\Sigma X_A = 250$		$\Sigma x_A^2 = 242$	$\Sigma X_B = 190$		$\Sigma x_B^2 = 154$
	Mean $(\bar{X}_A) = 25$			Mean $(\bar{X}_B) = 19$		

$$t = \frac{25 - 19}{\sqrt{\frac{242 + 154}{(10 + 10 - 2)}\left(\frac{1}{10} + \frac{1}{10}\right)}} =$$

$$t = \frac{6}{\sqrt{(22.0)(.2)}} =$$

$$t = \frac{6}{\sqrt{4.4}} =$$

$$t = \frac{6}{2.1} = 2.86$$

This formula looks rather complex and intimidating, but it boils down to simple components that can be calculated with elementary arithmetic. Let us work through one example with data shown in Table 16-1.

The first column of numbers presents the scores of the experimental group on a measure of attitudes toward the elderly. The mean score for group A is 25. In column 4, similar scores are shown for the control group, whose mean is 19. Is this six-point difference significant? What is the probability that a difference of this size is due to chance alone? The calculation of the t-statistic will enable such questions to be answered. In columns 2 and 5, deviation scores are obtained for each subject: 25 is subtracted from each score in group A and 19 is subtracted from each score in group B. Then, each deviation score is squared (columns 3 and 6), and the squared deviation scores are added. We now have all of the components for the formula presented above, as follows:

$$\overline{X}_A = 25 \text{ (mean of group A)}$$
$$\overline{X}_B = 19 \text{ (mean of group B)}$$
$$\Sigma x_A^2 = 242 \text{ (sum of group A squared deviation scores)}$$
$$\Sigma x_B^2 = 154 \text{ (sum of group B squared deviation scores)}$$
$$n_A = 10 \text{ (number of subjects in group A)}$$
$$n_B = 10 \text{ (number of subjects in group B)}$$

When these numbers are used in the t-equation, the value of the t-statistic is computed to be 2.86.

In order to ascertain whether this t-value is statistically significant, we need to consult a table that specifies the probability points associated with different t-values for the theoretical t-distributions. To make use of such a table, the researcher must have two pieces of information—the probability level sought (*i.e.*, the degree of risk of making a Type-I error that one is willing to accept) and the number of degrees of freedom available. For independent samples, the formula for degrees of freedom is as follows:

$$df = n_A + n_B - 2$$

A table of t-values is presented in Table A of the Appendix. The left-hand column lists various degrees of freedom, and the top row specifies different probability values. If we use as our decision-making criterion a probability (p) level of .05, we find that with 18 degrees of freedom the tabled value of t is 2.10. This value establishes an upper limit to what is "probable," if the null hypothesis were true; values in excess of 2.10 would be considered "improbable." Thus, our calculated t of 2.86 is improbable, that is, statistically significant. We are now in a position to say that the students in the experimental group scored significantly higher than those in the control group on the scale of attitudes toward the elderly. The probability that the mean difference of six points was the result of chance factors is less than 5 in 100 ($p < .05$). The null hypothesis is rejected, therefore, and the research hypothesis retained.

There are certain two-group situations for which the t-test for independent samples is not appropriate. For example, if pretreatment and posttreatment measures are obtained for a single sample, then one would need to compute a t-test for paired samples, using a different formula. If the researcher is working with very small groups,* or if the distribution of the dependent variable is markedly skewed, then a nonparametric test (such as the median test, the Mann–Whitney U test, or the Wilcoxon signed-rank test) may be more appropriate. The calculation of these tests is described in most texts on introductory statistics.

Analysis of Variance

The procedure known as *analysis of variance* (ANOVA) is one of the most commonly used statistical tests reported in research journals. Like the t-test, ANOVA is a parametric procedure used to test the significance of differences between means. ANOVA is not restricted to two-group situations: the means of three or more groups can also be compared.

The statistic computed in an ANOVA test is the *F-ratio* statistic. The computation of an F-ratio is somewhat more complex than that for a t-statistic. A brief overview of the logic of ANOVA might prove helpful.

Consider the raw scores shown in Table 16-1. The 20 scores—10 for each group—vary from one person to another. Some of that variability can be attributed to individual differences in feelings toward the elderly. Some of that variability could also be due to measurement error (unreliability), while some of it could be the result of the subjects' mood on that day, and so forth. The research question is "Can a significant portion of the variability be attributed to the independent variable, which in this case is exposure or nonexposure to a workshop on the elderly?"

Analysis of variance decomposes the total variability of a set of data into two components: (1) the variability resulting from the independent variable and (2) all other variability, such as individual differences, measurement unreliability, and so on. Variation *between* treatment groups is contrasted with variation *within* groups, to yield an F-ratio. If the differences between groups receiving different treatments is large relative to random fluctuations within groups, then it is possible to establish the probability that the treatment is related to, or resulted in, the group differences.

---

*We used a t-test in the above attitude-toward-the-elderly study, despite the small sample size, for exemplary purposes.

One-way ANOVA

Suppose that we were interested in comparing the effectiveness of different therapies to help people stop smoking. One group of smokers will undergo behavior modification therapy, which is based on reinforcement theory. A second group will be treated by means of hypnosis. A third group will serve as a control group and will receive no special treatment. The dependent variable in this experiment will be the average daily cigarette consumption during the week following completion of the therapies. Thirty subjects who smoke at least one package of cigarettes daily are randomly assigned to one of the three conditions. The null hypothesis for this study is that the population means for posttreatment cigarette smoking will be the same for all three groups, while the research hypothesis predicts inequality of means. Table 16-2 presents some hypothetical data for such a study.

For each of the three groups, the raw score for each subject is shown. Below the scores, the means have been calculated. The mean number of daily posttreatment cigarettes consumed is 20, 25, and 28 for groups A, B, and C, respectively. These means are different, but are they significantly different? Or are these differences attributable to random fluctuations?

The underlying concepts and terms for a one-way ANOVA will be briefly explained without working out the computations for the example at hand. Again, the reader is urged to consult a statistics text for formulas and more detailed explanations. In calculating an F-statistic, the total variability within the data is broken down into two sources, as mentioned above. The portion of the variance resulting from group membership (*i.e.*, from exposure to different treatments) is arrived at by calculating a com-

Table 16-2. Data for One-way ANOVA Example

GROUP A	GROUP B	GROUP C
X_A	X_B	X_C
28	22	29
10	31	40
17	26	23
20	30	35
25	34	28
19	25	20
24	12	17
18	19	38
23	24	24
16	27	26
$\Sigma X_A = 200$	$\Sigma X_B = 250$	$\Sigma X_C = 280$
Mean $(\overline{X}_A) = 20$	Mean $(\overline{X}_B) = 25$	Mean $(\overline{X}_C) = 28$

ponent known as the *sum of squares between groups*, or SS_B. The SS_B represents the sum of squared deviations of the group means from the overall mean, and it reflects the variability in individual scores attributable to a group membership.

The second component is the *sum of squares within groups*, or SS_W, which is the sum of the squared deviations of each individual score from its own group mean. The SS_W indicates variability attributable to individual differences, measurement error, and so on.

It may be recalled from the last chapter that the formula for calculating a variance is $\Sigma x^2/n - 1$. The two sums of squares described above are analogous to the numerator of this equation. The sums of squares represent sums of squared deviations from means. Therefore, to compute the variance within and the variance between groups, we must divide by a quantity analogous to $(n - 1)$. This quantity is the degrees of freedom associated with each sum of squares. For between groups, $df = G - 1$, which is the number of groups minus one. For within groups, $df = (n_A - 1) + (n_B - 1) + \ldots (n_G - 1)$. That is, degrees of freedom within is found by adding together for each group the number of subjects less 1.

In an ANOVA, the variance is conventionally referred to as the *mean square*. The formula for the mean square between groups and the mean square within groups is as follows:

$$MS_B = \frac{SS_B}{df_B} \qquad MS_W = \frac{SS_W}{df_W}$$

The *F*-ratio is the ratio of these mean squares, or

$$F = \frac{MS_B}{MS_W}$$

All of these computations for the data in Table 16-2 are presented in Table 16-3.

The last step is to compare the obtained *F*-statistic with the value from a theoretical *F*-distribution. Table B in the Appendix contains the upper limits of "probable" values for distributions with varying degrees of freedom. The first part of the table lists these values for a significance level of

Table 16-3. ANOVA Summary Table

SOURCE OF VARIANCE	SS	df	MS	F	P
Between groups	326.7	2	163.4	3.90	<0.05
Within groups	1130.0	27	41.9		
Total	1456.7	29			

.05, while the second part lists those for a .01 significance level. Let us say that we have chosen the .05 probability level. To enter the table, we find the column headed by our between-groups df (2), and go down this column until we reach the row corresponding to the within-groups df (27). The tabled value of F with 2 and 27 degrees of freedom is 3.35. Since our obtained F-value of 3.90 exceeds 3.35, we reject the null hypothesis that the population means are equal. The differences in the average daily number of cigarettes smoked after treatment are beyond chance expectations. Differences of this magnitude would be obtained by chance alone in fewer than 5 samples out of 100. The data support the hypothesis that the therapies affect cigarette-smoking behaviors.

The ANOVA procedure does not allow us to say that each group differed significantly from all other groups. We cannot tell from these results if treatment A was significantly more effective than treatment B. Some researchers incorrectly use t-tests to compare the different pairs of means (A vs. B, A vs. C, B vs. C) when this type of information is required. There are methods known as *multiple comparison procedures* that should be used in such situations. The function of these procedures is to isolate the comparisons between group means that are responsible for the rejection of the ANOVA null hypothesis. Multiple comparison methods are described in most intermediate statistical textbooks.

Multifactor ANOVA

The type of problem described above is known as a one-way ANOVA because it involves the effect of one independent variable (the different therapies) on a dependent variable. In Chapter 5 it was pointed out that hypotheses are sometimes complex and make predictions about the effect of two or more independent variables on a dependent variable. The analysis of data from such studies is often performed by means of a multifactor ANOVA. In this section we will describe some of the principles underlying a two-way ANOVA.

Let us suppose that we were interested in determining whether the two therapies discussed above were equally effective in helping both men and women stop smoking. We could design an experiment with four groups: women and men would be randomly assigned, separately, to the two therapy conditions. After the experimental period, each subject would be required to report the average daily number of cigarettes smoked. Some fictitious data for this problem are shown in Table 16-4.

With two independent variables, there are three research hypotheses. First, we are testing (for both sexes) whether the behavior modification therapy is more effective than hypnosis as a means of reducing smoking or vice versa. Second, we are analyzing for sex differences in smoking behavior for persons exposed to either therapeutic treatment.

Table 16-4. Fictitious Data for a Two-way (2 × 2) ANOVA

FACTOR B—SEX	FACTOR A—TREATMENT		
	Behavior Modification (1)	Hypnosis (2)	
Female (1)	24	27	
	28	30	
	22	15	
	19	19	
	27	22	
	25 Mean = 22	23 Mean = 20	Female Mean = 21
	18	18	
	21	20	
	23	12	
	13	14	
Male (2)	10	36	
	21	31	
	17	28	
	20	32	
	13	25	
	16 Mean = 16	22 Mean = 30	Male Mean = 23
	18	19	
	13	30	
	15	35	
	17	42	
	Treatment 1 Mean = 19	Treatment 2 Mean = 25	Grand mean = 22

Third, we are examining the differential effect of the two treatments on males and females. This last hypothesis is the *interaction hypothesis*. Interaction is concerned with whether the effect of one independent variable is consistent for every level of a second independent variable. In other words, do the two therapies have the same effect on both sexes?

The data in Table 16-4 reveal the following: that, overall, subjects in treatment 1 smoked less than those in treatment 2 (19 vs. 25); that females smoked less than males (21 vs. 23); and that males smoked less when exposed to treatment 1, but females smoked less when exposed to treatment 2. By performing a two-way ANOVA on these data, it would be possible to ascertain the statistical significance of these differences.

Multifactor ANOVA is an extremely important analytic technique. Human behaviors, conditions, and feelings are complex, and the ability to examine the combined effects of two or more independent variables permits this complexity to be incorporated into research designs. Theoretically, any number of independent variables is possible, although in practice, studies with more than four factors are rare because of the prohibitive number of subjects required.

Nonparametric ANOVA

Strictly speaking, nonparametric tests do not analyze variance. There are, however, nonparametric procedures analogous to the parametric ANOVA for use with ordinal-level data or in situations in which a small sample size or markedly skewed distribution render parametric tests questionable. When the number of groups is greater than two, and a one-way test for independent samples is desired, one may use a statistic developed by statisticians named Kruskal and Wallis. The *Kruskal–Wallis test* is a generalized version of the Mann–Whitney *U* test, based on the assignment of ranks to the scores from the various groups.

The Chi-square Test

The *chi-square* statistic is used when we have categories of data and hypotheses about the proportions of cases that fall into the various categories. In the last chapter we discussed the construction of contingency tables to describe the frequencies of cases falling into different classes. The chi-square (χ^2) statistic is applied to contingency tables to test the significance of different proportions.

Consider the following example. A researcher is interested in studying the effect of planned nursing instruction on patients' compliance with a self-medication regimen. The experimental group of patients is instructed by nurses who are implementing a new instructional approach. A second (control) group of patients is cared for by nurses who continue their usual mode of instruction. The hypothesis being tested is that a higher proportion of subjects in the experimental group will report self-medication compliance than will subjects in the control group.

The chi-square statistic is computed by comparing two sets of frequencies—those observed in the collected data and those that would be expected if there were no relationship between two variables. Observed frequencies for the present example are shown in Table 16-5.

Table 16-5. Observed Frequencies for a Chi-square Example

	COMPLIANCE	NONCOMPLIANCE	TOTAL
Experimental	60	40	100
Control	30	70	100
Total	90	110	200

The chi-square statistic is computed by summing differences between observed and expected frequencies for each cell.* In this example there are four cells, and thus χ^2 will be the sum of four numbers. More specifically, $\chi^2 = 18.18$ in the present case. As usual, we need to compare this test statistic with the value from a theoretical chi-square distribution. A table of chi-square values for various degrees of freedom and significance levels is available in Table C in the Appendix. For the chi-square statistic, the degrees of freedom are equal to $(R - 1)(C - 1)$, or the number of rows minus 1 times the number of columns minus 1. In the present case, $df = 1 \times 1$, or 1. With one degree of freedom, the value that must be exceeded in order to establish significance at the .05 level is 3.84. The obtained value of 18.18 is substantially larger than would be expected by chance. Thus, we can conclude that a significantly larger proportion of patients in the experimental group than in the control group complied with self-medication instructions.

Correlation Coefficients

In the previous chapter the computation and interpretation of the Pearson product-moment correlation coefficient were explained. The Pearson r statistic is both descriptive and inferential. As a descriptive statistic, the correlation coefficient summarizes the magnitude and direction of a relationship between two variables. As an inferential statistic, r is used to test hypotheses about population correlations, which are ordinarily symbolized by the Greek letter rho, or ρ. The most commonly tested null hypothesis is that there is no relationship between two variables.

For instance, suppose we were studying the relationship between patients' self-reported level of stress (higher stress scores imply more stress) and the pH level of their saliva. With a sample of 50 subjects, we find that $r = -.29$. This value implies that there was a slight tendency for

---

*The formula for a χ^2 statistic is as follows:

$$\chi^2 = \Sigma \frac{(f_o - f_E)^2}{f_E}$$

where f_o = observed frequency for a cell

f_E = expected frequency for a cell

Σ = sum of the $(f_o - f_E)^2/f_E$ ratios for all cells

$$f_E = \frac{f_R f_C}{N}$$

where f_R = observed frequency for the given row

f_C = observed frequency for the given column

N = total number of subjects

people who received high stress scores to have lower pH levels than those with low stress scores. But we need to question whether this finding can be generalized to the population. Does the coefficient of $-.29$ reflect a random fluctuation, caused only by the particular group of subjects sampled, or is the relationship significant? The table of significant values in Table D of the Appendix allows us to make this determination. Degrees of freedom for correlation coefficients are equal to the number of subjects minus 2, or $(n - 2)$. With $df = 48$, the critical value for r lies between .273 and .288, or approximately .282. Since the absolute value of the calculated r is .29, the null hypothesis can be rejected. Therefore, we may conclude that there is a significant relationship between a person's self-reported level of stress and the acidity of her or his saliva.

The Pearson r is a parametric statistic. When the assumptions for a parametric test are violated, or when the data are inherently ordinal-level, then the appropriate coefficient of correlation is *Spearman's rho*.

Overview of Various Statistical Tests

As we have seen in the preceding section, the selection and use of a statistical test depends on several factors. In some cases nonparametric tests are more appropriate than parametric tests. For some research problems a two-way ANOVA, rather than a one-way ANOVA, will be required. To aid researchers in selecting a test statistic or evaluating statistical procedures used by researchers in the literature, a chart summarizing the major features of several commonly used tests is presented in Table 16-6.

Research Example

McCurren (1983) studied psychological distress and marital satisfaction in a sample of 100 infertile/sterile couples.* He hypothesized that levels of well-being and satisfaction would be related to whether the source of the fertility problem was the person himself/herself, or the person's partner. He also hypothesized that, overall, women would be more adversely affected than men by the fertility problem. McCurren administered a questionnaire to 100 couples who were patients at an infertility clinic—50 couples for whom infertility had been diagnosed as attributable to male factors and 50 to female factors. The questionnaire included three psychological scales, labeled as follows: (1) depression, (2) marital satisfaction, and (3) feelings of sex-role inadequacy. The scores on these three scales

---

*This example is fictitious.

Table 16-6. Summary of Statistical Tests

NAME OF PROCEDURE	TEST STATISTIC	DEGREES OF FREEDOM	PARAMETRIC (P) OR NONPARAMETRIC (NP)	PURPOSE	LEVELS OF MEASUREMENT Var. 1 (Independent)	Var. 2 (Dependent)
t-Test for independent samples	t	$N_{Group\ A} + N_{Group\ B} - 2$	P	To test the difference between the means of two independent groups	Nominal	Interval or Ratio
t-Test for dependent (paired) samples	t	N-1	P	To test the difference between the means of two related groups or sets of scores	Nominal	Interval or Ratio
Median Test	χ^2	(Rows-1) × (Columns-1)	NP	To test the difference between the medians of two independent groups	Nominal	Ordinal
Mann–Whitney U Test	U (Z)	N-1	NP	To test the difference in the ranks of scores of two independent groups	Nominal	Ordinal

Test	Statistic	Degrees of Freedom	P/NP	Purpose		
Wilcoxon Signed-Rank Test	Z	N-2	NP	To test the difference in the ranks of scores of two related groups or sets of scores	Nominal	Ordinal
ANOVA	F	Between: N of groups-1 Within: N of subjects − N of groups	P	To test the difference among the means of three or more independent groups, or of more than one independent variable	Nominal	Interval or Ratio
Kruskal–Wallis Test	H (χ^2)	N of groups-1	NP	To test the difference in the ranks of scores of three or more independent groups	Nominal	Ordinal
Chi-square Test	χ^2	(Rows-1) × (Columns-1)	NP	To test the difference in proportions in two or more groups	Nominal	Nominal
Pearson's Product-Moment Correlation	r	N-2	P	To test that a correlation is different from zero (*i.e.*, that a relationship exists)	Interval or Ratio	Interval or Ratio
Spearman's rho	ρ	N-2	NP	To test that a correlation is different from zero (*i.e.*, that a relationship exists)	Ordinal	Ordinal

were analyzed in three separate two-way (2 × 2) ANOVAs. The table below summarizes the results of the analyses.

| | Source of Fertility Problem | MEAN SCORES | | F-TEST RESULTS |
| | | Sex of Subject | | |
		Male	Female	
Depression	Self	20.1	29.1	Sex: $F = 5.9, p < .05$
	Partner	15.3	23.6	Source: $F = 6.7, p < .01$
				Sex × Source: $F = 1.9$, NS
Marital	Self	25.6	26.3	Sex: $F = 1.1$, NS
Satisfaction	Partner	28.7	24.9	Source: $F = 0.9$, NS
				Sex × Source: $F = 1.3$, NS
Sex-Role	Self	27.5	38.9	Sex: $F = 6.4, p < .05$
Inadequacy	Partner	19.5	22.8	Source: $F = 9.3, p < .01$
				Sex × Source: $F = 4.9, p < .05$

McCurren concluded on the basis of these data that his hypotheses were partially supported.

McCurren's choice of a two-way ANOVA was well suited to his research design, hypotheses, and measures. His design called for the collection of data from both partners of 100 couples, half of whom were diagnosed as having a male-based fertility problem and the other half a female-based one. His hypotheses involved both the sex-of-subject factor and source-of-problem factor. His measures involved two nominal-level independent variables (sex and source of problem) and interval-level dependent variables (the scale scores). He could have performed two separate *t*-tests for each of the three scales (the results would have been the same for the main effects), but then he would not have learned anything about interaction effects.

The results of McCurren's study indicate that the women were significantly more depressed and felt less adequate about their sex roles than their husbands (regardless of the problem source), consistent with his hypothesis. Also as hypothesized, the person who was the source of the fertility problem was more depressed and had greater feelings of sex-role inadequacy than the person's partner (regardless of gender). Differences relating to marital satisfaction were not statistically significant. That is, the observed differences on this scale were probably the result of random fluctuations only. Thus, McCurren's hypothesis regarding marital satisfaction was not supported by the data.

Although not specifically hypothesized, there was one more significant effect: on the sex-role inadequacy scale, the interaction between sex and source of partner was significant at the .05 level. An inspection of the means reveals that this interaction does *not* involve a cross-over effect. In the example shown in Table 16-4, it may be recalled, an interaction was observed when women responded more to the hypnosis treatment, while men responded more to the behavior modification treatment. In McCurren's data the interaction is somewhat different. We can interpret the results as follows: overall, the women had more negative sex-role feelings than the men; overall, the people who were the source of the fertility problem felt worse about sex-role adequacy than those whose partners were the source; *but* the women were significantly more bothered than their husbands by feelings of sex-role inadequacy when they themselves were the source of the problem.

Note that, because this is an ex post facto study, there is nothing in the data to establish causal relationships. McCurren cannot conclude that depression and feelings of sex-role inadequacy are a consequence of an infertility problem or of being the responsible party in a couple's fertility problem. The direction of causality, after all, might be reversed: people who are depressed may have a psychogenic block that inhibits fertility. Statistical significance tells us nothing about whether there is a cause-and-effect relationship; it only tells us that there is a high probability that a "real" relationship exists in the population.

Summary

Inferential statistics allow a researcher to make inferences about the characteristics of a population based on data obtained in a sample. The reason that we cannot make such inferences directly from the data is that sample statistics inevitably contain a certain degree of error as estimates of population parameters. *Inferential statistics* offer the researcher a framework for deciding whether or not the sampling error is too high to provide reliable population estimates.

The *sampling distribution of the mean* is a theoretical distribution of the means of many different samples drawn from the same population. When an infinite number of samples are drawn from a population, the sampling distribution of means follows a normal curve. Because of this characteristic, it is possible to indicate the probability that a specified sample value will be obtained. The *standard error of the mean* is the standard deviation of the theoretical sampling distribution of the mean. This index indicates the degree of average error of a sample mean from the population mean. The smaller the standard error of the mean, the more accurate are the estimates of the population value. Sampling distributions are the basis for inferential statistics.

The testing of hypotheses by statistical procedures enables researchers to make objective decisions about the results of their studies. The *null hypothesis* is a statement that no relationship exists between the variables and that any observed relationships are due to chance or sampling fluctuations. Failure to reject the null hypothesis means that any observed differences may be attributable to chance fluctuations. Rejection of the null hypothesis lends support to the research hypothesis.

It is possible to fail to reject a null hypothesis when, in fact, it should be rejected. Such an error is referred to as a *Type-II error*. If a null hypothesis is rejected when it should not be rejected, the error is termed a *Type-I error*. Researchers are able to control some of the risk of making an error by establishing a *level of significance*, which specifies the probability of making a Type-I error. The two most commonly used levels of significance are .05 and .01. A significance level of .01 means that in only 1 out of 100 samples would the null hypothesis be rejected when, in fact, it should have been retained.

Researchers report the results of hypotheses testing as being either statistically significant or nonsignificant. The phrase *statistically significant* means that the obtained results are not likely to be due to chance fluctuations at the specified level of probability.

Statistical tests are classified as parametric and nonparametric. *Nonparametric tests* require less stringent assumptions than parametric tests and usually are used when the level of data is either nominal or ordinal, the sample size is small, and the normality of the distribution cannot be assumed. *Parametric tests* involve the estimation of at least one parameter, the use of interval-level or ratio-level measures, and assumptions about the variables under consideration. Parametric tests are more powerful than nonparametric tests and generally are preferred.

The most common parametric procedures are the *t-test* and *analysis of variance* (ANOVA), both of which can be used to test the significance of the difference between group means. The *t*-test can only be applied to two-group situations, while the ANOVA procedure can handle three or more groups, as well as more than one independent variable. The nonparametric test that is used most frequently is the *chi-square test*, which is used in connection with hypotheses relating to differences in proportions. Pearson's *r* can be used to test hypothesized relationships between two variables measured on at least an interval scale.

Study Suggestions

1. A researcher has administered a job-satisfaction scale to a sample of 50 primary nurses and 50 team nurses. The mean score on this scale was found to be 35.2 for the primary nurses and 33.6 for the team nurses. A *t*-statistic was computed and was found to be 1.89. Interpret this result, using the table for *t*-values in the Appendix.

2. Answer the following, given that (a) there are three groups of nursing school students, with 50 in each group; (b) the probability level is .05; (c) the value of the test statistic is 4.43; and (d) the mean scores on the test to measure motivation to attend graduate school are 25.8, 29.3, and 23.4 for groups A, B, and C, respectively:

    a. What test statistic would be used?

    b. How many degrees of freedom are there?

    c. Is the test statistic statistically significant?

    d. What does the test statistic mean?

3. What inferential statistic would you choose for the following sets of variables? Explain your answers. (Refer to Table 16-6.)

    a. Variable 1 is grade-point averages for 100 students; variable 2 is Graduate Record Examination scores for the same 100 students.

    b. Variable 1 is the patient's marital status; variable 2 is the patient's level of preoperative stress.

    c. Variable 1 is whether an amputee has a leg removed above or below the knee; variable 2 is whether or not the amputee has shown signs of aggressive behavior during rehabilitation.

Chapter 17
The Computer and
Data Analysis

The use of computers in scientific research is substantial and inevitably growing. One of the most important applications of the computer in scientific investigations is the analysis of data. While many other important applications have been developed, the discussion here will be geared to the person seeking to make sense of the information obtained during the course of a research project.

The purpose of this chapter is to introduce the reader to some of the basic principles of computer operations. While computers are electronically complex machines, the underlying logic of computers is not difficult to comprehend. It is hoped that an acquaintance with some of the basic characteristics of high-speed computers will be sufficient to demonstrate that computer analysis is within the reach of all readers of this book.

Powers and Limitations of Computers

High-speed computers are machines of tremendous power. Without any doubt, they are indispensable to modern scientists because of the characteristics we describe below. Computers are not, however, on the verge of making human intelligence obsolete. Respect for the computer's potency must be balanced by a recognition of its limitations.

The most noteworthy characteristic of electronic digital computers is unquestionably their remarkable speed. A computer can perform more arithmetic in 1 second than a human could perform working 40-hour weeks for several years.

Not only are computers fast, but they also are accurate. Highly complex calculations can be performed without error. By contrast, human "calculators" are fallible. An additional advantage of computers is that they are dependably accurate. They can work hour after hour without making a mistake. Computers do, of course, break down occasionally. Nevertheless, they behave for the most part as our faithful servants. They do exactly what they are told to do, day in and day out, no matter how boring or repetitive the task might be.

Computers also have several shortcomings. One of the most conspicuous limitations of the computer is its utter and complete stupidity. Computers are sometimes referred to as "giant brains," but they have absolutely no innate intelligence. They do only those operations that they are told to do by human beings. The computer's inability to think can result in many frustrating experiences for its users.

Computer time is quite costly, despite the downward trend of computer prices. Although costs vary markedly from one installation to another, it is not unusual for computer time to cost 10 dollars per minute. Of course, the computer could perform an enormous quantity of operations in 1 minute.

Another limitation is the detail with which instructions must be described. When a human being is confronted with the task $2 + 2 = X$, the solution is (at the conscious level at least) straightforward and simple. A computer normally requires several instructions to process such computations. Every logical and arithmetic operation must be "explained" to the computer in detail, a feature that makes most tasks seem more complex than they would to human beings. Fortunately, the average researcher does not have to worry about such matters for analyzing data. The detailed instructions are developed by computer experts who have taken pains to simplify the use of computers.

Overview of Computer Functioning

A computer system is an elaborate complex consisting of numerous components that perform specialized functions. The components of a computer system can be classified as either hardware or software. *Hardware* is a term that refers to the physical electronic equipment that stores, processes, and controls information. *Software* refers to the instructions and procedures required to operate the computer. In this section, several aspects of both hardware and software will be reviewed.

Computer Hardware

A schematic diagram of computer hardware is presented in Figure 17-1. Essentially, the computer consists of five types of components— input devices, a control unit, memory, an arithmetic/logic unit, and output devices. Information is fed into the computer through some type of *input device.* The information read in through an input device is composed of data and instructions about how the data are to be processed. After the computer has performed its necessary calculations, the resulting

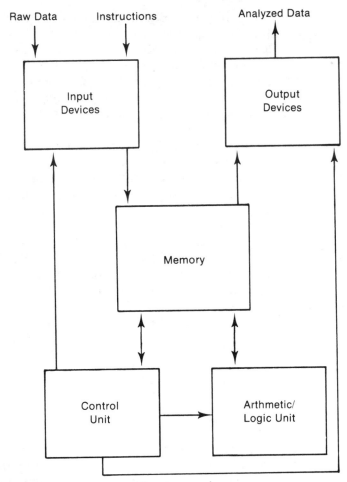

Figure 17-1. Scheme of computer components and interrelationships

information comes out through an *output device.* Input/output (sometimes abbreviated I/O) devices are normally the only parts of the machine with which a researcher comes in contact. For this reason, I/O devices are the only parts of the computer described in detail here.

Input devices convert alphabetical and numerical characters to a form amenable to storage in the computer's memory. A variety of input devices exist, and most computer installations have more than one type of device available for use. One type of input medium is the *punched card.* These cards contain 80 columns and 12 rows for storing information (either data or program instructions). The information is coded on the card in machine-readable form through a process known as *keypunching.* A keypunch machine is quite similar to a typewriter, except that as the keypunch operator types onto the keyboard, holes are punched onto successive columns of the card. A punched code corresponds to each number, letter, and symbol of the keyboard. The input device that accepts punched cards is called a *card reader.*

Data and instructions are increasingly being transmitted to the computer by direct communication devices. These devices transmit information through electronic impulses and permit the user to communicate directly with the computer without the use of cards. Direct communication devices take the form of a teletype, terminal, or console with a keyboard onto which the user types the relevant information.

Data and instructions can also be stored for input into the computer on *magnetic tape* (on reels similar to those used for a tape recorder) or *magnetic disks* (flat, spinning objects with magnetizable surfaces, analogous to a record). Tapes and, especially, disks are more dependable than cards for storing information. Both have the added advantage of being erasable for reuse.

The most common output medium is a permanent readable record of the results of the analysis. The *line printer* is typically a principal output device for the computer. The copy produced by printers is usually called the *printout* or *printed output.*

Various visual display devices are often used to output information in direct communication systems. *Cathode ray tube* (CRT) devices are becoming increasingly common in many settings, including hospitals. The information transmitted on a CRT is not permanent, but may be photographed.

Computer Software

The software components of a computer include the instructions for performing operations and the documentation for those instructions. A set of instructions is referred to as a *program.* The ability for a computer to solve problems is dependent upon computer programs, which specify clearly and precisely what operations the machine is to perform and how to perform them.

In order to give the computer a set of commands, people must be able to communicate with the machine. Computers, unfortunately, do not "speak" or understand natural languages such as English. Direct machine language that a computer *can* comprehend is extremely complex and learned only by computer experts. Happily, various *programming languages* have been developed that are reasonably easy to learn and that are structured in a manner comfortable to human communicators.

Various programming languages are available to computer users. Many of these languages have been developed for a specific type of application. The language most commonly used in scientific applications is FORTRAN, which is an acronym for FORmula TRANslation. The language known as PL/1 (Programming Language 1) is becoming increasingly popular in the scientific community. It includes many features of FORTRAN, but has additional new features and capabilities that make it attractive for use with scientific and social scientific problems. One of the simplest languages for beginning programmers to learn is BASIC (Beginners All-Purpose Symbolic Instruction Code).

Most researchers can make use of computers without having to learn a computer language. This is because there are standard programs available for most types of statistical analysis. It would be inefficient to have every researcher write a program to compute an average or percentage when a single program could be used by thousands of people. Available computer programs for data analysis are described below.

Available Programs

A great boon to researchers is the widespread availability of ready-made programs to perform standard statistical analyses. The computer centers at universities are particularly likely to have a variety of software packages available to their users, as well as a professional staff that is accessible for consultation.

Many computer facilities have a variety of simple, easy-to-use statistical programs in their general library. Many such "canned" programs can be run from an interactive terminal. The use of these programs requires no expertise at all on the part of the researcher. For example, a researcher could obtain some basic descriptive statistics about a set of data by typing in a simple instruction, such as RUN TALLY. The terminal would ask questions that would then guide the researcher in providing the necessary information to the computer.

These simple library programs are excellent heuristic devices for a user who is first learning to work with a computer. When a researcher has a large number of cases or a large number of variables, or desires a sophisticated statistical procedure, however, a more complex statistical software package may be required.

The most widely used software packages include the Biomedical Computer Programs or BMD (Dixon & Brown, 1983); the Statistical Package for the Social Sciences, or SPSS (Nie et al., 1979); Osiris (Institute for Social Research, 1973); and Statistical Analysis System, or SAS (SAS Institute, 1982). Each of these packages contains programs to handle a broad variety of statistical analyses.

Researchers using packaged programs do not need to know a programming language, but they still must be able to communicate to the computer some basic information about what their variables are and how the data are to be analyzed. This is accomplished by means of certain commands that are unique to each software package. To illustrate the kinds of commands the researcher would need to know, an example of a set-up for an SPSS task will be presented. SPSS was chosen because it is widely available and is fairly easy to learn.

Let us suppose that we have collected data on two variables from a sample of 100 subjects. The two variables are the person's height in inches and weight in pounds. These data have been keypunched onto cards, a separate card having been punched for individual subjects. The result is a deck of 100 cards, each of which contains the person's height in columns 1 and 2 and weight in columns 3 through 5. A sample card for a subject who is 65 inches tall and who weighs 115 pounds is presented in Figure 17-2.

In order to use SPSS to analyze the data, we must tell the computer how we have set up the deck of punched cards, just as we had to communicate this information to the reader in the preceding paragraph. The following instructions would be punched onto keypunch cards (or entered on a terminal), with one command per card or line:

VARIABLE LIST	HEIGHT, WEIGHT
INPUT FORMAT	FIXED (F2.0, F3.0)
INPUT MEDIUM	CARD
N OF CASES	100
FREQUENCIES	GENERAL = HEIGHT, WEIGHT
STATISTICS	ALL
READ INPUT DATA	

The first line tells the computer that there are two variables, which are designated as height and weight. SPSS permits up to eight characters for variable names. The INPUT FORMAT line is somewhat more complex. The instruction "FIXED" signifies that the data for the variables are in a fixed, specified location for each subject. The information in parentheses designates that fixed location: the first variable, height, takes up two columns on the data cards (F2.0) and the next variable, weight, takes up three columns on the data cards (F3.0). The input format line, in other words, tells the computer where to "look" to find the information on a person's height and weight. The INPUT MEDIUM line simply informs the computer that the data are to be read from punched cards rather than another input medium. Next comes the N OF CASES line, which specifies the number of subjects in the study. The following two lines, taken together, instruct the computer what statistical analysis to perform. These instructions will produce, for both the height and weight variables, a frequency distribution. In addition, the computer will print many basic descriptive statistics, such as the mean, median, standard deviation, and so forth. If we wanted more complex analyses performed, we would only need to replace the FREQUENCIES/STATISTICS lines with other instructions. The final line, READ INPUT DATA, tells the computer to begin reading the

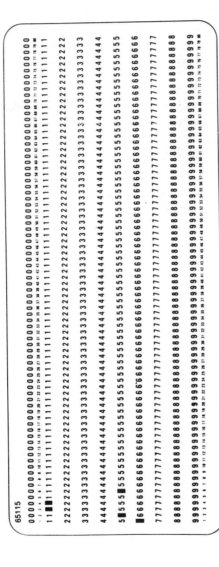

Figure 17-2. Example of a keypunch card with data. (Courtesy of International Business Machines Corporation)

actual data, which in the present case consist of our 100 cards with data punched in the first five columns.

Hopefully, this simple example has made it clear that a researcher need not be a computer whiz or mathematical genius in order to make use of a computer. SPSS has many features that were not described here, but these features are not difficult to understand either. Similarly, other packaged programs have commands that must be learned by users but that are designed to be easy to learn by persons with no or minimal computer skills.

Preparing Data for Computer Analysis

If a computer is to be used to analyze data, it is essential that the information be converted to a machine-readable form. Computers cannot process verbatim responses to open-ended questions, nor the field notes of a participant observer. It is similarly difficult for a computer to read and analyze information with verbal labels such as "male or female" or "agree or disagree." *Coding* is the process by which research information is transformed into symbols compatible with computer analysis. It is possible to code information using alphabetical symbols. For example, the code for females could be F and the code for males could be M. However, a completely numerical coding scheme is preferable since many packaged programs cannot handle alphabetical coding. Below we discuss some aspects of the coding process.

Coding

Some variables are inherently quantitative and do not need to be coded. Examples include such variables as age, weight, body temperature, and number of siblings. However, sometimes the researcher may ask for information of this type in a way that *does* call for the development of a coding plan. If a researcher asks respondents to indicate whether they are younger than 30, between the ages of 31 and 49, or over 50, then the responses would have to be coded before being entered into the computer.

In many situations, data that are not inherently quantitative can be coded prior to data collection. Closed-ended questions on self-report instruments are one example, as in the following illustration:

From what type of program did you receive your basic nursing
preparation?
( ) 1. Diploma school
( ) 2. Associate-degree program
( ) 3. Baccalaureate-degree program

Thus, if a nurse received his or her nursing preparation from a diploma school, the response to this question would be coded "1."

Sometimes respondents may have the option of checking off more than one answer in reply to a single question, as in the following illustration:

To which of the following journals do you subscribe?
(   ) *American Journal of Nursing*
(   ) *Nursing Forum*
(   ) *Nursing Outlook*
(   ) *Nursing Research*

With questions of this type, it is not possible to adopt a simple 1–2–3–4 code because subjects may check several, or none, of the responses. The most appropriate procedure for such multiple-response questions is to treat each journal on the list as a separate question. In other words, the researcher would code the responses as though the question were four separate questions: "Do you subscribe to the *American Journal of Nursing?* Do you subscribe to *Nursing Forum? . . .*" A checkmark beside a journal would be treated as though the reply were "yes." In effect, the question would be turned into four dichotomous variables, with a code (perhaps "1") signifying a "yes" response and another code (perhaps "2") signifying a "no" response.

Data from open-ended questions, unstructured observations, and projective tests usually are not directly amenable to computer analysis. When this type of information is to be analyzed by the computer, it is necessary to categorize and code it. The researcher should first scan all of the responses, or a sizeable sample of them, to get a feel for the nature of the replies. The categorization scheme should be designed to reflect both the researcher's theoretical and analytic goals as well as the substance of the information. The amount of detail in the categorization scheme can vary considerably, but too much detail is usually better than too little detail. In developing a coding scheme for unstructured information, the only "rule" is that the coding categories should be both mutually exclusive and collectively exhaustive.

One final issue concerns the coding of missing information. Missing data can be of various types. A person responding to an interview question may be undecided, refuse to answer, or say "don't know." An observer coding behavior may get distracted during a 10-second sampling frame, may be undecided about an appropriate categorization, or may observe behavior unlisted on the observation schedule. In some cases it may be important to distinguish between various types of missing data by specifying separate codes, while in another case a single code may suffice. This decision must be made with the conceptual aims of the research in mind. The choice of what number to use as the missing data code is fairly arbitrary, but the number must be the one that has not been assigned to an actual piece of information. Many researchers follow the convention of coding missing data as 9, since this value is normally out of the range of codes for true information. Others use blanks to indicate missing information.*

Whenever coding is performed by more than one person, it is imperative that precise instructions be developed for the coders. Coders, like observers and interviewers, must be properly trained. Intercoder reliability checks are strongly recommended.

One final comment concerns the need for proper documentation. The decisions that a researcher makes about coding, field width, placement of data in columns, and so on should be documented in full. The researcher's own memory should not be trusted to store all of the required information. Several weeks after coding, the researcher may no longer remember if men were coded 1 and women 2, or vice versa. Documentation often takes the form of a codebook. A *codebook* is a listing of each variable, the column(s) in which the variable has been entered, and the codes associated with the various aspects or attributes of the variable. The codebook is often prepared before coding so that it can be used as a guide by coders. Additional documentation is required if any type of transformation has been effected after the data have been entered. For instance, researchers often combine two or more variables to form a composite index or scale. Scale construction, item reversals, recodes, and other types of changes to the data should be recorded in full.

Data Entry

For most types of computer analysis, the coded data are transferred to punch cards through the process of keypunching, or onto a disk file by means of a console or terminal. Normally, data are entered into the computer according to some predesignated plan, some aspects of which are discussed below. We highlight the use of keypunch cards not because they are the most common method of data entry, but because they are tangible entities that are conceptually easy to deal with.

The researcher must plan the layout of information in advance of the data entry. It is usually preferable to adopt what is known as a *fixed format,* which places the values for any specific variable in the same location (card column) for every case. Some packaged programs also permit data to be entered in a *free format,* in which there is no necessary correspondence between the variables entered in any particular column from one case to the next. However, it is often safer to use a fixed format since it is

---

*The use of blanks for missing values may be problematic, because in many cases the computer program will not distinguish between blanks and zeros without some specific instruction. If zero is a legitimate code for an actual response, the researcher should be careful in using blanks for missing data.

more widely acceptable. Moreover, fixed format is usually preferable for beginning researchers since it permits an easier check for errors.

With fixed format, the researcher must specify in which columns all items of information are to be entered. Many variables will require no more than one column. That is, any code whose maximum value is one digit can be assigned to a single column. Examples include male/female, agree/disagree, and yes/no/maybe. Other variables, such as age, weight, and blood pressure measures, must occupy more than one column. Anytime the maximum value of a variable exceeds 9, the researcher must be sure to reserve two (or more, if the number is larger than 99) columns. The space allocated to a particular variable is referred to as a *field.*

The researcher must be careful in dealing with a variable whose values are of different widths. For example, if we were recording a person's weight, we would need two digits for persons weighing under 100 pounds, and three digits for those weighing 100 pounds or more. Since the maximum value would be three digits long, then three columns would be required. To record the weight of a 95-pound person, we would have to occupy the full three columns, so it would be necessary to enter 095. This procedure is known as *right-justifying* the data. Whenever a number smaller than the corresponding field is entered in fixed format, the number should be punched as far to the right as possible in the designated field. In the above example, if columns 1, 2, and 3 were reserved for the weight measurement, 95 should be punched in columns 2 and 3. If, instead, 95 were punched in columns 1 and 2, the value would be read typically as 950.

In designing the layout for the data on the punch cards, the researchers should allocate space for recording an identification number. Each individual case (*i.e.,* the information from a single questionnaire, test, observation, and so forth) should be assigned a unique identifying number, and this number should be entered along with the actual data. This procedure will permit the investigator to go back to the original source if there are any difficulties with the data. The numbering is completely arbitrary and is used only as a label.

Sometimes a researcher will find that one 80-column card or one line on a terminal is inadequate. There is no restriction on the number of cards that may be used for a given case or subject. In fact, it is quite common to require two or three cards to record all of the data for each subject. When multiple cards are needed, the identification number for a particular case should be entered onto all cards for that case.

A number of procedures are available to facilitate the actual data-entry process. The first is to transfer codes from the original source (such as a questionnaire) onto a specially prepared coding sheet. These sheets, which are available commercially, are ruled off into a grid with 80 columns and 20 to 40 rows. The columns correspond to the columns on the punch card, and each row represents a single card. A second procedure, known as *edge-coding,* is to use a margin on the original source to write the appropriate numerical codes for the person entering the data.

Data entry is a tedious and exacting task that is usually subject to numerous errors. Therefore, it is necessary to verify or check the entered data to correct the mistakes that are inevitably made. Even after verification, the data usually will contain a few errors. These errors could be due to data-entry mistakes but could also arise from coding or reporting problems.

Data are not ready for analysis until they have been cleaned. *Data cleaning* involves editing to check for *outliers* or wild codes. Using a computer printout of the frequency counts associated with every value for every variable, the researcher checks for undefined code values. The variable "sex" would have three defined code values—for example, 1 for female, 2 for male, and 9 for not reported. If it were discovered that a code of 5 were entered in the column specified for sex, then it would be clear that an error had been made. The computer could be instructed to list the identification number of the culpable case, and the error could be corrected by checking the appropriate code on the original source. Data cleaning is basically a systematic hunt for deviant cases. Editing of this type will never reveal mistakes that look "respectable" or plausible. If the gender of a man is mispunched as a 1, the mistake may never be detected.

Coding for Computer Analysis: A Hypothetical Example

Perhaps the coding and data-entry processes can be best understood by reference to a detailed example. Figure 17-3 presents a questionnaire that was contrived solely for the purpose of illustrating many of the points made in the preceding sections. This hypothetical instrument should by no means be taken as a good example of questionnaire design. The intent was to include a variety of question types to demonstrate how different coding problems could be handled.

In the left-hand margin of the questionnaire are the numerical codes to be entered into the computer. The first code—001—represents the right-justified identification number assigned to the respondent who completed the questionnaire. The three-digit number implies that at least 100 (but fewer than 1000) respondents participated in the study. Following the identification number are the codes corresponding to the subject's responses. In question 2, part B, the missing values code of 9 signifies the subject's failure to respond. With regard to question 5, each individual symptom is treated for data-analysis purposes as a separate question, with a check of "X" being coded as "1," and no check coded as "2." It might also be noted that the subject's height, reported in question 10, has been translated to inches.

The data-entry person using edge-coded questionnaires such as this

001	This questionnaire is part of a study on health-related habits and attitudes. We hope you will help us by answering the following questions.
	1. Overall, how would you describe your health in comparison with that of others your **age**?
2	( ) above average health
	(x) average health
	( ) below average health
	2. Have you been hospitalized within the past two years?
	( ) yes ┐
2	(X) no ↓
	If yes: how many times have you been hospitalized?
	( ) once
9	( ) two times
	( ) more than two times
	3. Do you smoke cigarettes?
1	(X) yes ┐
	( ) no ↓
	If yes, how many cigarettes do you usually smoke per day?
1	(X) 1 pack or less
	( ) between one and two packs
	( ) two packs or more
	4. How often do you drink alcoholic beverages?
4	( ) never (X) 2 or 3 times a month
	( ) 10 times a year or less ( ) about once a week
	( ) about once a month ( ) several times a week
	( ) nearly every day
	5. Below is a list of some common somatic complaints. Please check off those symptoms which have bothered you within the past month or so.
1	(x) headache
2	( ) indigestion
1	(x) constipation
2	( ) diarrhea
2	( ) insomnia
2	( ) lower back pains
2	( ) lack of appetite
	6. Which of the following statements best describes your health care practices?
	( ) I go for regular physical checkups as a preventive health care measure.
2	(X) I see a health care professional only when I have a specific complaint.
	( ) I have to be extremely ill before I will see a health care professional.
	7. Please indicate how important the following things are to you by placing an "X" under the appropriate column:

	Extremely important	Somewhat important	Not too important
1 Abundant leisure time	X		
3 A long life			X
2 Financial success and security		X	
1 Good family relationships	X		
2 Good health		X	
2 Lots of friends, popularity		X	

38	8. What is your present age? ___38___ years.
135	9. How much do you weigh? ___135___ pounds.
66	10. How tall are you? ___5___ feet, ___6___ inches.
1	11. What is your sex?
	(X) female
	( ) male

Figure 17-3. Example of a questionnaire with edge coding

SMOKE DO YOU SMOKE CIGARETTES?				
CATEGORY LABEL	CODE	ABSOLUTE FREQ	RELATIVE FREQ (PCT)	ADJUSTED FREQ (PCT)
YES	1.	76	50.7	51.7
NO	2.	68	45.3	46.3
	3.	2	1.3	1.4
	8.	1	0.7	0.7
	9.	3	2.0	MISSING
	TOTAL	150	100.0	100.0

Figure 17-4. Hypothetical data for data-cleaning example

would simply follow the numbers in the left-hand margin, entering them in consecutive columns. The total number of columns required to store the information from this fictitious questionnaire is 31. If there were 150 respondents and keypunch cards were used, there would be 150 cards, all with punches in the first 31 columns and no punches in the remaining 49 columns.

This example can also be used to illustrate the data-cleaning procedure. Figure 17-4 presents a computer printout of the frequency counts corresponding to all values punched for question 3—"Do you smoke cigarettes?" Of the 150 cases, 76 responses were entered as "1" or "yes" (in the second column under "ABSOLUTE FREQ"), and 68 responses were entered as "2" or "no." Three respondents apparently failed to answer (entered as "9"). The printout tells us that in two cases a "3" was incorrectly entered for question 3, and in one case an "8" was entered. This computer listing has informed us that there are incorrect entries for three cases in column 7. After identifying the ID numbers for these cases, the correct information would be looked up and the necessary changes made. After all the data have been cleaned, the data analysis could begin.

Data Analysis by Computer: A Hypothetical Example

In this concluding section we work through a fictitious example of a study to illustrate how the computer can be used to generate descriptive and inferential statistics. The intent of this section is to make the concepts of statistical analysis and computer processing less abstract by illustrating them with some data, and to familiarize the reader with printout from a standard software package, SPSS.

Suppose that a nurse researcher were interested in improving the childbirth outcomes among a group of young, low-income pregnant women. A program of intensive health care, nutritional counseling, and contraceptive counseling is developed, and an experiment is designed to test the effect of the program: half of a sample of pregnant girls under age 20, assigned randomly, will receive the special treatment, and the other half will be assigned to a group receiving routine care. The two outcomes that the researcher is primarily interested in are the birthweight of the infant and whether or not the young woman becomes pregnant again within 18 months of delivery. Some fictitious data for this example are presented in Table 17-1.

Figure 17-5 presents a frequency distribution printout for the birthweight variable. Under the term "CODE," each birthweight mentioned one or more times by the respondents is listed, in ascending order. In the next column, "ABSOLUTE FREQ," the number of occurrences of each birthweight is indicated. Thus, there was one 76-ounce baby, two 89-ounce babies, and so on. The next column, "RELATIVE FREQ," indicates the percentage of birthweights in each class: 3.3% of the babies weighed 76 ounces at birth, 6.7% weighed 89 ounces, and so on. The next column, "ADJUSTED FREQ," shows the percentage in each category after removing any missing data. In this example, birthweights were obtained for all 30 cases, but if one piece of data had been missing, the adjusted frequency for the 76-ounce baby would have been 3.4% (1 divided by 29 rather than 30). The last column, "CUM FREQ" (cumulative frequency), adds the adjusted frequency for a given row to the adjusted frequency for all preceding rows. Thus, we can tell by looking at the row for 99 ounces that 33.3% of the babies weighed *under* 100 ounces in this example.

The bottom of this printout provides a number of the descriptive statistics discussed in Chapter 15. The MEAN is equal to 104.7, while the MEDIAN is 102.5 and the MODE is 99. The RANGE is 52 (which is equal to the MAXIMUM of 128 minus the MINIMUM of 76). The standard deviation (STD DEV) is 10.955, while the VARIANCE is 120.010 (10.955^2). Two brief commands to the computer produced this printout, plus similar information for the remaining three variables.

In addition to descriptive statistics, SPSS can be used to calculate inferential statistics. One of our research hypotheses is the following: The babies of the experimental subjects will have higher birthweights than the babies of the control subjects. Birthweight, the dependent variable, is measured on a ratio scale. Therefore, the *t*-test for independent samples is used to test our hypothesis.*

---

*We use parametric tests here, despite the small Ns, for exemplary purposes. Normally the Ns would be considerably larger.

Table 17-1. Fictitious Data on Low-income Pregnant Young Women

GROUP (1 = experimental; 2 = control)	WEIGHT OF INFANT (in ounces)	REPEAT PREGNANCY (1 = yes; 0 = no)
1	107	1
1	101	0
1	119	0
1	128	1
1	89	0
1	99	0
1	111	0
1	117	1
1	102	1
1	120	0
1	76	0
1	116	0
1	100	1
1	115	0
1	113	0
2	111	1
2	108	0
2	95	0
2	99	0
2	103	1
2	94	0
2	101	1
2	114	0
2	97	0
2	99	1
2	113	0
2	89	0
2	98	0
2	102	0
2	105	0

Figure 17-6 presents the SPSS printout for the *t*-test. The left side of the printout presents some basic descriptive statistics for the birthweight variable, separately for the two groups. Thus, the mean birthweight of the babies in group 1 (the experimental group) was 107.5 ounces, compared with 101.9 ounces for the babies in group 2 (the control group). These data, then, are consistent with our research hypothesis: the weight of the experimental-group subjects is higher than the weight of the control-group subjects. But does the difference reflect the impact of the experimental intervention or does it merely represent random fluctuations? To answer this, we examine the results of the *t*-test, shown on the right side

WEIGHT   BIRTHWEIGHT OF BABY

CATEGORY LABEL	CODE	ABSOLUTE FREQ	RELATIVE FREQ (PCT)	ADJUSTED FREQ (PCT)	CUM FREQ (PCT)
	76.	1	3.3	3.3	3.3
	89.	2	6.7	6.7	10.0
	94.	1	3.3	3.3	13.3
	95.	1	3.3	3.3	16.7
	97.	1	3.3	3.3	20.0
	98.	1	3.3	3.3	23.3
	99.	3	10.0	10.0	33.3
	100.	1	3.3	3.3	36.7
	101.	2	6.7	6.7	43.3
	102.	2	6.7	6.7	50.0
	103.	1	3.3	3.3	53.3
	105.	1	3.3	3.3	56.7
	107.	1	3.3	3.3	60.0
	108.	1	3.3	3.3	63.3
	111.	2	6.7	6.7	70.0
	113.	2	6.7	6.7	76.7
	114.	1	3.3	3.3	80.0
	115.	1	3.3	3.3	83.3
	116.	1	3.3	3.3	86.7
	117.	1	3.3	3.3	90.0
	119.	1	3.3	3.3	93.3
	120.	1	3.3	3.3	96.7
	128.	1	3.3	3.3	100.0
	TOTAL	30	100.0	100.0	

MEAN	104.700	STD ERR	2.000	MEDIAN	102.500
MODE	99.000	STD DEV	10.955	VARIANCE	120.010
KURTOSIS	.473	SKEWNESS	-.254	RANGE	52.000
MINIMUM	76.000	MAXIMUM	128.000		

VALID CASES   30   MISSING CASES   0

Figure 17-5. SPSS computer printout: frequency distribution

of the printout. SPSS calculated that the value of t is 1.44. With 28 degrees of freedom, this value is not significant. The two-tailed probability (p-value) for this t-value is .16. This means that in 16 samples out of 100 one could expect to find a difference in weights at least this large as a result of chance alone. Therefore, we cannot conclude that the special intervention was effective in improving the birthweights of the experimental group.* The null hypothesis is accepted.

A second research hypothesis may be stated as follows: subjects in the experimental group will be less likely to have a repeat pregnancy 18 months after delivering their babies than control-group subjects. To test this hypothesis, which involves two nominal-level variables, we would instruct the computer to perform a cross-tabulation, as shown in the contingency table in Figure 17-7. This cross-tabulation resulted in four cells—an experimental group with no repeat pregnancy (upper left cell); a control group with no repeat pregnancy (upper right); an experimental group with repeat pregnancy (lower left cell); and a control group with repeat pregnancy (lower right cell). Each cell contains four pieces of information, which we will explain for the first cell. The first number is the number of girls in that cell. Ten experimental subjects did *not* have a repeat pregnancy within 18 months of their delivery. The next number is the *row* percentage: 47.6% of the girls who did not become pregnant again were in the experimental group (10 divided by 21). The next figure represents the *column* percent: 66.7% of the experimentals did not become pregnant (10 divided by 15). The last figure is the *overall* percentage of girls in that cell (10 divided by 30 equals 33.3%). This order need not be memorized. It is shown in the upper left corner of the table:

COUNT

ROW PCT

COL PCT

TOT PCT

Thus, this table indicates that a somewhat higher percentage of experimental-group subjects (33.3%) than control-group subjects (26.7%) experienced a repeat pregnancy. The row totals on the far right indicate that, overall, 30% of the sample (N = 9) had a subsequent pregnancy.

The data collected for this study conflict with the second research hypothesis: more experimental-group subjects than control-group subjects experienced a repeat pregnancy within 18 months postpartum. Even though we can tell at a glance that the hypothesis was not supported, we should test to see whether the group difference is statistically significant. Perhaps there is some aspect of the program that increases the likelihood of another early pregnancy. To test the hypothesis, the SPSS cross-tabulation program would be instructed to compute the chi-squared statistic.

---

*The difference in weights is fairly sizeable and in the right direction. The researcher might wish to pursue this study by increasing the sample size or by controlling some other variables, such as the mother's age, through analysis of covariance. Analysis of covariance is described in texts on intermediate or advanced statistics.

GROUP 1 - GROUP   1.
GROUP 2 - GROUP   2.

VARIABLE	NUMBER OF CASES	MEAN	STANDARD DEVIATION	STANDARD ERROR		POOLED VARIANCE ESTIMATE		
						T VALUE	DEGREES OF FREEDOM	2-TAIL PROB.
WEIGHT BIRTHWEIGHT OF BABY								
GROUP 1	15	107.5333	13.378	3.454		1.44	28	.160
GROUP 2	15	101.8667	7.239	1.869				

Figure 17-6. SPSS computer printout: T test

FILE NONAME (CREATION DATE = 12/ 9/81)

REPEAT REPEAT PREGNANCY WITHIN 18 MONTHS CROSSTABULATION OF BY GROUP

	GROUP		
COUNT ROW PCT COL PCT TOT PCT	EXPERIME 1. I	CONTROL 2. I	ROW TOTAL
REPEAT			
NO REPEAT PREG 0.	10 / 47.6 / 66.7 / 33.3	11 / 52.4 / 73.3 / 36.7	21 / 70.0
REPEAT PREG 1.	5 / 55.6 / 33.3 / 16.7	4 / 44.4 / 26.7 / 13.3	9 / 30.0
COLUMN TOTAL	15 / 50.0	15 / 50.0	30 / 100.0

Figure 17-7. SPSS computer printout: contingency table

Although this is not shown in Figure 17-7, the computed value is 0.159. With one degree of freedom, this value is not significant. Thus, we must conclude on the basis of this evidence that the experimental intervention had no effect on either subsequent early pregnancies or the birthweight of the subjects' infants. The program may have had other beneficial effects (e.g., improving the self-confidence or dietary practices of the young mothers), but there is no way of knowing this if these variables were not measured.

Summary

The advantages of computers to researchers include their speed, accuracy, and dependability. On the other hand, computers are costly and require considerable attention to detail on the part of users.

The components of a computer system are broadly categorized as either hardware or software. The term *hardware* refers to the physical equipment that stores, processes, and controls information. *Software* refers to the instructions and procedures required to operate the computer.

The five essential components of computer hardware are the *input device, memory, control unit, arithmetic/logic unit,* and *output device.* The input device is the means by which the researcher feeds information into the computer. The most commonly used input media include *punched cards, magnetic tape, magnetic disk,* and *direct communication* by means of a terminal or console. The most commonly used output media are the paper *printout* (which is a permanent, readable record of the results of the analysis produced by a line printer) and displays from *cathode ray tubes.*

Computer software consists primarily of *programs,* which are sets of instructions informing the computer what to do. *Programming languages* make it possible for humans to communicate with computers. FORTRAN, PL/1, and BASIC are examples of programming languages. Many packaged software programs exist for the researcher who is not greatly skilled in a programming language. SPSS, which was used to illustrate a computer-performed statistical analysis, is among the most widely used software package for data analysis.

Information collected in a research project must be converted to machine-readable form if a computer is to be used. *Coding* is the procedure of transforming research data into symbols compatible with computer analysis. Preferably, the coding scheme adopted is completely numerical. If the data are inherently quantitative (such as a person's weight), or if a precategorization scheme was used to collect the data, the coding task is straightforward. For uncategorized data, such as responses to open-ended questions, a coding system must be developed for analytic purposes. Special codes should be developed to signify missing data.

The researcher usually must plan in advance the layout of information prior to entering data into the computer. In a *fixed-format* arrangement, which is commonly used for research data, each variable is entered onto the same column for every case. The width of the *field* (the space allocated to a particular variable) is determined by the maximum numerical value for that variable. The data should always be *right-justified*, or entered as far to the right as possible in the designated field. It is wise to identify each case with an identification number, which is typically entered onto the first few columns for the case. The researcher's coding decisions should always be carefully documented, usually in the form of a *codebook.*

There are several available procedures for performing the actual data entry task. The researcher may transfer the codes from the original source onto specially prepared *coding sheets,* which are ruled off into grids of 80 columns (one column per column on a punch card) and about 20 rows (one row for each punch card). A second procedure is to use an *edge-coding* scheme, in which the numerical codes to be entered are written onto the margin of the original source.

Data entry is susceptible to a high rate of error. Records, therefore, should be checked or *verified* for errors. Even after the data are verified, they almost inevitably contain a few errors. Because of this fact, data should be *cleaned* before proceeding with the desired analyses. The cleaning process is primarily a check for *outliers* or numerical values that are not part of the coding scheme.

Study Suggestions

1. Visit a computer center. Check what types of input and output devices the computer has. If possible, learn how to operate a keypunch machine or a terminal. Ask someone what software packages are available for doing statistical analyses.

2. Suppose you had data from 50 subjects on the following four variables—age, sex (coded 1 for females, 2 for males), number of cigarettes smoked per day, and number of days absent from work in the past year. Write out SPSS instructions that would produce a frequency listing for these four variables. (Note: first determine in which columns the data would be punched.)

3. Complete the questionnaire in the study by Hocking and her coworkers entitled "Willingness of Psychiatric Nurses to Assume the Extended Role" (*Nursing Research,* 1976, *25,* 44–48). Then code your own or a fellow student's responses.

4. If you have access to a keypunch machine or terminal, enter the data presented in Figure 17-3. Enter the same data *twice*, then verify for accuracy by comparing the two lines of numbers.

5. What field width would you need for the following variables— marital status, annual income, body temperature, white blood cell count, religious affiliation, heart rate, annual days absent from work, Apgar score, and time to first postsurgical voiding?

Part VI
Final Steps in the Research Process

Chapter 18
Evaluating and Interpreting Research Findings

The "bottom line" of a scientific investigation is the conclusions reached by the researcher on the basis of the data analysis. At the end of the study the researcher (as well as those reading a research report) must decide what the answer is to the research question or if the research hypothesis has been supported. An even more basic, and critical, question is "Has this study adequately addressed and answered the research question or tested the research hypothesis?"

We have stressed throughout this book that the research process involves numerous decisions, each of which could affect the quality of the study. The interpretation of research findings should always take into consideration an evaluation of the researcher's methodological decisions. For example, if an investigator finds that there are no differences between samples of physicians and nurse practitioners with respect to their use of touch to communicate with patients, can we conclude with confidence that physicians use touch as much as nurse practitioners? We would be foolish to do so without a critical evaluation of every component of the study. Special attention should be paid to the five major decisions described in Chapter 3. Of course, as we have repeatedly stressed, even high-quality, sophisticated research is subject to some error; no single study can ever prove or disprove a hypothesis.

Evaluating Methodological Decisions

A scientific study is an amalgam of both substantive or theoretical concerns (the research problem) and methodological decisions (the methods chosen to solve the problem). In a text such as this we cannot hope to do justice to guiding an evaluation of the substantive side. Such an evaluation must be based on your nursing experience and knowledge. Questions that should be addressed include the following: Is this an interesting and important research question? Could the answer have implications for the

345

field of nursing? Does the research hypothesis make sense? Is the research question supported by theory?

On the methodological side, we can offer more help. Whether you have just conducted a study or whether you are reading the results of someone else's data analysis, you should pause before interpreting the findings and, as objectively as possible, evaluate each major methodological decision for clues to why the results might have turned out the way they did. Findings do not always reflect the true state of affairs; therefore, a proper interpretation depends on how accurate that reflection is.

Below we offer some questions to guide both producers and consumers of research through a critique of the five principal methodological decisions. Two preliminary comments arc in order. First, we highlight these five areas because they are critical to the issue of interpretation, which is the topic of this chapter. Normally, many other aspects of a research report would be evaluated, such as the adequacy of the literature review and theoretical framework, the correctness of the wording of the hypothesis, the appropriateness of the style of the report, and so on. A complete critique of a fictitious study is presented in the next chapter.

Second, the function of critical evaluations of a study's methods is not to dogmatically hunt for and expose mistakes. A good critique objectively identifies adequacies and inadequacies, virtues as well as faults. Sometimes the need for such balance is obscured by the terms "critique" and "critical appraisal," which connote unfavorable observations. The merits of a researcher's methodological decisions are as important as the limitations in coming to conclusions about the findings. Therefore, the critique should reflect a thoughtful, objective, and balanced consideration of the study's methods.

Evaluating Research Designs

An assessment of a study's research design concerns both whether the appropriate design was chosen and, once chosen, whether it was properly executed. Some guiding questions from both perspectives are presented below.

General Design Issues

Does the design account for all research hypotheses?

Is the general approach (*i.e.*, experimental, quasi-experimental, or nonexperimental) the best approach for testing the research hypotheses?

Is the setting of the study (field vs. laboratory) appropriate for the research question?

Does the design control for threats to the internal validity of the study?

What procedures are used to control for individual differences, and are these procedures the most effective ones possible?

Were steps taken to control external factors and to ensure constancy of conditions?

Have steps been taken to prevent contamination of treatments between groups?

If a cross-sectional design is used, would a longitudinal design be more appropriate?

If a longitudinal design is used, are methods for reestablishing contact with subjects and reducing attrition problems adequate?

Experimental Designs

Were subjects assigned to groups by a completely random process?

Is the specific design appropriate?

Were pretreatment data collected? Should they have been?

Was there differential loss of subjects (attrition) in the experimental and control groups and, if so, what effect might this have?

Quasi- and Pre-experimental Designs

Was the most powerful design used, given that an experimental design was not used?

If a comparison group was used, how confident can we be that groups are initially equivalent?

If no comparison groups were used, is there a sound rationale for the omission? Were pretreatment data collected? Should they have been?

Nonexperimental Studies

Is there a comparison group? Should there have been?

What steps, if any, were taken to produce comparable comparison groups? Are these steps adequate?

How similar are the comparison groups? To what extent is self-selection a problem?

Has the best possible design been used (e.g., prospective vs. retrospective)?

Evaluating the Population Chosen

As indicated in Chapter 3, a researcher can, to a certain extent, control extraneous variables through a careful specification of the population. The generalizability of the research findings is also linked to the population.

Given the research problem and limitations on resources, is the target population appropriately designated?

Would a more limited population specification have controlled for important sources of extraneous variation not covered by the research design?

Is there a difference between the accessible and target population? If so, is it reasonable to assume that the accessible population is a representative subset of the target population? If not, what are the potential biases?

Evaluating Data-Collection Procedures

Like the assessment of the research design, a critique of data collection concerns the suitability of the chosen approach and the care with which that approach was implemented.

General Data-Collection Issues

Are the data-collection methods the most appropriate way possible to measure the critical variables?

If the instruments are new or adapted from other sources, have they been properly pretested?

Have the instruments been assessed for reliability and validity? If yes, was the appropriate method used to make the assessments?

Are the instruments sufficiently reliable and valid?

Self-Report Techniques

Was the method of data collection (personal interview vs. telephone interview vs. questionnaire) appropriate?

Do the questions adequately cover the complexities of the problem under investigation?

Are open-ended and closed-ended questions used effectively and with an appropriate admixture?

Are the questions simply and clearly phrased?

Do the questions tend to bias responses in a certain direction?

Is the schedule of an appropriate length?

Are the directions for the interviewers or respondents clear?

Are the qualifications and training of the interviewers adequate?

Is the ordering of questions on the schedule meaningful and appropriate?

In closed-ended questions, do the responses adequately cover the alternatives?

Was confidentiality or anonymity assured to respondents?

Were appropriate steps taken to prevent a low response rate?

Were appropriate steps taken to minimize response-set biases?

If a scale was used, is it sufficiently long? Were steps taken to counterbalance positive and negative items? Was a new scale constructed when an existing one would have been preferable?

Observational Techniques

Is the degree of structure used in the observation consistent with the aims of the study?

Is the unit of behavior adopted appropriate for the problem being studied?

Is the degree of concealment used consistent with the aims of the study and with ethical principles?

Is the category system (if any) adequately comprehensive?

Are the observers required to make an inordinate amount of inferences?

Are the observers required to code too many complex behaviors in too short a time frame?

Is the method of sampling behaviors appropriate?

Have the observers been sufficiently trained to use the observational methods?

Was interobserver reliability calculated and is it sufficiently high?

Are potential biases stemming from the observer or the person being observed minimized?

Is the problem of subject reactivity appropriately handled?

Evaluating the Sampling Design

The most important considerations in evaluating a sampling design are its representativeness and the adequacy of its size for supporting subsequent data analysis. These concerns are reflected in the following questions:

Was a probability or nonprobability sampling design used? Could a more rigorous design have been employed?

To what potential biases does the chosen sampling plan give rise?

Was the sampling plan properly implemented?

How representative of the accessible and target population is the sample likely to be?

Was the response rate sufficiently high? Were steps taken to estimate the nature of any nonresponse biases?

Given the heterogeneity of the population, was the sample size sufficiently large?

Evaluating the Analysis

The results of a study are affected not only by the methods of collecting the data but also by the procedures used to analyze them. The data analysis should be consistent with the objectives of the study, the research design, the measurement level of the data, and with the assumptions underlying the use of a particular statistical test. Once these criteria are satisfied, it is desirable to use as powerful a procedure as possible. Beginning researchers may have some difficulty in handling this part of the critique if their statistical skills are weak, but many of the questions below are sufficiently general that an elementary knowledge of statistics should prove adequate for routine appraisals.

Were the data analyzed qualitatively, quantitatively, or both? Was the type of analysis appropriate for the types of data that were collected?

Are the descriptive statistics used appropriate for the data? Were a sufficient number of descriptive statistics calculated to adequately summarize the major characteristics of the sample?

Were only descriptive statistics computed? Should inferential statistics have been calculated?

Are the statistics used appropriate for the level of measurement of the variables?

Are parametric tests used when the assumptions for parametric tests are patently violated?

Are nonparametric tests used when more powerful parametric tests would probably have been appropriate?

Is information thrown away unnecessarily by converting measures of a relatively high measurement level to lower-level measures (e.g., converting height in inches to the dichotomy "tall/short")?

Are the tests of significance appropriate for testing the research hypotheses?

Are statistical results clearly organized and comprehensible? Is there any evidence of bias in the reporting of the findings?

It must be admitted that the answers to many of the above questions will call upon the reader's judgment as much as, or even more than, his or her knowledge. An evaluation of whether or not the most appropriate data-collection procedure was used for the research problem necessarily involves a degree of subjectivity. Issues concerning the appropriateness of various strategies and techniques are topics about which even experts disagree. One should strive to be as objective as possible and to indicate one's reasoning for the judgments made. Clearly it is easier to be objective about someone else's study than about one's own. For this reason, researchers often ask colleagues or advisors to comment on or critique methodological decisions. It is useful to do this both before implementing those decisions and before interpreting the study findings.

Interpretation of Results

The interpretation of a study's results involves a consideration of the quality of the study's methods, but technical concerns alone are insufficient. Interpretation of data involves imbuing the numbers with meaning, and this task cannot be done mechanically. To be sure, statistical and research skills are required for interpreting the findings of a study, but there is also a need for creativity, intellectual insights, logical reasoning, and knowledge of prior relevant research. These are not attributes that can be learned in a textbook. This section will offer some general guidelines for helping the researcher with interpretation, but it should be recognized that these guidelines tell only half the story of this challenging task.

When statistics are used to test research hypotheses, there are only four possible outcomes: (1) the hypotheses can be supported at a significant level; (2) the results of statistical tests can be nonsignificant; (3) significant results in a direction *opposite* to that hypothesized can be obtained;

and (4) the results can be mixed. We use this scheme to organize our comments about interpretation.

Interpreting Hypothesized Results

When the tests of statistical significance support the original research hypotheses, the task of interpreting the results is somewhat easier than when the hypotheses are rejected. In a sense, the interpretation has been partly accomplished beforehand in such a situation, because the researcher has already had to bring together prior research findings, a theoretical framework, and logical reasoning in the development of the hypotheses. This groundwork can then form the context within which interpretations are made.

Even when the study hypotheses are supported by the data, there is still a need for circumspection and critical appraisal. A few cautionary suggestions should be kept in mind.

First, it is preferable to be somewhat conservative in drawing conclusions from the data. The intrusion of personal viewpoints and subjective judgments is inevitable in making sense of research results, but they must be held in check insofar as possible. It is sometimes tempting to go far beyond the data in developing explanations for what the results mean, but conscientious scientists normally avoid doing so. A simple example might help to explain what is meant by "going beyond the data." Suppose a nurse researcher hypothesized that a relationship existed between a pregnant woman's level of anxiety about the labor and delivery experience and the number of children she has already borne. Her data revealed that a negative relationship between anxiety levels and parity (r = −.40) did indeed exist. The researcher, therefore, concluded that increased experience with childbirth causes decreasing amounts of anxiety. Is this conclusion supported by the data? The conclusion appears to be logical but, in fact, there is nothing within the data that leads directly to this interpretation. An important, indeed critical, research precept is *correlation does not prove causation.* The finding that two variables are related offers no evidence suggesting which of the two variables—if either—caused the other. In the present example, perhaps causality runs in the opposite direction, that is, that a woman's anxiety level influences how many children she bears. Or perhaps a third variable not examined in the study, such as the ethnic or religious background of the woman, "causes" or influences both anxiety and number of children.

Alternative explanations for the findings should always be considered. If these competing interpretations can be ruled out on the basis of the data or previous research findings, so much the better. However, every angle should be examined to see if one's pet explanation has been given adequate competition.

The fact that statistical significance was attained in testing the hypothesis does not necessarily mean that the results were important or of value to the nursing community and their clients. Statistical significance indicates that the results were unlikely to be a function of chance. This means that the observed group differences or observed relationships were probably real but not necessarily important. With large samples, even modest relationships are statistically significant. For instance, with a sample of 500, a correlation coefficient of .10 is significant at the .05 level, but a relationship of this magnitude probably has little practical value. Therefore, attention must be paid to the numerical values obtained in an analysis in addition to the significance level when assessing the implications of the findings.

The support of research hypotheses with empirical evidence never constitutes proof of their veracity. Hypothesis testing, as we have seen, is probabilistic. There always remains a possibility that the obtained relationships were due to chance (*i.e.,* a Type-I error might have been made). Therefore, one must be tentative about both the results and the interpretations given to those results. Care should also be taken in considering whether the results can be generalized beyond the study sample, particularly if a nonrandom sampling plan has been used. In sum, even when the findings are in line with expectations, restraint should be exercised in drawing conclusions.

Interpreting Nonsignificant Results

The retention of the null hypothesis is particularly problematic from an interpretative point of view. The statistical procedures described in Chapter 16 are geared toward disconfirmation of the null hypothesis. The failure to reject a null hypothesis could occur for one or more reasons, and the researcher does not usually know which of these reasons pertains. First, the null hypothesis could actually be true. The nonsignificant result, in this case, would accurately reflect the absence of a relationship among the research variables. On the other hand, the null hypothesis could be false, in which case a Type-II error would have been made. The retention of a false null hypothesis can be attributed to several things, such as internal validity problems, the selection of a deviant sample, the use of a weak statistical procedure, or too small a sample. Unless the researcher has special justification for attributing the nonsignificant findings to one of these factors, interpreting such results is a tricky business.

In any event, there is never justification for interpreting a retained null hypothesis as proof of a *lack* of relationship among variables. The safest interpretation is that nonsignificant findings represent a lack of evidence for either truth or falsity of the hypothesis. Thus, one can see that if the researcher's actual research hypothesis states that no differences or no relationships will be observed, traditional hypothesis-testing procedures will never permit the required inferences.

When no significant results are found, there is sometimes a tendency to be overcritical of the research strategy and methods and undercritical of the theory or logical reasoning on which the hypotheses were based. It is important to look for and identify flaws in the research methods, but it is equally important to search for conceptual shortcomings.

Interpreting Unhypothesized Significant Results

There probably is nothing more puzzling than to obtain results opposite to those hypothesized. For instance, a nurse researcher might hypothesize that individualized patient teaching of breathing techniques is more effective than group instruction, but the results might reflect that the group method was better. Or a positive relationship might be predicted between a nurse's age and level of job satisfaction, but a negative relationship might be found.

It should go without saying that researchers should not alter the hypothesis after the results are "in." Although some researchers may view such situations as awkward or embarrassing, there is really little basis for such feelings. The purpose of research is not to corroborate the scientist's notions, but to arrive at truth and enhance understanding. There is no such thing as a study in which the results "came out the wrong way," if the "wrong way" is the truth.

In the case of unhypothesized significant findings, it is less likely, though not impossible, that the methods are flawed than that the reasoning or theory is incorrect. As always, the interpretation that the researcher gives to the findings should involve comparisons with other research, a consideration of alternate theories, and a critical scrutiny of the design, data collection, and analysis. The final result of such an examination should be a tentative explanation for the unexpected findings, together with suggestions for how such explanations could be tested in other research projects.

Interpreting Mixed Results

The interpretive process is often confounded by mixed results. The investigator may find some hypotheses supported by the data, while others are not. Or a hypothesis may be accepted when one measure of the dependent variable is used but rejected when using a different measure of the same variable. Of all the situations mentioned, mixed results are probably the most prevalent.

When only some results run counter to a theoretical position or conceptual scheme, the research methods are probably the first aspect of the study deserving of scrutiny. Differences in the validity and reliability of the various measures could account for such discrepancies, for example. On the other hand, mixed results could be indicative of how a theory needs to be qualified, or of how certain constructs within the theory need to be reconceptualized.

In sum, the interpretation of research findings is a demanding task but offers the possibility of unique intellectual rewards. The researcher must in essence play the role of a scientific detective, trying to make pieces of the puzzle fit together so that a coherent picture emerges.

Other Issues in Interpretation

In addition to trying to make sense of the statistical analysis, several other considerations emerge in interpreting study outcomes. The first concerns the generalizability of the results (*i.e.,* the study's external validity). Researchers are rarely interested in discovering relationships among variables for a specific group of people at a specific point in time. The aim of research is typically to reveal enduring relationships, the understanding of which can be used to improve the human condition. If a nursing intervention under investigation is found to be successful, others will want to adopt the procedure. Therefore, an important interpretive question is whether the intervention will "work" or whether the relationships will "hold" in other settings with other people. Part of the interpretation process involves asking the question "To what groups, environments, and conditions can the results of the study be applied?"

A second issue concerns the use of the interpretation as a springboard for additional research. Interpretations are necessarily speculative: they represent one's best guess—albeit an educated guess—about what the data really mean. Therefore, the interpretation represents a good starting point for suggesting further lines of inquiry. Is a replication needed, and, if so, with what groups? Are methodological refinements needed to really test the hypothesis? If observed relationships are significant, what do we need to know next in order for the information to be maximally useful?

Finally, the interpretive task is not complete without considering the implications of the findings for nursing. Do the findings have implications for what is taught to nursing students, or for how nursing content should be taught? Are the results of potential use to clinical nurses? Typically, the results of an investigation can have several applications, and this should be kept in mind in trying to formulate an interpretation of the study's results. Of course, if the study is seriously flawed it may be that the results are not usable within the nursing profession. But they will probably be useful, nevertheless, in designing an improved new study for the same research question.

In this chapter we do not follow the pattern established in the preceding chapters of presenting a fictitious research example that highlights points made within the chapter. An entire (fictitious) research report is presented in Chapter 19, however, together with a critique. The critique examines the methodological decisions made by the researcher and discusses the researcher's interpretation of the findings.

Summary

The interpretation of a study's findings basically is a search for the broader meaning and implications of the results of an investigation. The results of the data analysis need to be scrutinized and reflected upon, with consideration given to the objectives of the project, the specific hypotheses that were tested, prior research findings, and the shortcomings of the methods used to answer the research questions.

With respect to the study's technical aspects, special attention should be paid to critically evaluating the five major methodological decisions (the design, population specification, data collection, sampling plan, and analyses.) Some guidelines for evaluating these decisions were presented in this chapter.

The results of a study can either support the researcher's hypotheses, result in nonsignificant findings, result in opposing evidence, or provide mixed findings. Whether the hypotheses are supported or not, it is important to be objective, to avoid the temptation of reading too much into the results, to be critical of both conceptual and methodological weaknesses, and to consider alternative explanations for the obtained findings. The primary interpretive task is to consider the intrinsic meaning of the observed results, but additional concerns involve the generalizability of the findings and the implications of the results for the nursing profession and future research endeavors.

Study Suggestions

1. Read an article in a recent issue of *Nursing Research*. Compare your interpretation of the findings with that of the author.

2. Suppose that a researcher has found that women who experienced severe cramps during menstruation were significantly more likely to smoke cigarettes than women who did not experience the discomforts of menstrual cramps. Suggest two or three different ways that this finding might be interpreted.

3. Read an article in *Nursing Research* and evaluate the five major methodological decisions the researcher made. Prepare a two- to three-page written critique summarizing the major technical strengths and weaknesses of the study.

Chapter 19
Research Reports

No scientific project is ever complete until a research report has been written. The most brilliant piece of work is of little value to the scientific community unless that work is known. The reporting of results adds to the general store of knowledge and is a scientist's responsibility. It is also to the researcher's advantage to have research findings known by others, because proper credit should be given to the work that has been completed.

Research reports are written for different audiences and for different purposes. A thesis or dissertation not only communicates the research strategy and results, but also serves as documentation of the student's thoroughness and ability to perform scholarly empirical work. Theses and dissertations, therefore, are rather lengthy documents. Journal articles, on the other hand, are typically short because they must compete with other reports for limited journal space and because they will be read by busy professionals.

Despite these differences, the general form and content of research reports is quite similar. The major distinction lies in the amount of detail reported. The section below discusses the content that is normally included in a research report.

The Content of a Research Report

Most research reports contain four major sections—introduction, methods, results, and discussion. Sometimes the introductory materials are covered in two or more sections (e.g., in separate literature review and conceptual framework sections), but there are nevertheless some standard topics covered in a research report, despite some variations in how the material is organized and presented. The description below is meant to provide producers of research some guidelines for what to include, and

357

consumers of research some guidelines for what to look for in a scientific report.

The Introduction

The purpose of the *introductory section* of a research report is to acquaint readers with the research problem on which the investigation has focused. A precise and unambiguous problem statement, phrased in question form, is of immense value in communicating the major objectives of the study. If formal hypotheses have been developed, they should also be identified in the introduction.

The researcher should explain enough of the background of the study to make clear the reasons that the problem was considered worth pursuing. The justification of a nursing research problem should ideally include both the practical and theoretical significance of the study. This ideal is not always feasible. Not all studies have a direct bearing on theoretical issues, nor should they all necessarily be expected to have such a bearing in a practicing profession such as nursing. With the present state of knowledge, no one should feel apologetic if a study can solve a practical problem but is not linked to an existing theory. Artificial attempts to contrive theoretical relevance do nothing to advance scientific knowledge and should be avoided. Of course, studies that are framed within a theoretical context are most likely to make enduring contributions to general knowledge about nursing and the nursing process. The introductory section should make explicit such theoretical rationales when they exist.

The statement of the problem should also be accompanied by a summary of related research, so that the research may be seen in perspective. The review of the literature helps to clarify the theoretical and practical foundations of the research problem. It also helps readers, who often are less familiar with research on a given topic than the investigator, to understand the context in which the study was initiated.

Finally, the introductory section should incorporate definitions of the concepts under investigation, and a specification of underlying assumptions. Sometimes complete operational definitions are reserved for the "methods" section, but a reader should have a fairly good idea early in the report what the researcher had in mind with regard to such terms as "grief," "stress," "therapeutic touch," and so forth.

In sum, the purpose of the introduction is to set the stage for a description of what was done and what was discovered. The introductory section should answer the following questions: (1) What did the researcher want to know? (2) Why did he or she want to know it? and (3) What is the likely significance of such a study?

The Methods Section

The scientific reader needs to know what has been done to solve the problem. The *methods section* should have as its goal a description of what was done to collect and analyze the data in sufficient detail such that another researcher could replicate the study if desired. In theses and reports to funding agencies, this goal should always be satisfied. In journal articles it is often necessary to condense the methods section. For example, it may be impossible to include a complete quesionnaire, interview schedule, or observation schedule. Nevertheless, the degree of detail should permit a reader to evaluate the manner in which the research problem was addressed.

The methods section is often subdivided into several parts. The reader needs to know, first of all, who the subjects participating in the study were. The description of the subjects normally includes the specification and description of the population from which the sample was drawn. If the target and accessible populations are not identical, then both populations should be discussed. The method of sample selection, together with the reasons for the selection of this sampling design, need to be clearly delineated so that the reader can estimate the generalizability of the findings. It is advisable to describe the basic characteristics of the subjects, such as their age, sex, and other relevant attributes, and to indicate, if known, the degree to which these characteristics are representative of the population. For instance, if it is known that a sample of nurses tends to underrepresent those who have not received a bachelor's degree or a higher degree, then this fact should be pointed out.

The design of the study is often given more detailed coverage in an experimental project than in a nonexperimental one. In an experiment, the researcher should indicate what variables were being manipulated, how subjects were assigned to groups, the nature of the experimental intervention, and the specific design adopted. In any type of study, it is essential to identify what steps were taken to control the research situation in general and extraneous variables in particular.

A critical component of the methods section is the description of the instruments used to measure the target variables. In rare cases, this description may be accomplished in three or four sentences, such as when a standard physiological measure has been utilized. More often, a detailed explanation of the instruments and a rationale for their use are required in order to communicate to the reader the manner in which the variables were operationalized. When it is not feasible to include the actual research instrument within the report, its form and content should be outlined in as much detail as possible. It is insufficient to merely say "A questionnaire containing questions on the research problem was administered to the subjects." How many questions did the instrument include?

Were the items open-ended or closed-ended? What were the major sections of the instrument and how were these sections organized? Whenever the instrument is not incorporated in the report, it is courteous to indicate from whom a copy of the complete instrument could be obtained. If the measuring devices were constructed specifically for the research project, the report should describe how they were developed, the methods used for pretesting, revisions made as a result of pretesting, coding and scoring procedures, and guidelines for interpretation. Any information relating to the validity and reliability of the instruments should also be mentioned.

A procedure section provides information about what steps were followed in actually collecting the data. In an experiment, how much time elapsed between the intervention and the measurement of the dependent variable? In an interview study, where were the interviews conducted and how long, on the average, did each one last? In an observational study, what was the role of the observer vis-à-vis the subjects? When questionnaires are used, how were they delivered to respondents, and were follow-up procedures used to increase the response rate? Any unforeseen events occurring during the collection of data that could affect the findings should be described and assessed. Those reading a report must be in a position to evaluate the quality of the data obtained, and a description of research procedures assists in this evaluation.

A delineation of the statistical analyses and, when applicable, the computer programs used to handle the data is sometimes incorporated into the methods section and sometimes put with the results of the analyses. From the reader's point of view, it is usually preferable to explain the analytic approach in the methods section so that he or she will be able to judge the appropriateness of the research methods taken as a whole. It is not necessary to give computational formulas or even references for commonly used statistical procedures. For unusual procedures, or unusual applications of a common procedure, a technical reference justifying the approach should be noted.

The Results Section

The *results section* summarizes the results of the analyses. If both descriptive and inferential statistics have been used, the descriptive statistics ordinarily come first. The researcher must be careful to report all results as accurately and completely as possible, whether or not the hypotheses were supported. If there are too many analyses for inclusion in the report, the criterion used to select analyses should be their relevance to the overall objectives of the study.

When the results of several analyses are to be presented, it is frequently useful to summarize the findings in a table. Good tables, with precise headings and titles, are an important way to economize on space and to avoid dull, repetitious statements. Important findings can then be highlighted in the text. Figures that present the results in graphic form are used less as an economy than as a means of dramatizing important findings and relationships. Tables and figures should be numbered for easy reference.

Although we will discuss style in a later section, it is difficult to avoid the mention of style here. The write-up of statistical results is often a difficult task for beginning researchers, because they are unsure both about what should be said and about the style in which to present it. A few suggestions may prove helpful. First, the research report should never claim that the data "proved," "verified," "confirmed," or "demonstrated" that the hypotheses were correct or incorrect. Hypotheses are "supported" or "not supported," "accepted" or "rejected." Second, the presentation of results should be written in the past tense. For example, it is inappropriate to say "Nurses who receive special training perform triage functions significantly better than those without training." In this sentence, "receive" and "perform" should be changed to "received" and "performed." The present tense implies that the results are unquestionably generalizable to all nurses, when in fact the statement pertains only to a particular sample whose behavior was observed in the past. Finally, when the results of statistical tests are reported, three pieces of information are normally included—the value of the calculated statistic, the number of degrees of freedom, and the significance level. For instance, the following might be stated: A chi-square test revealed that patients who were exposed to the experimental intervention were significantly less likely to develop decubitus ulcers than patients in a control group ($\chi^2 = 8.23$, $df = 1$, $p < .01$). The researcher who is writing up a results section for the first time would profit from using as a model a research report published in a professional journal.

The Discussion Section

A bare report of the statistical findings is never sufficient in a research report. The meaning that a researcher gives to the results plays a rightful and important role in the report. The *discussion section* is typically devoted to a consideration of interpretations, limitations, and recommendations.

The interpretation of the results, as discussed in the previous chapter, involves the "translation" of statistical findings into practical and conceptual meaning. The interpretative process is a global one, encompassing the investigator's knowledge of the results, the methods, the sample characteristics, related research findings, and theoretical issues. Included with the interpretations should be a statement of the population to which the results can be reasonably be generalized. The researcher should justify the interpretations, explicitly stating why alternative explanations have been ruled out. If the findings conflict with those of earlier research investigations, tentative explanations should be offered.

Although the readers should be told enough about the methods of the study to identify its major weaknesses, report writers themselves should point out the limitations. The researcher is in the best position to detect and assess the impact of sampling deficiencies, design problems, instrument weaknesses, and so forth, and it is a professional responsibility to alert the reader to these difficulties. Moreover, if the writer shows that he or she is aware of the study's limitations, then the reader will know that these limitations were not ignored in the development of the interpretations.

The implications derived from a study are usually speculative and, therefore, should be couched in tentative terms. For instance, the kind of language appropriate for a discussion of the interpretations is illustrated by the following sentence: The results suggest that it may be possible to facilitate nurse–physician interaction by modifying the medical student's stereotype of the nurse as the physician's handmaiden. The speculative nature of the researcher's interpretation should be demonstrated in another way. The interpretation is, in essence, a hypothesis and as such can presumably be tested in another research project. The discussion section, thus, should include recommendations for investigations that would help to test this hypothesis, as well as suggestions for other research to answer questions raised by the findings of the study.

Other Aspects of the Report

Every research report should have a title. The phrases "Research Report" or "Report of a Nursing Research Investigation" are not adequate. The title should indicate to prospective readers the nature of the study. Insofar as possible, the dependent and independent variables should be named in the title. It is also desirable to indicate the population studied. However, the title should be brief (no more than about 15 words), so the writer must balance clarity with brevity. Some examples of titles include the following:

The Effect of Advance Information on Pain Perception in Hospitalized Children

Attitudes Toward Preventive Medicine in the Urban Working Class

Educational Preparation: Its Effects on Role Conflict Among Nurses

If the title gets too unwieldly, its length can often be reduced by omitting unnecessary terms, such as "A Study of . . . " or "An Investigation to Examine the Effects of . . . " and so forth. The title should communicate clearly and concisely the phenomena that were researched.

Journals and theses often require the preparation of an abstract to precede the main body of the report. *Abstracts* are brief descriptions of the problem, methods, and findings of the study, written so that a reader can assess whether the entire report should be read. Abstracts typically are as short as 100 or 200 words. Since the abstract may be the only part of the report that is read, the writer should describe only that which is essential in order for the reader to grasp what the study was all about. Sometimes a report concludes with a brief summary, which usually substitutes for the abstract.

The Style of a Research Report

Good scientific writing need not sound stuffy or pedantic, but certain stylistic constraints are imposed on the report writer. These constraints are designed primarily to enhance the objectivity of research reports. A scientific report is not an essay but rather a factual account of how and why a problem was studied and what results were obtained. The report should not include overtly subjective statements, emotionally laden statements, or exaggerations. When opinions are stated, they should be clearly identified as such, with proper attribution if the opinion was expressed by another writer. The personality and point of view of the authors should intrude as little as possible and the overall tone should be one of impersonality. In keeping with the goal of objective reporting, personal pronouns such as "I," "my," and "we" are often avoided, since the passive voice and impersonal pronouns do a better job of conveying impartiality. However, some journals are beginning to break with this tradition and are encouraging a greater balance between active and passive voice and first-person and third-person narration. If a direct presentation can be made without sacrificing objectivity, a more readable and lively product usually will result.

The use of nonsexist language in the preparation of scientific reports is being increasingly encouraged. The use of awkward or wordy constructions (*e.g.,* "Each subject was instructed that he or she should schedule his or her next appointment himself or herself.") can often be avoided simply by using the plural ("Subjects were instructed to schedule their next appointment themselves.").

It is not easy to write simply and clearly, but these are important goals of scientific writing. The use of pretentious words or technical jargon does little to enhance the communicative value of the report, although colloquialisms should be avoided. The style should be concise and straightforward. If writers can add elegance to their reports without interfering with clarity and accuracy, so much the better, but the product is not expected to be a literary achievement. Needless to say, this does not imply that grammatical and spelling accuracy should be sacrificed. The research report should reflect scholarship, not pedantry.

A common flaw in the reports of beginning researchers is inadequate organization. The overall structure is relatively inflexible and, therefore, should pose no difficulties, but the organization within sections and subsections needs careful attention. Sequences should be in an orderly progression with appropriate transition. Themes or ideas should be neither introduced too abruptly nor abandoned suddenly. Continuity and logical thematic development are critical to good communication.

First drafts of research reports are almost never perfect. The assistance of a colleague or an adviser can be invaluable in improving the quality of a scientific paper. Objective criticism can often be achieved by simply putting the report aside for a few days and then rereading it with a fresh outlook.

Types of Research Documents

Most research documents are similar in terms of content and style, although certain characteristics and requirements vary. Below we highlight some of the features of three important types of documents—proposals, theses and dissertations, and journal articles.

Research Proposals

A *research proposal* is a written document specifying what the investigator proposes to study and is, therefore, written before the project has commenced. Proposals serve to communicate the research problem, its significance, and planned procedures for solving the problem to some interested party.

Proposals are written for various reasons. A student enrolled in a research class is often expected to submit a brief plan to the professor before data collection actually begins. Most universities require a formal proposal and a proposal hearing for students about to engage in research for a thesis or dissertation. Funding agencies that sponsor research almost always award funds on a competitive basis and use proposals as a basis for their funding decisions.

A proposal is actually very much like a research report, with three important distinctions. First, a proposal is written in the future tense: it explains what researchers *will* do rather than what they did. Second, a proposal obviously does not contain results and discussion sections, since data have not yet been collected. However, a detailed description of the study problem, relevant literature, theoretical context, and proposed methods are normally included in a research proposal. Finally, proposals normally include evidence or supporting statements to document that the study is well-conceived, is well-designed, and can be accomplished according to the proposed plan. In studies for which funding is being sought, such documentation would normally include a description of the researcher's qualifications, a detailed work plan showing when specific tasks would be accomplished, a budget with justification for expenditures, and a description of the facilities available for the research.

Proposals represent the means for opening communication between researchers on the one hand and parties interested in the conduct of research on the other. Those "parties" may be funding agencies, faculty advisors, or institutional officers, depending on the circumstances. An accepted proposal is a two-way contract: those accepting the proposal are effectively saying "We are willing to offer our (emotional or financial) support, as long as the investigation proceeds as proposed," and those writing the proposal are saying "If you will offer support, I will conduct the project as proposed." Therefore, the proposal offers some assurance that neither party will be disappointed.

Student Research Reports

Most doctoral degrees are granted upon the successful completion of an empirical research project. Empirical theses are sometimes required of master's-degree candidates as well. And, increasingly, students enrolled in a research-methods course are being required to conduct a small individual or group research project as well.

Theses, dissertations, and, to a lesser extent, class project reports typically document completely the steps performed in carrying out the research investigation. Faculty members overseeing the project must be able to judge whether the student has understood the research problem both substantively and methodologically. The majority of doctoral dissertations are between 100 and 250 pages long, double-spaced. Small-scale student projects are normally summarized in 20 to 40 pages.

Each faculty member or school may have a preferred format for their students' reports; however, the format is normally similar to that described in the first section of this chapter on report content. One possible exception is that a separate section or chapter may be required for the literature review.

Journal Articles

Progress in nursing research is dependent upon researchers' efforts to share their work with others. Dissertations are rarely read by more than a handful of people. They are too lengthy and too inaccessible for widespread use. Publication in a professional journal ensures the broadest possible circulation of scientific findings. From a personal point of view, it is exciting and professionally advantageous to have one or more publications. Students should definitely not rule out the possibility of publishing the results of their studies in a professional journal.

Journal articles follow the standard format described earlier but are typically brief (15–25 typed pages, double-spaced) because journal space is limited. Since readers are particularly interested in the findings of a research project, a relatively large proportion of the journal report normally is devoted to the results and discussion sections.

Several nursing journals accept research articles for publication. *Nursing Research*, which is currently published six times annually, is the major communications outlet for research in the field of nursing. Other nursing journals that focus primarily on publishing empirical studies are *Advances in Nursing Science*, *Research in Nursing and Health*, and *Western Journal of Nursing Research*. Nursing journals that are not devoted exclusively or even primarily to research but that accept research reports for publication include the *American Journal of Nursing*, *Nursing Forum*, *Nursing Outlook*, *Journal of Obstetrical and Gynecological Nursing*, *Journal of Advanced Nursing*, and *Journal of Gerontological Nursing*. Many journals that do not focus directly on nursing also publish articles by nurse authors, such as *The Journal of Public Health*, *Journal of School Health*, *Perceptual and Motor Skills*, *Family Planning Perspectives*, and numerous others. The prospective author should check through recent issues of journals under consideration for guidance about the journals' stylistic requirements and content coverage. Many publications make an explicit statement about the type of papers they are seeking.

Papers that are submitted for publication are not always accepted. If a manuscript is not found acceptable, the authors are usually sent copies of the reviewers' comments or a summary of the reasons for its rejection. This information can be used to revise a manuscript before submitting it to another journal. A rejection by one journal should not discourage researchers from sending the manuscript to another journal. The competition for journal space is quite keen and a rejection does not necessarily mean that a study is unworthy of publication. Although it is considered unethical to submit an article to two journals simultaneously, manuscripts may need to be reviewed by several journals before final acceptance.

A Research Report: Presentation and Critique

We conclude this book with a presentation of a fictitious research report and a critique of various aspects of the report. This example is designed to highlight features about the form and content of both a written description of a scientific investigation and a written evaluation of the study's worth. To economize on space, we have prepared a relatively brief report, but one that hopefully incorporates the essential elements necessary for a meaningful appraisal.

The Report

The Role of Health-Care Providers in Teenage Pregnancy
by Florence Moreland, 1983

Background. Of the 20 million teenagers living in the United States today, approximately one in five is sexually active by age 14; 50% have had sexual intercourse by age 19 (Kelman and Zander, 1978).* Despite increased availability of contraceptives to teenagers, the number of teenage pregnancies has risen at an alarming rate over the past few years. Over one million girls under age 20 become pregnant each year and, of these, 600,000 become teenage mothers (U.S. Bureau of the Census, 1980). Dr. Robert Woodsome, director of the Obstetrical Department of an inner-city Detroit hospital, has commented, "Pregnancy among adolescents is one of the most stubborn problems facing obstetrical staff today." (Woodsome, 1975).

Public concern regarding the teenage pregnancy epidemic stems not only from the rising number of involved teenagers, but also from the extensive research that has documented the adverse consequences of early parenthood. In the health arena, pregnant teenagers have been found to receive less prenatal care (Tremain, 1975), to be more likely to develop toxemia (Schendley, 1976; Walters, 1973), to be more likely to experience prolonged labor (Curran, 1979), to be more likely to have low-birthweight babies (Tremain, 1975; Beach, 1976), and to be more likely to have babies with low Apgar scores (Beach, 1976) than older mothers. The long-term consequences to the teenagers themselves are also extremely bleak: teenage mothers get less schooling, are more likely to be on public assistance, are likely to earn lower wages, and are more likely to get divorced if they marry than their peers who postpone parenthood (Jamail, 1974; Weissbach, 1976; North, 1978; Smithfield, 1979).

The one million teenagers who become pregnant each year are caught up in a tough emotional decision—to carry the pregnancy to term and keep the baby, to have an abortion, or to deliver the baby and surrender it for adoption. Despite the widely reported adverse consequences of young parenthood cited above, most young women today are opting for delivery and childrearing (Jaffrey, 1978; Henderson, 1977).

The purpose of this study was to test the effectiveness of a special inter-

---

*All references are fictitious, although most of the information in this fictitious study is based on real studies and is, therefore, accurate.

vention based in an outpatient clinic of a Chicago hospital in improving the health outcomes of a group of pregnant teenagers. Specifically, it was hypothesized that pregnant teenagers who were in the special program would receive more prenatal care, would be less likely to develop toxemia, would be less likely to have a low-birthweight baby, would spend fewer hours in labor, would have babies with higher Apgar scores, and would be more likely to use a contraceptive 6 months postpartum than pregnant teenagers not enrolled in the program.

The theoretical model on which this research was based is an ecological model of personal behavior (Brandenburg, 1979). A schematic diagram of the ecological model is presented in Figure 19-1. In this framework, the actions of the person are the focus of attention, but those actions are believed to be a function not only of the person's own characteristics, attitudes, and abilities, but also a function of other influences in their environment. Environmental influences can be differentiated according to their proximal relationship with the target person. Health-care workers and institutions are, according to the model, more distant influences than family, peers, and boyfriends. Yet it is assumed that these less immediate forces are real and can intervene to change the behaviors of the target person. Thus, it is hypothesized that pregnant teen-

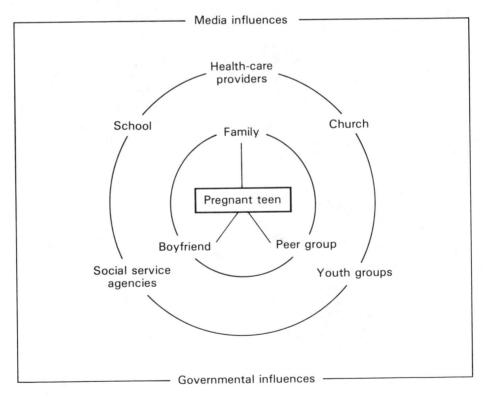

Figure 19-1. Model of ecological contexts

agers can be influenced by increased exposure to a health-care team providing a structured program of services designed to promote improved health outcomes.

Methods. A special program of services for pregnant teenagers was implemented in the outpatient clinic of an inner-city public hospital in Chicago. The intervention involved nutrition education and counseling, parenting education, instruction on prenatal health care, preparation for childbirth, and contraceptive counseling.

All teenagers with a confirmed pregnancy attending the clinic were asked if they wanted to participate in the special program. The goal was to enroll 150 pregnant teenagers during the program's first year of operation. A total of 276 teenagers attending the clinic were invited to participate; of these, 59 had an abortion or miscarriage and 108 declined to participate, yielding an experimental group sample of 109 girls.

To test the effectiveness of the special program, a comparison group of pregnant teenagers was needed. Another inner-city hospital agreed to cooperate in the study. Staff obtained information on the labor and delivery outcomes of the 120 teenagers who delivered at the comparison hospital, where no special teen-parent program was available. For both experimental- and comparison-group subjects a follow-up telephone interview was conducted 6 months postpartum to determine if the teenagers had adopted birth control.

The independent variable in this study was the teenager's program status: experimental-group members participated in the special program while comparison-group members did not. The dependent variables were the teenagers' labor–delivery and postpartum contraceptive outcomes. The operational definitions of the dependent variables were as follows:

Prenatal Care—Number of visits made to a physician/nurse during the pregnancy, exclusive of the visit for the pregnancy test
Toxemia—Presence versus absence of preeclamptic toxemia as diagnosed by a physician
Labor Time—Number of hours elapsed from the first contractions until delivery of the baby, to the nearest half hour
Low Infant Birthweight—Birthweights of less than 2500 grams versus those of 2500 grams or greater
Apgar Score—Infant Apgar score taken at 3 minutes after birth
Contraceptive Use Postpartum—Self-reported use of any form of birth control 6 months postpartum versus self-reported nonuse

The two groups were compared on these six outcome measures using *t*-tests and chi-square tests.

Results. The teenagers in the sample were, on average, 17.6 years old at the time of delivery. The mean age was 17.1 in the experimental group and 18.0 in the comparison group.

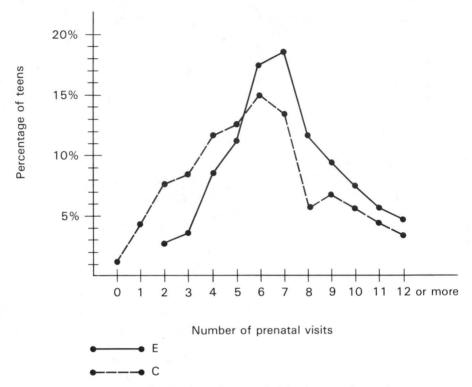

Figure 19-2. Frequency distribution of prenatal visits, by experimental versus comparison group. (*E* = experimental group; *C* = comparison group)

By definition, all of the teenagers in the experimental group had received prenatal care. Two of the teenagers in the comparison group had had no health-care treatment prior to delivery. The distribution of visits for the two groups is presented in Figure 19-2. The experimental group had a higher mean number of prenatal visits than the comparison group, as shown in Table 19-1, but the difference was not statistically significant at the 0.05 level, using a t-test for independent groups.

In the sample as a whole, about one girl in ten was diagnosed as having preeclamptic toxemia. The difference between the two groups was in the hypothesized direction, with 1.6% more of the comparison-group teenagers developing this complication. However, the group difference in percentages was not significant using a chi-square test.

The hours spent in labor ranged from 3.5 to 29.0 in the experimental group and from 4.5 to 33.5 in the comparison group. On average, teenagers in the experimental group spent 14.3 hours in labor, compared to 15.2 hours for comparison-group teenagers. The difference was not statistically significant.

With regard to low-birthweight babies, a total of 43 girls out of 229 in the

Table 19-1. Summary of Experimental/Comparison-Group Differences

| OUTCOME VARIABLE | GROUP | | DIFFERENCE | TEST STATISTIC |
	Experimental (N = 109)	Comparison (N = 120)		
Mean number of prenatal visits	7.1	5.9	1.2	$t = 1.83$, df = 227, NS
Percentage with toxemia	10.1%	11.7%	−1.6%	$X^2 = 0.15$, df = 1, NS
Mean hours spent in labor	14.3	15.2	−0.9	$t = 1.01$, df = 227, NS
Percentage with low-birth-weight baby	16.5	20.9	−4.4%	$X^2 = 0.71$, df = 1, NS
Mean Apgar score	7.3	6.7	0.6	$t = 0.98$, df = 227, NS
Percentage adopting contraception postpartum	81.7%	62.5%	19.2	$X^2 = 10.22$, df = 1, $p < .01$

sample gave birth to babies who weighed under 2500 grams (5.5 pounds).* More of the comparison-group teenagers (20.9%) than experimental-group teenagers (16.5%) had low-birthweight babies but, once again, the group difference was not significant.

The 3-minute Apgar score in the two groups was quite similar—7.3 for the experimental group and 6.7 for the comparison group. This small difference was nonsignificant.

Finally, the teenagers were compared with respect to their adoption of birth control 6 months after delivering their babies. For this variable, teenagers were coded as users of contraception if they were either using some method of birth control at the time of the follow-up interview or if they were nonusers but were sexually inactive (*i.e.*, were using abstinence to prevent a repeat pregnancy). The results of a chi-square test revealed that a significantly higher percentage of experimental-group teenagers (81.7%) than comparison-group teenagers (62.5%) were using birth control after delivery. This difference was significant beyond the .01 level.

Discussion. The results of this evaluation were disappointing, but not discouraging. There was only one outcome for which a significant difference was observed. The experimental program significantly increased the percentage of teenagers who used birth control after delivering their babies. Thus, one highly

---

*All mothers gave birth to live infants; however, there were two neonatal deaths within 24 hours of birth in the comparison group.

important result of participating in the program is that an early repeat pregnancy will be postponed. There is abundant research that has shown that repeat pregnancy among teenagers is especially damaging to their educational and occupational attainment, and leads to particularly adverse labor and delivery outcomes in the higher-order births (Klugman, 1974; Jackson, 1976).

The experimental group had more prenatal care, but not significantly more. Perhaps part of the difficulty is that the program can only begin to deliver services once pregnancy has been diagnosed. If a teenager does not come in for a pregnancy test until her fourth of fifth month, this obviously puts an upper limit on the number of visits she will have; it also gives less time for her to eat properly, avoid smoking and drinking, and take other steps to enhance her health during pregnancy. Thus, one implication of this finding is that the program needs to do more to encourage early pregnancy screening. Perhaps a joint effort between clinic personnel and school nurses in neighboring middle schools and high schools could be launched to publicize the need for a timely pregnancy test and to inform teenagers where such a test could be obtained.

The two groups performed similarly with respect to the various labor and delivery outcomes chosen to evaluate the effectiveness of the new program. The issue of timeliness is again relevant here. The program may have been delivering services too late in the pregnancy for the instruction to have much impact on the health of the mother and her child. This interpretation is supported, in part, by the fact that the one variable for which timeliness was *not* an issue (postpartum contraception) was, indeed, positively affected by program participation. Another possible implication is that the program itself should be made more powerful, for example, by lengthening or adding to instruction sessions.

Given that the experimental–comparison differences were all in the hypothesized direction, it is also tempting to criticize the sample size. A larger sample (which was originally planned) might have yielded some significant differences.

In summary, the experimental intervention is not without promise. A particularly exciting finding is that participation in the program resulted in better contraceptive use, which will presumably lower the incidence of repeat pregnancy. It would be interesting to follow these teenagers 2 years after delivery to see if the groups differ in the rates of repeat pregnancy. It appears that more needs to be done to get these teenagers into the program early in their pregnancy. Perhaps then the true effectiveness of the program would be demonstrated.

Critique of the Research Report

Below we present some comments regarding the quality of various aspects of the above fictitous research report. Students are urged to read the report and formulate their own opinions about its strengths and weaknesses prior to reading this critique. An evaluation of a study is necessarily partly subjective. Therefore, it should be expected that students will disagree with some of the points made below. Other students will also criticize some aspects of the study that we do not comment on. However, we believe that some of the most serious methodological flaws of the study are highlighted in our critique.

Title. The title for the study is misleading. The research does *not* investigate the role of health-care professionals in serving the needs of pregnant teenagers. A more appropriate title would be "Health-Related Outcomes of an Intervention for Pregnant Teenagers."

Background. The background section of the report consists of three distinct elements that can be analyzed separately—a literature review, statement of the problem, and description of a theoretical framework.

The literature review is relatively clearly written and well-organized. It serves the important function of establishing a need for the experimental program by documenting how widespread the problem of teenage pregnancy is and what some of the adverse consequences of teenage parenthood are.

However, the literature review could be improved. First, an inspection of the citations suggests that the author is not as up-to-date on research relating to teenage pregnancy as she might have been. All but one reference is from the 1970s, often the early and mid-70s. Second, there is material in the literature-review section that is not relevant and should be removed. For example, the paragraph on the options with which a pregnant teenager is faced (paragraph 3) is not germane to the research problem. Another example is the quote by Dr. Woodsome; it adds little in documenting the need for special programs for teenagers and is only one person's opinion.

A third, and more critical, flaw is what the review does *not* cover. Given the research problem, there are probably four main points that should be addressed in the review: (1) How widespread is teeange pregnancy? (2) What are the social, economic, and health consequences of early pregnancy? (3) What has been done (especially by nurses) to address the problems associated with teenage parenthood? and (4) How successful have other interventions been? The review adequately handles the first question: the need for concern is established. The second question is covered in the review, but perhaps more depth is needed here. The entire study is based on an assumption of negative health outcomes in teenage mothers. The author has strung together a series of references without giving the reader any clues about how reliable the information is. The author would have more convincingly made her point if she added a sentence such as "For example, in a carefully executed prospective study involving nearly 8,000 pregnant women, Beach (1976) found that low maternal age was significantly associated with higher rates of prematurity and other negative neonatal outcomes." The third and fourth points that should have been covered are totally absent from the review. Surely the author's experimental program does not represent the first attempt to address the needs of pregnant teenagers. How is Moreland's intervention different from or better than other interventions? What reason does she have to believe that such an intervention will be successful? Moreland has provided a rationale for addressing the problem, but no rationale for the manner in which she has addressed it. If, in fact, little has been written about other interventions, then the review should say so.

The problem statement and hypothesis were stated succinctly and clearly. The hypothesis is complex (there are multiple dependent variables) and directional (it predicts better outcomes among teenagers participating in the special program).

The third component of the background section of the report is the theoretical framework. In our opinion, the theoretical framework chosen does little to enhance the research. The hypothesis is not generated on the basis of the model, nor does the intervention itself grow out of the model. One gets the feeling that the model was slapped on as an afterthought to try to make the study seem more "sophisticated." Actually, if more thought had been given to this conceptual framework, it might have proven useful. According to this model, the most immediate and direct influences on a pregnant teenager are her family, friends, and sexual partner. One programmatic implication of this is that the intervention should involve one or more of these influences. For example, a workshop for the teenagers' parents could have been developed to reinforce the teenagers' need for adequate nutrition and prenatal care. A research hypothesis that could have been tested in the context of the model is that teenagers who are missing one of the direct influences would be more susceptible to the influence of the less-proximal health-care providers (i.e., the program). For example, it might be hypothesized that pregnant teenagers who no longer have contact with the babies' fathers or those who do not live with both parents will have to depend on alternative sources of social support (such as health-care personnel) during the pregnancy. Thus, it is not that the theoretical context is far-fetched, but rather that it was not convincingly linked to the actual research problem. Perhaps an alternative theoretical context would have been better. Or perhaps the researcher should have simply been honest and admitted that her research was practical, not theoretical.

Methods. The design used to test the research hypothesis was a widely used preexperimental design. Two groups, in which their equivalence is assumed but not examined, are compared on several outcome measures. The design is one that has serious problems, because the pretreatment comparability of the groups is undetermined.

The most serious threat to the internal validity of the study is selection bias. Selection bias can work both to mask true treatment effects or to create the illusion of a program effect when none exists. This is because selection bias can be either positive (*i.e.,* the experimental group can have pretreatment advantages) or negative (*i.e.,* the experimental group can be initially disadvantaged vis-à-vis the comparison group). In the present study, it is possible that the two hospitals served clients of a different social class, for example. If the average income of the families of the experimental-group teenagers was higher, then these teenagers would probably have a better opportunity for adequate prenatal nutrition than the comparison-group teenagers (the reverse might also be true). Or the comparison hospital might serve younger teenagers, or a higher percentage of married teenagers, or a higher percentage of pregnant teenagers attending a special school-based program. None of these extraneous variables has been controlled.

Another way in which the design was vulnerable to selection bias is the high refusal rate in the experimental group. Of the 217 eligible teenagers, 50% declined to participate in the special program. We cannot assume that the 109 girls who participated were a random sample of the eligibles. Again, biases could be either positive or negative. A positive selection bias would be created if the "best" teenagers (*i.e.,* the most motivated to have a healthy pregnancy or become good mothers) self-selected themselves into the experimental group. A negative selection bias would result if the most needy teenagers (*i.e.,* those from the poorest households or from families offering little support) elected to participate in the program. In the comparison group, hospital records were used primarily to collect the data, so that this self-selection problem could not occur (except for refusals to answer the contraceptive questions 6 months postpartum).

The researcher could have taken a number of steps to either control selection biases or, at the very least, estimate their direction and magnitude. The following are among the most critical extraneous variables to control: subjects' social class (or family income), age, race/ethnicity, parity, participation in another pregnant-teenager program, marital status, and prepregnancy experience with contraception (for the postpartum contraception outcome). The researcher should have attempted to gather information on these variables from experimental- and comparison-group teenagers *and* from eligible teenagers in the experimental hospital who declined to participate in the program. To the extent that these three groups are similar on these variables, credibility in the internal validity of the study would be enhanced. If sizeable differences are observed, the researcher would at least know or suspect the direction of the biases and could factor that information into her interpretation and conclusions.

Had the researcher gathered information on the extraneous variables, another possibility would have been to match experimental- and comparison-group subjects on one or two variables, such as social class and age.

Matching is not an ideal method of controlling extraneous variables, but it is preferable to doing nothing. Pair-matching would have probably resulted in some wastage. For example, if there were no match in the comparison group for a 13-year-old teenager from a middle-income family, then data from that experimental teenager would be dropped from the study. Of course, matching on two variables does not equate the two groups in terms of the other extraneous variables; that is one of the shortcomings of matching.

Another strategy the researcher could have adopted would be to gather outcome data for the 108 eligible refusers attending the clinic where the special program was offered. In other words, a second comparison group could have been created. Researchers sometimes use two comparison groups because it has been learned, through methodological research, that different comparison groups frequently contain different types of biases. Thus, if an experimental group can be shown to be significantly different from two different comparison groups, then the researcher can be more confident in the internal validity of the study.

So far we have focused our attention on the research design, but other aspects of the study are also problematic. Let us consider the decision the researcher made about the population. The target population is not explicitly defined by the researcher, but one can infer that the target population is pregnant girls under age 20 who carry their infants to delivery. The accessible population presumably is pregnant teenagers from Chicago's inner city. Is it reasonable to assume that the accessible population is representative of the target population? No, it is not. It is likely that the accessible population is quite different from the overall population in terms of family income, race/ethnicity, access to health care, family intactness, and many other characteristics. A more narrowly defined target population is called for.

By delimiting the target population, the researcher could have controlled numerous extraneous variables. For example, the specification could have excluded multigravidas, or very young teenagers (under 15), or married teenagers. Such a specification would have limited the generalizability of the findings, but would have enhanced the internal validity of the study by increasing the comparability of the two groups.

The sample was a sample of convenience, the least effective sampling design. There is no way of knowing whether the sample represents the accessible and target populations. While probability sampling from the accessible population would have been difficult, if not impossible, to accomplish, the researcher could have taken some steps to improve her sampling design. A quota sampling plan would have offered some improvement. For example, if the researcher knew that among Chicago's teenage parents 50% were white, 35% were black, and 15% were Hispanic, then it might have been possible to enhance the representativeness of the samples by establishing these percentages as quotas for the study (but not necessarily for the program).

Sample size is a difficult issue. Many of the results reported were in the hypothesized direction but were nonsignificant. When this is the case, the adequacy of the sample size is always suspect, as Moreland pointed out. Each group had about 100 subjects. In many cases this sample size would be considered adequate, but in the present case it is not. One of the difficulties in testing the effectiveness of new interventions is that, generally, the experimental group is not being compared with a "no-treatment" group. Although the comparison group in this example was not getting the special program services, it cannot be said that this group was getting no services at all. Some comparison-group members may have had ample prenatal care during which the health-care staff may have provided much of the same information as that taught in the special program. The point is not that the new program was not needed, but rather that unless an intervention is extremely powerful and innovative, the incremental improvement will typically be rather small. Whenever relatively small effects are anticipated, the sample must be very large in order for differences to be statistically significant. Although it is beyond the scope of this book to explain the calculations, it can be shown that in order to detect a significant difference between the two groups with respect, say, to the incidence of toxemia, a sample of over 5000 would have been needed.

The fourth major methodological decision concerns measurement of the research variables. For the most part, the researcher did a good job in selecting objective, reliable, and valid outcome measures. Also, her operational definitions were clearly worded and unambiguous. Two comments are in order. First, it might have been better to operationalize two of the variables differently. Infant birthweight might have been more sensitively measured as actual weight (a ratio-level measurement) rather than being transformed to a dichotomous (normal-level) variable. The contraceptive variable could also have been operationalized to yield a more sensitive (i.e., more discriminating) measure. Rather than measuring contraceptive use as a dichotomy, Moreland could have created an ordinal scale based either on the frequency of use (e.g., 0%, 1%–25%, 26%–50%, 51%–75%, and 76%–100% of the time) or on the effectiveness of the type of birth control used.

A second consideration is whether the outcome variables adequately captured the effects of program activities. It might have been easier, with a sample of 229 teenagers, to capture group differences in, say, nutritional habits than in infant birthweight. None of the outcome variables measured the effects of parenting education. In other words, the researcher could have added several more direct measures of the effect of the special program.

In summary, the researcher failed to really give the new program a fair test. Moreland should have taken a number of steps to control extraneous variables and should have attempted to get a larger sample (even if this meant waiting for additional subjects to enroll in the program). In addition to concerns about the internal validity of the study, its generalizability is also questionable.

Results. Moreland did a good job of presenting the results of the study. The presentation was straightforward and succinct, and was enhanced by the inclusion of a good table and figures. The style of this section was also appropriate: it was written in the past tense and was objective and well-organized.

The statistical analyses were also reasonably well done. The descriptive statistics (means and percentages) were appropriate for the level of measurement of the variables. The author did not, however, provide any information on the variability of measures, except for noting the range for the "time spent in labor" variable. Figure 19-2 suggests that the two groups did differ in variability: the comparison group was more heterogeneous than the experimental group with regard to prenatal care.

The two types of inferential statistics used (the t-test and chi-square test) were also appropriate given the level of measurement of the outcome variables and the sample size. The results of these tests were efficiently presented in a single table. It should be noted that there are more powerful statistics available that could have been used to control extraneous variables (e.g., analysis of covariance), but since no data were collected on many of the extraneous variables (social class, ethnicity, parity, and so on), these techniques could not have been used even if the researcher had the technical skills to do so.

Discussion. Moreland's discussion section fails almost entirely to take the study's limitations into account in interpreting the data. The one exception was her acknowledgment that the sample size was too small. She seems unconcerned about the many threats to the internal or external validity of her research.

Moreland lays almost all the blame for the nonsignificant findings on the program rather than on the research methods. She feels that two aspects of the program should be changed—(1) recruitment of teenagers into the program earlier in their pregnancy and (2) strengthening program services. Both recommendations might be worth pursuing, but there is little in the data to suggest these modifications.

With nonsignificant results such as those that predominated in this study, there are two possibilities to consider: (1) the results are accurate; the program is not effective for those outcomes examined (though it might be effective for other measures); and (2) the results are false; the existing program *is* effective for the outcomes examined, but the test failed to demonstrate it. Moreland concluded that the first possibility was correct, and therefore recommended that the program be changed. Equally plausible—perhaps even more plausible—is the possibility that the study methods were too weak to demonstrate the program's true effects.

We do not have enough information about the characteristics of the sample to conclude with certainty that there were substantial selection biases. We do, however, have a clue that selection biases were operative in a direction that would make the program look less effective than it actually is. Moreland noted in the beginning of the results section that the average age of teenagers in the experimental group was 17.1, compared with 18.0 in the comparison group. Age is inversely related to positive labor and delivery outcomes (indeed, that is the basis for having a special program for teenage mothers). Therefore, the experimental group's performance on the outcome measures was possibly depressed by the youth of that group. Had the two groups been equivalent in terms of age, the group differences might have been larger and could have reached statistical significance. Other uncontrolled pretreatment differences could also have masked true treatment effects.

For the one significant outcome, we cannot rule out the possibility that a Type-I error was made—that is, that the null hypothesis was in fact true. Again, selection biases could have been operative. The experimental group might have contained many more girls who had had preprogram experience with contraception; it might have contained more highly motivated teenagers, or more single teenagers, or more teenagers who had already had multiple pregnancies than the comparison group. There is simply no way of knowing whether the significant outcome reflects true program effectiveness or merely initial group differences.

Aside from Moreland's disregard for the problems of internal validity, the author definitely overstepped the bounds of scholarly speculation by reading too much into her data. She unquestioningly assumed that the program has caused contraceptive improvements: "the experimental program significantly increased the percentage of teenagers who used birth control . . ." Worse yet, she goes on to conclude that repeat pregnancies will be postponed in the experimental group, although she does not know whether teenagers used an effective contraception, whether they used it all the time, or whether they used it correctly.

As another example of "going beyond the data," Moreland became overly invested in her notion that teenagers need greater and earlier exposure to the program. It is not that her hypothesis has no merit; the problem is that she builds an elaborate rationale for program changes with no apparent empirical support. She probably had information on when in the pregnancy the teenagers entered the program, but that information was not shared with readers. Her argument about the need for more publicity on early screening would have had more clout if she had reported that the majority of teenagers entered the program during the fourth month of their pregnancies or later. Additionally, she could have martialed more evidenced in support of her proposal if she had been able to show that earlier entry into the program was associated with better health outcomes. For example, she could have compared the outcomes of teenagers entering the program in their first, second, and third trimesters.

In conclusion, the study is not without some merits. As Moreland noted, there *is* some reason to be modestly optimistic that the program *could* have some beneficial effects. However, the existing study is too seriously flawed to reach any conclusions, even tentatively. A replication with improved research methods is clearly needed to solve the research problem.

Summary

The research project is not complete until the results have been communicated in the form of a report. Despite some differences in the length, purposes, and audience of different types of research reports, the general form and content is similar. In general, the four major sections of a research report are the introduction, methods, results, and discussion.

The purpose of the *introductory section* is to acquaint the readers with the research problem. This section includes the problem statement, the research hypothesis, a justification of the importance or value of the research, a summary of relevant related literature, the identification of a theoretical framework, a statement of underlying assumptions, and definitions of the concepts being studied. The *methods section* acquaints the reader with what the researcher did to solve the research problem. This section normally includes a description of the subjects, how they were selected, the target and accessible populations, the study design, the instruments used to collect the data, the procedures used, and the techniques used to analyze the data. In the *results section,* the findings obtained from the analyses are summarized. Finally, the *discussion* section of a research report presents the researcher's interpretations of the results, together with a consideration of the study's limitations and recommendations for future research.

Scientific communications should be written as simply and clearly as possible. Emotionally laden statements, overtly subjective statements, and exaggerations should be excluded from research reports. The report should be well-organized and written with a minimum of technical jargon. The presentation should be professional, but not pompous or pedantic.

Three types of research documents were discussed. A *research proposal* is a written description of a researcher's plans for the conduct of a scientific investigation. For theses, dissertations, and other student reports, there is typically extensive documentation of the conceptual underpinnings and methodological decisions of the study, since the document serves to communicate not only the study findings, but also evidence of the student's skills. Journal articles, which are typically brief, serve the important function of communicating to a wide audience of nurses the knowledge gained as a result of the research.

Study Suggestions

1. Suggest titles for the fictitious research studies described at the end of Chapters 5 through 17 of this book.

2. Prepare an abstract for the fictitious research report presented in this chapter. Compare your abstract with that of one of your classmates.

3. Read an article in a recent issue of *Nursing Research.* Comment on the appropriateness of the author's style.

Glossary

accessible population: The population of subjects available for a particular study; often a nonrandom subset of the target population.

accidental sampling: Selection of the most readily available persons (or units) as subjects in a study; also known as *convenience sampling*.

analysis of covariance: A statistical procedure used to test the effect of one or more treatments on different groups while controlling for one or more extraneous variables (covariates); also referred to as ANCOVA.

analysis of variance: A statistical procedure for testing the effect of one or more treatments on different groups by comparing the variability between groups to the variability within groups; also referred to as ANOVA.

anonymity: Protection of the participants in a study such that even the researcher cannot link them with the information provided.

applied research: Research that concentrates on finding a solution to an immediate practical problem.

assumptions: Basic principles that are accepted as being true on the basis of logic or reason, without proof or verification.

attribute variables: Preexisting characteristics of the entity under investigation, which the researcher simply observes and measures.

attrition: The loss of participants during the course of a study; can introduce an unknown amount of bias by changing the composition of the sample initially drawn—particularly if more subjects are lost from one group than another; can thereby be a threat to the internal validity of a study.

basic research: Research designed to extend the base of knowledge in a discipline for the sake of knowledge production or theory construction, rather than for solving an immediate problem.

bias: Any influence that produces a distortion in the results of a study.

bivariate statistics: Statistics derived from the analysis of two variables simultaneously for the purpose of assessing the empirical relationship between them.

case study: A research method that involves a thorough, in-depth analysis of a person, group, institution, or other social unit.

causal relationship: A relationship between two variables such that the presence or absence of one variable (the "cause") determines the presence or absence, or value, of the other (the "effect").

cell: The intersection of a row and column in a table with two or more dimensions. In an experimental design, a cell is the representation of an experimental condition in a schematic diagram.

central tendency: A statistical index of the "typicalness" of a set of scores that comes from the center of the distribution of scores. The three most common indices of central tendency are the mode, the median, and the mean.

chi-square test: A test of statistical significance used to assess whether or not a relationship exists between two nominal-level variables. Symbolized as χ^2.

closed-ended question: A question that offers respondents a set of mutually exclusive and jointly exhaustive alternative replies, from which the one that most closely approximates the "right" answer must be chosen.

cluster sampling: A form of multistage sampling in which large groupings ("clusters") are selected first (e.g., nursing schools), with successive subsampling of smaller units (e.g., nursing students).

codebook: The documentation used in data processing that indicates the location and values of all the variables in a data file.

coding: The process of transforming raw data into standardized form (usually numerical) for data processing and analysis.

coefficient alpha (Cronbach's alpha):   A reliability index that estimates the internal consistency or homogeneity of a measure composed of several items or subparts.

cohort study: A kind of trend study that focuses on a specific subpopulation (which is often an age-related subgroup) from which different samples are selected at different points in time (e.g., nursing students graduated in 1970-1974).

comparison group: A group of subjects whose scores on a dependent variable are used as a basis for evaluating the scores of the target group or group of primary interest. The term "comparison group" is generally used instead of "control group" when the investigation does not use a true experimental design.

computer: An electronic device that performs simple operations with extreme accuracy and speed.

computer program: A set of instructions to a computer.

concept: An abstraction based on observations of certain behaviors or characteristics (e.g., stress, death).

conceptual framework: Interrelated concepts or abstractions that are assembled together in some rational scheme by virtue of their relevance to a common theme (see also *theory*).

concurrent validity: The degree to which an instrument can distinguish individuals who differ on some other criterion measured or observed at the same time.

confidentiality: Protection of participants in a study such that their individual identities will not be linked to the information they provided and publicly divulged.

construct validity: The degree to which an instrument measures the concept under investigation.

content analysis: A procedure for analyzing written, verbal, or visual materials in a systematic and objective fashion, typically with the goal of quantitatively measuring variables.

content validity: The degree to which the items in an instrument adequately represent the universe of content.

control: The process of holding constant possible influences on the dependent variable under investigation.

control group: Subjects in an experiment who do not receive the experimental treatment and whose performance provides a baseline against which the effects of the treatment can be measured (see also *comparison group*).

convenience sampling: Selection of the most readily available persons (or units) as subjects in a study; also known as *accidental sampling*.

correlation: A tendency for variation in one variable to be related to variation in another variable.

correlation coefficient: An index that summarizes the degree of relationship between two variables. Correlation coefficients typically range from +1.00 (for a perfect direct relationship) to 0.0 (for no relationship) to −1.00 (for a perfect inverse relationship).

correlational research: Investigations that explore the interrelationships among variables of interest without any active intervention on the part of the researcher.

criterion variable (criterion measure):   The quality or attribute used to measure the effect of an independent variable; sometimes used instead of *dependent variable*.

✗**criterion-related validity:**   The degree to which scores on an instrument are correlated with some external criterion.

✓**cross-sectional study:**   A study based on observations of different age or developmental groups at a single point in time for the purpose of inferring trends over time.

crosstabulation: A determination of the number of cases occurring when simultaneous consideration is given to the values of two or more variables (e.g., sex—male/female—crosstabulated with smoking status—smoker/non-smoker). The results are typically presented in a table with rows and columns divided according to the values of the variables.

data: The pieces of information obtained in the course of a study (singular is datum).

degrees of freedom: A concept used in tests of statistical significance, referring to the number of sample values that cannot be calculated from knowledge of other values and a calculated statistic (e.g., by knowing a sample mean, all but one value would be free to vary); degrees of freedom (df) is usually $N - 1$, but different formulas are relevant for different tests.

dependent variable: The outcome variable of interest; the variable that is hypothesized to depend on or be caused by another variable (called the *independent variable*); sometimes referred to as the *criterion variable*.

✓**descriptive research:**   Research studies that have as their main objective the accurate portrayal of the characteristics of persons, situations, or groups, and the frequency with which certain phenomena occur.

descriptive statistics: Statistics used to describe and summarize the researcher's data set (e.g., mean, standard deviation).

dichotomous variable: A variable having only two values or categories (e.g., sex).

directional hypothesis: A hypothesis that makes a specific prediction about the direction (i.e., positive or negative) of the relationship between two variables.

double-blind experiment: An experiment in which neither the subjects nor those who administer the treatment know who is in the experimental or control group.

empiricism: The process wherein evidence rooted in objective reality and gathered through the human senses is used as the basis for generating knowledge.

error of measurement: The degree of deviation between true scores and obtained scores when measuring a characteristic.

ethics: The quality of research procedures with respect to their adherence to professional, legal, and social obligations to the research subjects.

evaluation research: Research that investigates how well a program, practice, or policy is working.

ex post facto research: Research conducted *after* the variations in the independent variable have occurred in the natural course of events; a form of nonexperimental research in which causal explanations are inferred "after the fact."

experiment: A research study in which the investigator controls (manipulates) the independent variable and randomly assigns subjects to different conditions.

experimental group: The subjects who receive the experimental treatment or intervention.

exploratory research: A preliminary study designed to develop or refine hypotheses, or to test and refine the data-collection methods.

external validity: The degree to which the results of a study can be generalized to settings or samples other than the ones studied.

extraneous variable: Variables that confound the relationship between the independent and dependent variables and that need to be controlled either in the research design or through statistical procedures (*e.g.*, in a study of the effect of a mother's age on the rate of premature deliveries, social class and ethnicity would be extraneous variables).

factorial design: An experimental design in which two or more independent variables are simultaneously manipulated; this design permits an analysis of the main effects of the independent variables separately, plus the interaction effects of these variables.

field study: A study in which the data are collected "in the field" from persons in their normal roles, rather than as subjects in a laboratory study.

follow-up study: A study undertaken to determine the subsequent development of persons with a specified condition or who have received a specified treatment.

frequency distribution: A systematic array of numerical values from the lowest to the highest, together with a count of the number of times each value was obtained.

generalizability: The degree to which the research procedures justify the inference that the findings represent something beyond the specific observations upon which they are based; in particular, the inference that the findings can be generalized from the sample to the entire population.

graphic rating scale: A scale in which respondents are asked to rate something (*e.g.*, a concept, issue, institution) along an ordered bipolar continuum (*e.g.*, "excellent" to "very poor").

Hawthorne effect: The effect on the dependent variable caused by subjects' awareness that they are "special" participants under study.

historical research: Systematic studies designed to establish facts and relationships concerning past events.

history: A threat to the internal validity of a study; refers to the occurrence of events external to the treatment but concurrent with it, which can affect the dependent variable of interest.

homogeneity: (1) In terms of the reliability of an instrument, the degree to which the subparts are internally consistent (*i.e.*, are measuring the same critical attribute). (2) More generally, the degree to which objects are similar (*i.e.*, characterized by low variability).

hypothesis: A statement of predicted relationships between the variables under investigation; hypotheses lead to empirical studies that seek to confirm or disconfirm those predictions.

independent variable: The variable that is believed to cause or influence the dependent variable; in experimental research, the independent variable is the variable that is manipulated.

inferential statistics: Statistics that permit us to infer whether relationships observed in a sample are likely to occur in a larger population of concern.

informed consent: An ethical principle that requires researchers to obtain the voluntary participation of subjects, after informing them of possible risks and benefits.

interaction effect: The effect on a dependent variable of two or more independent variables acting in combination (interactively) rather than as unconnected factors.

internal consistency: A form of reliability, referring to the degree to which the subparts of an instrument are all measuring the same attribute or dimension.

internal validity: The degree to which it can be inferred that the experimental treatment (independent variable), rather than uncontrolled, extraneous factors, is responsible for observed effects.

interrater reliability: The degree to which two raters, operating independently, assign the same ratings for an attribute being measured; such ratings normally occur in the context of observational research or in coding qualitative materials.

interval measure: A level of measurement in which an attribute of a variable is rank ordered on a scale that has equal distances between points on that scale (*e.g.*, Fahrenheit degrees).

intervention: (1) In experimental research, the experimental treatment or manipulation. (2) More generally, the structure the investigator imposes on the research setting prior to making observations.

interview: A method of data collection in which one person (an interviewer) asks questions of another person (a respondent); interviews are conducted either face-to-face or by telephone.

item: A term used to refer to a single question on a test or questionnaire, or a single statement on an attitude scale or other scale (*e.g.*, a final examination might consist of 100 items).

judgmental sampling: A type of nonprobability sampling method in which the researcher selects subjects for the study on the basis of personal judgment about which ones will be most representative or productive; also referred to as *purposive sampling*.

key informant: A person well-versed in the phenomenon of research interest and who is willing to share the information and insight with the researcher; key informants are often used in needs assessments.

known-groups technique: A technique for estimating the construct validity of an instrument through an analysis of the degree to which the instrument separates groups that are predicted to differ on the basis of some theory or known characteristic.

Likert scale: A type of composite measure of attitudes that involves summation of scores on a set of items (statements) to which respondents are asked to indicate their degree of agreement or disagreement.

literature review: A critical summary of research on a topic of interest, generally prepared to put a research problem in context or to identify gaps and weaknesses in prior studies so as to justify a new investigation.

longitudinal study: A study designed to collect data at more than one point in time, in contrast to a cross-sectional study.

manipulation: An intervention or treatment introduced by the researcher in an experimental or quasi-experimental study; the researcher manipulates the independent variable to assess its impact on the dependent variable.

matching: The pairing of subjects in one group with those in another group based on their similarity on one or more dimension, done in order to enhance the overall comparability of groups; when matching is performed in the context of an experiment, the procedure results in a randomized block design.

maturation: A threat to the internal validity of a study that results when factors influence the outcome measure (dependent variable) as a result of time passing.

mean: A descriptive statistic that is a measure of central tendency, computed by summing all scores and dividing by the number of subjects.

measurement: The assignment of numbers to objects according to specified rules to characterize quantities of some attribute.

median: A descriptive statistic that is a measure of central tendency, representing the exact middle score or value in a distribution of scores; the median is the value above and below which 50% of the scores lie.

methods (research): The steps, procedures, and strategies for gathering and analyzing the data in a research investigation.

mode: A descriptive statistic that is a measure of central tendency; the score or value that occurs most frequently in a distribution of scores.

model: A symbolic representation of concepts or variables, and interrelations among variables.

molar approach: A way of making observations about behaviors that entails studying large units of behavior and treating them as a whole.

molecular approach: A way of making observations about behavior that uses small and highly specific behaviors as the unit of observation.

mortality: A threat to the internal validity of a study, referring to the differential loss of subjects (attrition) from different groups.

multistage sampling: A sampling strategy that proceeds through a set of stages from larger to smaller sampling units (e.g., from states, to nursing schools, to faculty members).

multitrait-multimethod matrix approach: A method of establishing the construct validity of an instrument that involves the use of multiple measures for a set of subjects; the target instrument is valid to the extent that there is a strong relationship between it and other measures purporting to measure the same attribute (*convergence*) and a weak relationship between it and other measures purporting to measure a different attribute (*discriminability*).

N: Often used to designate the total number of subjects in a study (*e.g.*, "the total N was 500").

n: Often used to designate the number of subjects in a subgroup or in a cell of a study (*e.g.*, "each of the four groups had an n of 125, for a total N of 500").

needs assessment: A study in which a researcher collects data for estimating the needs of a group, community, or organization; usually used as a guide to resource allocation.

negative relationship: A relationship between two variables in which there is a tendency for higher values on one variable to be associated with lower values on the other (*e.g.*, as temperature increases, people's productivity may decrease); also referred to as an *inverse relationship.*

nominal measure: The lowest level of measurement that involves the assignment of characteristics into categories (*e.g.*, males, category 1; females, category 2).

nondirectional hypothesis: A research hypothesis that does not stipulate in advance the direction (*i.e.*, positive or negative) of the relationship between variables.

nonequivalent control group: A comparison group that was not developed on the basis of random assignment; when randomization is not used, there is no way of assuring the initial equivalence among different groups.

nonexperimental research: Studies in which the researcher collects data without introducing any new treatments or changes.

nonparametric statistics: A general class of inferential statistics that does not involve rigorous assumptions about the distribution of the critical variables; most often used when samples are small or when the data are measured on the nominal or ordinal scales.

nonprobability sampling: The selection of subjects or sampling units from a population using nonrandom procedures; examples include accidental, judgmental, and quota sampling.

normal distribution: A theoretical distribtuion that is bell-shaped and symmetrical.

null hypothesis: The hypothesis that states there is no relationship between the variables under study; used primarily in connection with tests of statistical significance as the hypothesis to be rejected.

observational research: Studies in which the data are collected by means of observing and recording behaviors or activities of interest.

obtained score: The actual score or numerical value assigned to a subject on a measure.

open-ended question: A question in an interview or questionnaire that does not restrict the respondents' answers to preestablished alternatives.

operational definition: The definition of a concept or variable in terms of the operations or procedures by which it is to be measured.

ordinal measure: A level of measurement that yields rank orders of a variable along some dimension.

outcome measure: A term sometimes used to refer to the dependent variable, (*i.e.*, the variable that the researcher is attempting to predict, explain, or understand).

outliers: Wild codes or numerical values that are not part of the coding scheme.

panel study: A type of longitudinal study in which the same subjects are used to provide data at two or more points in time.

parameter: A characteristic of a population (*e.g.,* the mean age of all United States citizens).

parametric statistics: A class of inferential statistics that involves (a) assumptions about the distribution of the variables, (b) the estimation of a parameter, and (c) the use of interval or ratio measures.

participant observation: A method of collecting data through the observation of a group or organization in which the researcher participates as a member.

pilot study: A small-scale version, or trial run, done in preparation for a major study.

population: The entire set of people (or objects) having some common characteristic(s) (*e.g.,* all RNs in the state of California); sometimes referred to as *universe.*

positive relationship: A relationship between two variables in which there is a tendency for high values on one variable to be associated with high values on the other (*e.g.,* as physical activity increases, pulse rate also increases).

predictive validity: The degree to which an instrument can predict some criterion observed at a future time.

preexperimental design: A research design that does not include controls to compensate for the absence of either randomization or a control group.

pretest: (1) The collection of data prior to the experimental intervention; sometimes referred to as *baseline data.* (2) The trial administration of a newly developed instrument to identify flaws or assess time requirements.

probability sampling: The selection of subjects or sampling units from a population using random procedures: examples include simple random sampling, cluster sampling, and systematic sampling.

probing: Eliciting more useful or detailed information from a respondent than was volunteered during the first reply.

problem statement: The statement that identifies the key research variables, specifies the nature of the population, and suggests the possibility of empirical testing.

projective techniques: Methods for measuring psychological attributes (values, attitudes, personality) by providing respondents with unstructured stimuli to which to respond.

proposal: A document specifying what the researcher proposes to study; it communicates the research problem, its significance, planned procedures for solving the problem, and, when funding is sought, how much the research will cost.

prospective study: A study that begins with an examination of presumed causes (*e.g.,* cigarette smoking) and then goes forward in time to observe presumed effects (*e.g.,* lung cancer).

purposive sampling: A type of nonprobability-sampling method in which the researcher selects subjects for the study on the basis of personal judgment about which ones will be most representative or productive; also referred to as *judgmental sampling.*

Q-sort: A method of scaling in which the subject sorts statements into a number of piles (usually 9 or 11) according to some bipolar dimension (*e.g.,* most like me/least like me; most useful/least useful).

qualitative analysis: The nonnumerical organization and interpretation of observations for the purpose of discovering important underlying dimensions and patterns of relationships.

quantitative analysis: The manipulation of numerical data through statistical procedures for the purpose of describing phenomena or assessing the magnitude and reliability of relationships among them.

quasi-experiment: A study in which subjects cannot be randomly assigned to treatment conditions, although the researcher does manipulate the independent variable and exercises certain controls to enhance the internal validity of the results.

quasi-statistics: An "accounting" system used to assess the validity of conclusions derived from qualitative analysis.

questionnaire: A method of gathering self-report information from respondents through self-administration of questions in a paper-and-pencil format.

quota sampling: The nonrandom selection of subjects in which the researcher prespecifies characteristics of the sample to increase its representativeness.

random-number table: A table of digits from 0 to 9 set up in such a way that each number is equally likely to follow any other; used in randomization of random sampling.

random sampling: The selection of a sample such that each member of a population (or subpopulation) has an equal probability of being included.

randomization: The assignment of subjects to treatment conditions in a random manner (*i.e.*, in a manner determined by chance alone); also known as *random assignment*.

range: A measure of variability, consisting of the difference between the highest and lowest values in a distribution of scores.

ratio measure: A level of measurement in which there are equal distances between score units and that has a true meaningful zero point; the highest level of measurement (*e.g.*, age).

reactivity: A measurement distortion arising from the subject's awareness of being observed, or, more generally, from the effect of the measurement procedure itself.

reliability: The degree of consistency or dependability with which an instrument measures the attribute it is designed to measure.

replication: The duplication of research procedures in a second investigation for the purpose of determining if earlier results can be repeated.

research: Systematic inquiry that uses orderly scientific methods to answer questions or solve problems.

research design: The overall plan for collecting and analyzing data, including specifications for enhancing the internal and external validity of the study.

response rate: The rate of participation in a survey; calculated by dividing the number of persons participating by the number of persons sampled.

response set bias: The measurement error introduced by the tendency of some people to respond to items in characteristic ways (*e.g.*, always agreeing), independently of the item's content.

retrospective study: A study that begins with the manifestation of the dependent variable in the present (*e.g.*, lung cancer) and then links this effect to some presumed cause occurring in the past (*e.g.*, cigarette smoking).

sample: A subset of a population selected to participate in a research study.

sampling: The process of selecting a portion of the population to represent the entire population.

sampling bias: Distortions that arise from the selection of a sample that is not representative of the population from which it was drawn.

sampling distribution: A theoretical distribution of a statistic using an infinite number of samples as a basis and the values of the statistic computed from these samples as the data points in the distribution.

sampling frame: A list of all the elements in the population, from which the sample is drawn.

scale: A composite measure of an attribute, consisting of several items that have a logical or empirical relationship to each other; involves the assignment of a score to place subjects on a continuum with respect to the attribute.

selection bias: A threat to the internal validity of the study that results from pre-treatment differences between experimental and comparison groups.

self-report: Any procedure for collecting data that involves a direct report of information by the person who is being studied (e.g., by interview or questionnaire).

semantic differential: A technique used to measure attitudes that asks respondents to rate a concept of interest on a series of seven-point bipolar rating scales.

significance level: The probability that an observed relationship could be caused by chance (i.e., because of sampling error); significance at the .05 level indicates the probability that a relationship of the observed magnitude would be found by chance only 5 times out of 100.

skewness: A quality of a set of scores relating to their asymmetrical distribution around a central point.

software: The instructions for performing operations made to a computer, and the documentation for those instructions.

Spearman-Brown prophecy formula: An equation for making corrections to a reliability estimate that was calculated by the split-half method.

split-half technique: A method for estimating the internal consistency (reliability) of an instrument by correlating scores on half of the measure with scores on the other half.

standard deviation: The most frequently used statistic for measuring the degree of variability in a set of scores.

standard error: The standard deviation of a sampling distribution.

statistic: An estimate of a parameter, calculated from sample data.

statistical significance: A term indicating that the results obtained in an analysis of sample data are unlikely to have been caused by chance, at some specified level of probability.

strata: Subdivisions of the population according to some characteristic (e.g., males and females); singular is stratum.

stratified random sampling: The random selection of subjects from two or more strata of the population independently.

subject: A person who participates and provides data in a study; subjects are sometimes designated as *ss*, as "there were 50 ss in the experiment."

survey research: A type of nonexperimental research that focuses on obtaining information about the status quo of some situation, often through direct questioning of a sample of respondents.

systematic sampling: The selection of subjects such that every *k*th (*e.g.*, every tenth) person (or element) in a sampling frame or list is chosen.

target population: The entire population in which the researcher is interested and to which he or she would like to generalize the results of a study.

test statistic: A statistic used to test for the statistical significance of relationships between variables; the sampling distributions of test statistics are known for circumstances in which the null hypothesis is true; examples include chi-square, F-ratio, *t*, and Pearson's *r*.

test–retest reliability: Assessment of the stability of an instrument by correlating the scores obtained on repeated administrations.

theory: An abstract generalization that presents a systematic explanation about the relationships among phenomena.

time sampling: In observational research, the selection of time periods during which observations will take place.

time-series design: A quasi-experimental design that involves the collection of information over an extended period of time, with multiple data-collection points both prior to and after the introduction of a treatment.

treatment: A term used to refer to an experimental intervention or manipulation.

trend study: A form of longitudinal study in which different samples from a population are studied over time with respect to some phenomenon (*e.g.*, a series of Gallup polls of political preferences).

true score: A hypothetical score that would be obtained if a measure were infallible; it is the portion of the observed score not due to random error or measurement bias.

t-test: A parametric statistical test used for analyzing the difference between two means.

Type-I error: A decision to reject the null hypothesis when it is true (*i.e.*, the researcher concludes that a relationship exists when in fact it does not).

Type-II error: A decision to accept the null hypothesis when it is false (*i.e.*, the researcher concludes that *no* relationship exists when in fact it does).

univariate statistics: Statistical procedures for analyzing a single variable for purposes of description.

validity: The degree to which an instrument measures what it is intended to measure.

variability: The degree to which values on a set of scores are widely different or dispersed (*e.g.*, one would expect higher variability of age of clients within a hospital than within a nursing home).

variable: A characteristic or attribute of a person or object that varies (*i.e.*, takes on different values) within the population under study (*e.g.*, body temperature, age, heart rate).

variance: A measure of variability or dispersion, equal to the square of the standard deviation.

References

American Nurses' Association Commission on Nursing Research: Generating a scientific basis for nursing practice: Research priorities for the 1980s. *Nursing Research*, 1980, *29*, 219.

Austin, J. K., McBride, A. B. and Davis, H. W.: Parental attitude and adjustment to childhood epilepsy. *Nursing Research*, 1984, *33*, 92–96.

Bales, R. F.: *Interaction process analysis.* Reading, Mass.: Addison–Wesley, 1950.

Becker, H. S.: *Sociological work: Method and substance.* Chicago: Aldine, 1970.

Borgatta, E. F.: A systematic study of interaction process scores, peer- and self-assessments, personality and other variables. *Genetic Psychology Monographs*, 1962, *65*, 219–291.

Bradburn, N. M. and Sudman, S.: *Improving interview method and questionnaire design.* San Francisco: Jossey Bass, 1979.

Campbell, D. T. and Fiske, D. W.: Convergent and discriminant validation by the multitrait–multimethod matrix. *Psychological Bulletin*, 1959, *56*, 81–105.

Campbell, D. T. and Stanley, J. C.: *Experimental and quasi-experimental designs for research.* Chicago: Rand McNally Publishing Co., 1963.

Cochran, W. G.: *Sampling techniques* (3rd ed.). New York: John Wiley and Sons, 1977.

Cohen, J.: *Statistical power analysis for the behavioral sciences.* (Rev. ed.). New York: Academic Press, 1977.

Dixon, W. J. and Brown, M. B. (Eds.): *BMDP–83: Biomedical computer programs, P-Series.* Berkeley: University of California Press, 1983.

Downs, F. and Fitzpatrick, J. J.: Preliminary investigation of the reliability and validity of a tool for the assessment of body position and motor activity. *Nursing Research*, 1976, *25*, 404–408.

Institute for Social Research: *Osiris III.* Ann Arbor: University of Michigan Press, 1973.

Keiser, G. J. and Bickle, I. M.: Attitude change as a motivational factor in producing behavior change related to implementing primary nursing. *Nursing Research*, 1980, *30*, 290–294.

Kerlinger, F. N.: *Foundations of behavioral research* (2nd ed.). New York: Holt, Rinehart and Winston, 1973.

King, I. M.: *Toward a theory for nursing.* New York: John Wiley and Sons, 1971.

King, I. M.: *A theory for nursing: Systems, concepts, process.* New York: John Wiley and Sons, 1981.

Lazarsfeld, P.: Foreword in H. Hyman, *Survey design and analysis*. New York: The Free Press, 1955.

Levine, M. L.: *Introduction to clinical nursing*. Philadelphia: F. A. Davis, 1969.

Nie, N. H. *et al.: Statistical package for the social sciences* (2nd ed.). New York: McGraw–Hill, 1979.

Nunnally, J.: *Psychometric theory*. New York: McGraw–Hill, 1978.

Polit, D. F. and Hungler, B. P.: *Nursing research: Principles and methods* (2nd ed.). Philadelphia: J. B. Lippincott, 1983.

Roy, C. and Roberts, S. L.: *Theory construction in nursing: An adaptation model*. Englewood Cliffs, N.J.: Prentice-Hall, 1981.

SAS Institute. *SAS user's guide basics*. Cary, N. C.: SAS Institute, 1982.

Seltiz, C., Wrightsman, L. S., and Cook, S. W.: *Research methods in social relations* (3rd ed.). New York: Holt, Rinehart and Winston, 1976.

Selye, H.: *The stress of life* (2nd ed.). New York: McGraw–Hill, 1978.

Stillman, M. J.: Women's health beliefs about breast cancer and breast self-examination. *Nursing Research*, 1977, *26*, 121–127.

Weick, K.: Systematic observational methods. In G. Lindzey and E. Aronson (Eds.). *The handbook of social psychology* (2nd ed.). Reading, Mass: Addison–Wesley, 1968, Volume II.

Appendix

Table A. Distribution of *t* Probability

df	p = .05	.02	.01	.001
1	12·706	31·821	63·657	636·619
2	4·303	6·965	6·925	31·598
3	3·182	4·541	5·841	12·941
4	2·776	3·747	4·604	8·610
5	2·571	3·365	4·032	6·859
6	4·447	3·143	3·707	5·959
7	2·365	2·998	3·499	5·405
8	2·306	2·896	3·355	5·041
9	2·262	2·821	3·250	4·781
10	2·228	2·764	3·169	4·587
11	2·201	2·718	3·106	4·437
12	2·179	2·681	3·055	4·318
13	2·160	2·650	3·012	4·221
14	2·145	2·624	2·977	4·140
15	2·131	2·602	2·947	4·073
16	2·120	2·583	2·921	4·015
17	2·110	2·567	2·898	3·965
18	2·101	2·552	2·878	3·922
19	2·093	2·539	2·861	3·883
20	2·086	2·528	2·845	3·850
21	2·080	2·518	2·831	3·819
22	2·074	2·508	2·819	3·792
23	2·069	2·500	2·807	3·767
24	2·064	2·492	2·797	3·745
25	2·060	2·485	2·787	3·725
26	2·056	2·479	2·779	3·707
27	2·052	2·473	2·771	3·690
28	2·048	2·467	2·763	3·674
29	2·045	2·462	2·756	3·659
30	2·042	2·457	2·750	3·646
40	2·021	2·423	2·704	3·551
60	2·000	2·390	2·660	3·460
120	1·980	2·358	2·617	3·373
∞	1·960	2·326	2·576	3·291

Table B. Significant Values of F

$p = .05$

df_B df_W	1	2	3	4	5	6	8	12	24	∞
1	161·4	199·5	215·7	224·6	230·2	234·0	238·9	243·9	249·0	254·3
2	18·51	19·00	19·16	19·25	19·30	19·33	19·37	19·41	19·45	19·50
3	10·13	9·55	9·28	9·12	9·01	8·94	8·84	8·74	8·64	8·53
4	7·71	6·94	6·59	6·39	6·26	6·16	6·04	5·91	5·77	5·63
5	6·61	5·79	5·41	5·19	5·05	4·95	4·82	4·68	4·53	4·36
6	5·99	5·14	4·76	4·53	4·39	4·28	4·15	4·00	3·84	3·67
7	5·59	4·74	4·35	4·12	3·97	3·87	3·73	3·57	3·41	3·23
8	5·32	4·46	4·07	3·84	3·69	3·58	3·44	3·28	3·12	2·93
9	5·12	4·26	3·86	3·63	3·48	3·37	3·23	3·07	2·90	2·71
10	4·96	4·10	3·71	3·48	3·33	3·22	3·07	2·91	2·74	2·54
11	4·84	3·98	3·59	3·36	3·20	3·09	2·95	2·79	2·61	2·40
12	4·75	3·88	3·49	3·26	3·11	3·00	2·85	2·69	2·50	2·30
13	4·67	3·80	3·41	3·18	3·02	2·92	2·77	2·60	2·42	2·21
14	4·60	3·74	3·34	3·11	2·96	2·85	2·70	2·53	2·35	2·13
15	4·54	3·68	3·29	3·06	2·90	2·79	2·64	2·48	2·29	2·07
16	4·49	3·63	3·24	3·01	2·85	2·74	2·59	2·42	2·24	2·01
17	4·45	3·59	3·20	2·96	2·81	2·70	2·55	2·38	2·19	1·96
18	4·41	3·55	3·16	2·93	2·77	2·66	2·51	2·34	2·15	1·92
19	4·38	3·52	3·13	2·90	2·74	2·63	2·48	2·31	2·11	1·88
20	4·35	3·49	3·10	2·87	2·71	2·60	2·45	2·28	2·08	1·84
21	4·32	3·47	3·07	2·84	2·68	2·57	2·42	2·25	2·05	1·81
22	4·30	3·44	3·05	2·82	2·66	2·55	2·40	2·23	2·03	1·78
23	4·28	3·42	3·03	2·80	2·64	2·53	2·38	2·20	2·00	1·76
24	4·26	3·40	3·01	2·78	2·62	2·51	2·36	2·18	1·98	1·73
25	4·24	3·38	2·99	2·76	2·60	2·49	2·34	2·19	1·96	1·71
26	4·22	3·37	2·98	2·74	2·59	2·47	2·32	2·15	1·95	1·69
27	4·21	3·35	2·96	2·73	2·57	2·46	2·30	2·13	1·93	1·67
28	4·20	3·34	2·95	2·71	2·56	2·44	2·29	2·12	1·91	1·65
29	4·18	3·33	2·93	2·70	2·54	2·43	2·28	2·10	1·90	1·64
30	4·17	3·32	2·92	2·69	2·53	2·42	2·27	2·09	1·89	1·62
40	4·08	3·23	2·84	2·61	2·45	2·34	2·18	2·00	1·79	1·51
60	4·00	3·15	2·76	2·52	2·37	2·25	2·10	1·92	1·70	1·39
120	3·92	3·07	2·68	2·45	2·29	2·17	2·02	1·83	1·61	1·25
∞	3·84	2·99	2·60	2·37	2·21	2·09	1·94	1·75	1·52	1·00

Table B (continued). Significant Values of F

$p = .01$

df_B / df_W	1	2	3	4	5	6	8	12	24	∞
1	4052	4999	5403	5625	5764	5859	5981	6106	6234	6366
2	98·49	99·00	99·17	99·25	99·30	99·33	99·36	99.42	99·46	99·50
3	34·12	30·81	29·46	28·71	28·24	27·91	27·49	27·05	26.60	26·12
4	21·20	18·00	16·69	15·98	15·52	15·21	14·80	14·37	13·93	13·46
5	16·26	13·27	12·06	11·39	10·97	10·67	10·29	9·89	9·47	9·02
6	13·74	10·92	9·78	9·15	8·75	8·47	8·10	7·72	7·31	6·88
7	12·25	9·55	8·45	7·85	7·46	7·19	6·84	6·47	6·07	5·65
8	11·26	8·65	7·59	7·01	6·63	6·37	6·03	5·67	5·28	4·86
9	10·56	8·02	6·99	6·42	6·06	5·80	5·47	5·11	4·73	4·31
10	10·04	7·56	6·55	5·99	5·64	5·39	5·06	4·71	4·33	3·91
11	9·65	7·20	6·22	5·67	5·32	5·07	4·74	4·40	4·02	3·60
12	9·33	6·93	5·95	5·41	5·06	4·82	4·50	4·16	3·78	3·36
13	9·07	6·70	5·74	5·20	4·86	4·62	4·30	3·96	3·59	3·16
14	8·86	6·51	5·56	5·03	4·69	4·46	4·14	3·80	3·43	3·00
15	8·68	6·36	5·42	4·89	4·56	4·32	4·00	3·67	3·29	2·87
16	8·53	6·23	5·29	4·77	4·44	4·20	3·89	3·55	3·18	2·75
17	8·40	6·11	5·18	4·67	4·34	4·10	3·79	3·45	3·08	2·65
18	8·28	6·01	5·09	4·58	4·25	4·01	3·71	3·37	3·00	2·57
19	8·18	5·93	5·01	4·50	4·17	3·94	3·63	3·30	2·92	2·49
20	8·10	5·85	4·94	4·43	4·10	3·87	3·56	3·23	2·86	2·42
21	8·02	5·78	4·87	4·37	4·04	3·81	3·51	3·17	2·80	2·36
22	7·94	5·72	4·82	4·31	3·99	3·76	3·45	3·12	2·75	2·31
23	7·88	5·66	4·76	4·26	3·94	3·71	3·41	3·07	2·70	2·26
24	7·82	5·61	4·72	4·22	3·90	3·67	3·36	3·03	2·66	2·21
25	7·77	5·57	4·68	4·18	3·86	3·63	3·32	2·99	2·62	2·17
26	7·72	5·53	4·64	4·14	3·82	3·59	3·29	2·96	2·58	2·13
27	7·68	5·49	4·60	4·11	3·78	3·56	3·26	2·93	2·55	2·10
28	7·64	5·45	4·57	4·07	3·75	3·53	3·23	2·90	2·52	2·06
29	7·60	5·42	4·54	4·04	3·73	3·50	3·20	2·87	2·49	2·03
30	7·56	5·39	4·51	4·02	3·70	3·47	3·17	2·84	2·47	2·01
40	7·31	5·18	4·31	3·83	3·51	3·29	2·99	2·66	2·29	1·80
60	7·08	4·98	4·13	3·65	3·34	3·12	2·82	2·50	2·12	1·60
120	6·85	4·79	3·95	3·48	3·17	2·96	2·66	2·34	1·95	1·38
∞	6·64	4·60	3·78	3·32	3·02	2·80	2·51	2·18	1·79	1·00

Table B (continued). Significant Values of *F*

p = .001

df_B df_W	1	2	3	4	5	6	8	12	24	∞
1	405284	500000	540379	562500	576405	585937	598144	610667	623497	636619
2	998·5	999·0	999·2	999·2	999·3	999·3	999·4	999·4	999·5	999·5
3	167·5	148·5	141·1	137·1	134·6	132·8	130·6	128·3	125·9	123·5
4	74·14	61·25	56·18	53·44	51·71	50·53	49·00	47·41	45·77	44·05
5	47·04	36·61	32·20	31·09	29·75	28·84	27·64	26·42	25·14	23·78
6	35·51	27·00	23·70	21·90	20·81	20·03	19·03	17·99	16·89	15·75
7	29·22	21·69	18·77	17·19	16·21	15·52	14·63	13·71	12·73	11·69
8	25·42	18·49	15·83	14·39	13·49	12·86	12·04	11·19	10·30	9·34
9	22·86	16·39	13·90	12·56	11·71	11·13	10·37	9·57	8·72	7·81
10	21·04	14·91	12·55	11·28	10·48	9·92	9·20	8·45	7·64	6·76
11	19·69	13·81	11·56	10·35	9·58	9·05	8·35	7·63	6·85	6·00
12	18·64	12·97	10·80	9·63	8·89	8·38	7·71	7·00	6·25	5·42
13	17·81	12·31	10·21	9·07	8·35	7·86	7·21	6·52	5·78	4·97
14	17·14	11·78	9·73	8·62	7·92	7·43	6·80	6·13	5·41	4·60
15	16·59	11·34	9·34	8·25	7·57	7·09	6·47	5·81	5·10	4·31
16	16·12	10·97	9·00	7·94	7·27	6·81	6·19	5·55	4·85	4·06
17	15·72	10·66	8·73	7·68	7·02	6·56	5·96	5·32	4·63	3·85
18	15·38	10·39	8·49	7·46	6·81	6·35	5·76	5·13	4·45	3·67
19	15·08	10·16	8·28	7·26	6·61	6·18	5·59	4·97	4·29	3·52
20	14·82	9·95	8·10	7·10	6·46	6·02	5·44	4·82	4·15	3·38
21	14·59	9·77	7·94	6·95	6·32	5·88	5·31	4·70	4·03	3·26
22	14·38	9·61	7·80	6·81	6·19	5·76	5·19	4·58	3·92	3·15
23	14·19	9·47	7·67	6·69	6·08	5·65	5·09	4·48	3·82	3·05
24	14·03	9·34	7·55	6·59	5·98	5·55	4·99	4·39	3·74	2·97
25	13·88	9·22	7·45	6·49	5·88	5·46	4·91	4·31	3·66	2·89
26	13·74	9·12	7·36	6·41	5·80	5·38	4·83	4·24	3·59	2·82
27	13·61	9·02	7·27	6·33	5·73	5·31	4·76	4·17	3·52	2·75
28	13·50	8·93	7·19	6·25	5·66	5·24	4·69	4·11	3·46	2·70
29	13·39	8·85	7·12	6·19	5·59	5·18	4·64	4·05	3·41	2·64
30	13·29	8·77	7·05	6·12	5·53	5·12	4·58	4·00	3·36	2·59
40	12·61	8·25	6·60	5·70	5·13	4·73	4·21	3·64	3·01	2·23
60	11·97	7·76	6·17	5·31	4·76	4·37	3·87	3·31	2·69	1·90
120	11·38	7·31	5·79	4·95	4·42	4·04	3·55	3·02	2·40	1·56
∞	10·83	6·91	5·42	4·62	4·10	3·74	3·27	2·74	2·13	1·00

Table C. Distribution of χ^2 Probability

df	p = .05	.02	.01	.001
1	3·841	5·412	6·635	10·827
2	5·991	7·824	9·210	13·815
3	7·815	9·837	11·345	16·268
4	9·488	11·668	13·277	18·465
5	11·070	13·388	15·086	20·517
6	12·592	15·033	16·812	22·457
7	14·067	16·622	18·475	24·322
8	15·507	18·168	20·090	26·125
9	16·919	19·679	21·666	27·877
10	18·307	21·161	23·209	29·588
11	19·675	22·618	24·725	31·264
12	21·026	24·054	26·217	32·909
13	22·362	25·472	27·688	34·528
14	23·685	26·873	29·141	36·123
15	24·996	28·259	30·578	37·697
16	26·296	29·633	32·000	39·252
17	27·587	30·995	33·409	40·790
18	28·869	32·346	34·805	42·312
19	30·144	33·687	36·191	43·820
20	31·410	35·020	37·566	45·315
21	32·671	36·343	38·932	46·797
22	33·924	37·659	40·289	48·268
23	35·172	38·968	41·638	49·728
24	36·415	40·270	42·980	51·179
25	37·652	41·566	44·314	52·620
26	38·885	42·856	45·642	54·052
27	40·113	44·140	46·963	55·476
28	41·337	45·419	48·278	56·893
29	42·557	46·693	49·588	58·302
30	43·773	47·962	50·892	59·703

Table D. Significant Values of the Correlation Coefficient

df	p = .1	.05	.02	.01	.001
1	·98769	·99692	·999507	·999877	·9999988
2	·90000	·95000	·98000	·990000	·99900
3	·8054	·8783	·93433	·95873	·99116
4	·7293	·8114	·8822	·91720	·97406
5	·6694	·7545	·8329	·8745	·95074
6	·6215	·7067	·7887	·8343	·92493
7	·5822	·6664	·7498	·7977	·8982
8	·5494	·6319	·7155	·7646	·8721
9	·5214	·6021	·6851	·7348	·8471
10	·4973	·5760	·6581	·7079	·8233
11	·4762	·5529	·6339	·6835	·8010
12	·4575	·5324	·6120	·6614	·7800
13	·4409	·5139	·5923	·6411	·7603
14	·4259	·4973	·5742	·6226	·7420
15	·4124	·4821	·5577	·6055	·7246
16	·4000	·4683	·5425	·5897	·7084
17	·3887	·4555	·5285	·5751	·6932
18	·3783	·4438	·5155	·5614	·6787
19	·3687	·4329	·5034	·5487	·6652
20	·3598	·4227	·4921	·5368	·6524
25	·3233	·3809	·4451	·4869	·5974
30	·2960	·3494	·4093	·4487	·5541
35	·2746	·3246	·3810	·4182	·5189
40	·2573	·3044	·3578	·3932	·4896
45	·2428	·2875	·3384	·3721	·4648
50	·2306	·2732	·3218	·3541	·4433
60	·2108	·2500	·2948	·3248	·4078
70	·1954	·2319	·2737	·3017	·3799
80	·1829	·2172	·2565	·2830	·3568
90	·1726	·2050	·2422	·2673	·3375
100	·1638	·1946	·2301	·2540	·3211

Index

Note: Page numbers in bold type refer to the glossary.

ch 9- 18

∂ ch 1 revisited